PHYSICIAN ASSISTANTS
IN AMERICAN MEDICINE

RODERICK S. HOOKER, PA, MBA

Physician Assistant
Kaiser Permanente
Portland, Oregon

JAMES F. CAWLEY, MPH, PA-C

Professor of Prevention and Community Health
School of Public Health and Health Services
Professor of Health Care Sciences
School of Medicine and Health Sciences
The George Washington University
Washington, D.C.

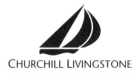

CHURCHILL LIVINGSTONE

New York, Edinburgh, London, Madrid, Melbourne, San Francisco, Tokyo

Library of Congress Cataloging-in-Publication Data

Hooker, Roderick S.
    Physician assistants in American medicine / Roderick S. Hooker,
James F. Cawley.
      p. cm.
    Includes bibliographical references and index.
    ISBN 0-443-05731-1 (alk. paper)
    1. Physicians' assistants—Vocational guidance. 2. Physicians'
assistants—United States.   I. Cawley, James F.   II. Title.
    [DNLM: 1. Physician Assistants. 2. Delivery of Health Care-
-trends—United States.   W 21.5 H784p 1997]
    R697.P45H66 1997
    610.69'53'02373—dc21
    DNLM/DLC
    for Library of Congress   97–8216
                                              CIP

ISBN 0-443-05731-1

© Churchill Livingstone Inc. 1997

Distributed in the United Kingdom by Churchill Livingstone, Robert Stevenson House, 1–3 Baxter's Place, Leith Walk, Edinburgh EH1 3AF, and by associated companies, branches, and representatives throughout the world.

Medical knowledge is constantly changing. As new information becomes available, changes in treatment, procedures, equipment and the use of drugs become necessary. The editors/authors/contributors and the publishers have, as far as it is possible, taken care to ensure that the information given in this text is accurate and up to date. However, readers are strongly advised to confirm that the information, especially with regard to drug usage, complies with the latest legislation and standards of practice.

The Publishers have made every effort to trace the copyright holders for borrowed material. If they have inadvertently overlooked any, they will be pleased to make the necessary arrangements at the first opportunity.

Production Editor: *Elizabeth A. Plowman*
Production Supervisor: *Kathleen R. Smith*
Cover Design: *Jeannette Jacobs*
Desktop Coordinator: *Jo-Ann Demas*

Printed in the United States of America

First published in 1997   7 6 5 4 3 2 1

To my wife, Donna Lux Hooker, and my mother, Shirley H. Hooker. To my children, Lindsay and Tyler—they could be writing this book today had they paid more attention at dinner.

Roderick S. Hooker

To Susanne D. Cawley and the memories of Patrick B. Cawley and Roberta M. Cawley. Also, to Andrea B. Cawley and Patti Gerhardt.

James F. Cawley

Foreword

As medical care in the United States moves forward in an environment characterized by rapid change and the realignments and adjustments related to "managed care," physician assistants have become key players. The physician assistant profession provides high quality health care at a lower cost than does the conventional practice utilizing physicians exclusively. It is likely that collaborative teams containing physicians, physician assistants, and other health care professionals will emerge from the current realignments as the dominant practice model and that these teams will provide excellent and convenient care to a wider segment of our population than was possible in the past.

The physician assistant profession is still new, and regrettably, there are many who know little about its characteristics, roots, traditions, and utility across all branches and specialties of medical care. *Physician Assistants in American Medicine* will meet a real need, by providing an authoritative and current source of information about the profession while reflecting its unique philosophy and relationship to the medical profession.

While other books have been written about the profession, most have been written by physicians, educators, and/or academicians who have only observed the profession. This is a book written by individuals who were primarily educated into the profession and have practiced within it.

Each of the authors has a unique perspective, and these viewpoints fit together well for the purposes of writing a comprehensive description of the field. Both entered the profession with health care experience typical of the physician assistant

practice, one in primary care and the other in specialty care. Each has pursued further education as needed for their expanded careers. Both have become leaders in the profession and are widely recognized as its spokesmen and as representatives through appointment to panels and task forces studying the profession and its relationship with other health professions. It is in this context that I have become acquainted with both authors and have come to respect their knowledge, integrity, perspective, and wisdom.

This volume is both timely and authoritative. The authors have used the remarkable data set gathered and updated each year by the American Academy of Physician Assistants. They have also extensively utilized sources such as the early conceptual and educational leaders of the new profession, most of whom are still alive and available, and they have included those who have not left a trail of publications. They have also consulted with a wide network of fellow physician assistants, who have been willing to review and provide critical input to this volume.

Physician Assistants in American Medicine should prove to be an invaluable collection of useful and necessary information about this new and emerging field, and its authors are to be congratulated on their foresight and effort in making it available.

E. Harvey Estes, Jr., M.D.
Emeritus Professor of Community
and Family Medicine
Duke University Medical Center

Director
Kate B. Reynolds Community Practitioner Program
North Carolina Medical Society Foundation Inc.

Preface

We set out to write a book about one type of health care worker, the physician assistant. While their numbers are relatively small, their presence in American health care is significant from a number of standpoints. Almost one-quarter of general and family practice physicians report employing or working with a physician assistant (Gonzalez 1995). As we will reveal, physician assistants have many extraordinary attributes.

Our experiences and professional expertise are complementary in background—Jim Cawley with training in political science and Rod Hooker with a background in biology. We both trained as physician assistants in the mid-1970s and have been ardent observers of physician assistants in health care delivery and how they interact with other medical personnel. Mr. Cawley is an academic and educator; Mr. Hooker works in the private sector as a clinician and researcher. We both, however, are medical social researchers with a keen interest in human behavior and have had the rare privilege of observing the physician assistant movement from a relatively early beginning. Mr. Hooker has focused on the use of providers in group practice and managed care settings, while Mr. Cawley has sought the national picture of health care personnel utilization. We both have a deep respect for history and are committed to recording it accurately.

The impetus for *Physician Assistants in American Medicine* began in 1991 when a series of phone calls sparked an interest in documenting the history of physician assistants for which we had observed almost a quarter century of the profession. Both of us were invited to write a paper for the silver jubilee of the profession in the *Journal of the American Academy of Physician Assistants* (October 1992 edition). During this we realized a comprehensive reference for physician assistants was needed. We envisioned a document that could serve both colleagues and students alike. Thus, we have sought to develop both a reference and a textbook, anchored firmly in the past, and one that will have the opportunity for future editions.

Paradoxically this book is both narrow in focus and broad in scope. On one hand it examines a small element of the health care workforce—physician assistants. But at the same time, they are described in the context of the broad range of health care delivery. While we make no pretense of being complete, we have made a concerted effort to cover the most important issues in the field. This writing occurred within the spirit of a true partnership, with both authors contributing to theory, analysis, and editing. Since neither can take credit for having done more than the other in bringing this book to bear, we assign no order in authorship.

A few caveats are necessary when reading this book. First, in a field as quickly changing as health care, information about the supply of services is inevitably somewhat outdated by the time it is published. We have tried to shape this book so it will be both historically accurate and timely and lend itself to easy updating. Regarding our sources of information, we have used national data wherever possible; however, this information is sometimes limited. The Membership and Research Division staff at the American Academy of Physician Assistants (AAPA) have graciously given us a great deal of their time and information. While we are grateful for this data, we must caution the reader that information about the distribution of physician assistants and some of their activities comes from this one source, the AAPA, the professional society of physician assistants. Also, the utilization of physician assistants in the United States is in considerable flux and it is not clear what patterns will emerge as a result of new opportunities and efforts to reform health care.

We have attempted to be thorough in assembling studies and information done in the past decade. We also spared no effort to reach as far back as we could to include important historical documents to help anchor the roots of this profession. Our efforts to assemble such work, such as documents sponsored by the federal government and state governments and foundations, was aided by networking with a great many people. To this end we are grateful to our friends and colleagues who have helped us in locating these documents. We also conducted an extensive computer-bibliographical search to identify material in the published literature, including dissertations, and we sought the advice of colleagues about work in progress. Although we may have missed some items, we are satisfied that we have garnered sufficient data to depict the field as a whole.

The profession most often compared to physician assistants is nurse practitioners. Throughout this book we include information on nurse practitioners where appropriate, such as in demographics and reimbursement issues.

Some of that literature is meaningful, but from a historical standpoint the nurse practitioners literature tends to reflect that graduates are nurses first and clinicians second. That, plus the fact that the physician assistant profession has reached a critical mass, compels us to devote this book to understanding the physician assistant profession first, and how it relates to all health occupations second. Prior to the mid-1980s the literature was fragmented and it was not always clear which profession was being discussed. As a consequence many studies were performed on both professions with the data aggregated. Now, the gaps in our understanding of physician assistant behavior is closing and the depth of material on physician assistants alone justifies this work.

Our intent in writing *Physician Assistants in American Medicine* is to create a document that will serve both as a textbook and a reference source for any number of actors in the health care arena: clinicians, policy makers, students, educators, and administrators. It contains more than 700 references and we hope this bibliography will guide others to more in-depth reading. We are grateful to the many colleagues who generously gave their time to review select parts of this book. Their comments, criticisms, and suggested changes were quickly incorporated wherever possible, but we take sole responsibility for any errors or misstatements contained in this text.

Roderick S. Hooker, PA, MBA
James F. Cawley, MPH, PA-C

Acknowledgments

We have too many friends who have been in some way responsible for shaping this book to list all of them. Some special attention needs go to Archie Golden, Richard K. Riegelman, Richard Johnson, Donald Freeborn, and the late Jane Record, special mentors whom we emulate. They taught us ideals of excellence that we can only strive to achieve. Steve Crane, Marilyn Fitzgerald, Nicole Gara, Nancy Hughes, Kevin Kraditor, and others at the American Academy of Physician Assistants helped immensely in innumerable ways. Eric Schuman, Joe Marzucco, Reginald Carter, Glen Combs, Richard Rohrs, Bert Simon, Jeff Heinrich, Bruce Fichandler, Walter Stein, and Virginia Fowlkes edited some of our chapters and pointed out areas for improvement. Special thanks goes to Donna Lux Hooker who patiently edited some of the most awkward lines ever written.

About the Authors

Roderick S. Hooker, PA, MBA, is a physician assistant with Kaiser Permanente in Portland, Oregon and an Associate Professor in the School of Physician Assistant Studies at Pacific University in Forest Grove, Oregon. Prior to training at the St. Louis University Physician Assistant Program, he was a biologist and health worker with the Peace Corps in Tonga. His background includes serving as a corpsman in the U.S. Navy and an emergency room technician. He has been involved in health services research since 1980 and has an interest in managed care and health economics. Mr. Hooker is an adjunct researcher with the Kaiser Permanente Center for Health Research and is on the adjunct faculty of the University of Washington and Pacific University. He is a doctoral candidate in health policy at Portland State University studying outcomes of care.

James F. Cawley is Director, Physician Assistant/Master of Public Health Program, Professor of Prevention and Community Health in the School of Public Health and Health Services, and Professor of Health Care Sciences in the School of Medicine and Health Sciences at the George Washington University. After earning his Bachelor's degree and an MPH in epidemiology from Johns Hopkins University, he has held faculty positions in physician assistant programs at Johns Hopkins University, the State University of New York at Stony Brook, and Yale University. Since 1981 he has taught in the Physician Assistant program at the George Washington University and has conducted research and published extensively on the physician assistant profession and health work force issues. He has held numerous leadership positions within the physician assistant profession. In 1994 he was selected by the Bureau of Health Professions to chair the Advisory Group on Physician Assistants and the Workforce (AGPAW) of the Council on Graduate Medical Education (COGME) and was principal author of AGPAW's Final Report to the Council published by the Department of Health and Human Services. He has consulted on physician assistant work force issues with numerous colleges and universities, governmental agencies, and private organizations nationwide, and is presently a doctoral candidate at the George Washington University with a concentration in health policy.

Contents

The Physician Assistant: A Timeline of the Profession

1650 Feldshers, originally German military medical assistants, are introduced into Russian armies by Peter the Great in the 17th century.

1778 Congress provided for a number of hospital mates to assist physicians in the provision of patient care modeled after the "loblolly boys" of the British Royal Navy.

1803 Officiers de Santé are introduced in France by Fourcroy to help alleviate health personnel shortages in the military and civilian sectors. Abolished in 1892.

1891 Establishment of the first company for "medic" instruction at Fort Riley, Kansas.

1940 Community Health Aids introduced in Alaska to improve the village health status of Eskimos and other Native Americans.

1959 U.S. Surgeon General identifies shortage of medically trained personnel.

1961 Charles Hudson, in an editorial in the *Journal of the American Medical Association*, calls for a "mid-level" provider from the ranks of former military corpsmen.

World Health Organization begins introducing and promoting health care workers in developing countries (e.g., Me'decin Africain, Dresser, Assistant Medical Officer, and Rural Health Technician).

1965 First physician assistant (PA) class enters Duke University, North Carolina.

1966 Barefoot Doctors in China arise in response to Chairman Mao's purge of the elite and intellectual, sending many physicians into the fields to work, leaving peasants without medical personnel.

Child Health Associate Program begins at University of Colorado.

Allied Health Professions Personnel Act (PL-751) promotes the development of programs to train new types of primary care providers.

1967 First class of PA graduates.

1968 Alderson-Broaddus (West Virginia) program officially enrolls its first class.

American Academy of Physician Assistants (AAPA) is established.

Health Manpower Act (PL-90-490) funds the training of a variety of health providers.

Physician Assistants, Volume 1, is published.

1969 Medex program launched at University of Washington (Seattle, Washington); first class enters.

1970 Kaiser Permanente becomes first HMO to employ a PA.

1971 American Medical Association recognizes the PA profession, and begins work on national certification and codification of its practice characteristics.

Comprehensive Health Manpower Training Act (PL-92-157) contracts for physician assistant education and deployment.

1972　*The Physician's Assistant: Today and Tomorrow* by Sadler, Sadler, and Bliss, is published; first book written on the PA profession.

The Association of Physician Assistant Programs is established.

Alderson-Broaddus' first four-year program graduates its first class.

"The Essentials" Accreditation standards for PA programs are adopted and the Joint Review Committee on Educational Programs for Physician Assistants (JRC-PA) is formed to evaluate compliance with the standards.

Federal support for physician assistant education enacted by Health Resources Administration (HRA).

1973　First AAPA Annual Conference held at Sheppard Air Force Base, Texas, with 275 attendees.

AAPA and Association of Physician Assistant Programs (APAP) establish a national office in Washington, DC.

National Commission on Certification of Physician Assistants is established.

National Board of Medical Examiners administers the first Certifying Examinations for Primary Care Physician Assistants.

1974　AAPA becomes an official organization on the Joint Review Committee on Educational Programs for physician assistants. The committee reviews physician and surgeon assistant programs and makes accreditation recommendations to the Committee on Allied Health Education and Accreditation.

The American College of Surgeons become a sponsoring organization of the JRC-PA.

1975　*The Physician Assistant: A National and Local Analysis*, by Ford, is published.

1976　Federal support of PA education continues under grants from Health Professions Educational Assistance Act (PL 94-484).

1977　*The New Health Professionals: Nurse Practitioners and Physician's Assistants*, by Bliss and Cohen, is published.

The Physician's Assistant: A Baccalaureate Curriculum, by Myers, is published.

AAPA Education and Research Foundation (later renamed Physician Assistant Foundation) incorporated to recruit public and private contributions for student financial assistance and to support research on the PA profession.

Rural Health Clinic Services Act (PL 95-210) passed by Congress provides Medicare reimbursement of PA and Nurse Practitioner services in rural clinics.

Health Practitioner (later renamed *Physician Assistant*) journal begins publication; later distributed to all PAs as the official AAPA publication.

1978　*The Physician's Assistant: Innovation in the Medical Division of Labor*, by Schneller, is published.

AAPA House of Delegates becomes policy-making legislative body of the Academy.

Air Force begins appointing PAs as commissioned officers.

1979　Graduate Medical Education National Advisory Council estimates a surplus of physicians and nonphysician providers in the near future.

1980　The AAPA Political Action Committee established to support candidates for federal office who support the PA profession.

1981　*Staffing Primary Care in 1990: Physician Replacement and Cost Savings*, by Record, documents that PAs in HMO settings provide 79 percent of the care of a primary care physician, at 50 percent of the cost.

The Art of Teaching Primary Care, by Golden and Hager, is published.

1982 *Physician Assistants: Their Contribution to Health Care*, by Perry and Breitner, is published.

1984 *First Annual Report on Physician Assistant Educational Programs in the United States*, by Oliver and the Association of Physician Assistant Programs, is published.

Alternatives in Health Care Delivery, edited by Carter and Perry, is published.

1985 AAPA's first Burroughs Wellcome Health Policy Fellowship created and first fellow, Marshall Sinback, named.

Membership of AAPA surpasses 10,000 mark. Membership categories expanded to include physicians, affiliates, and sustaining members.

AAPA and APAP begin first joint project providing PA graduates with a national job bank service: PA JOB FIND.

1986 AAPA succeeds in legislative drive for coverage of PA services in hospitals and nursing homes, and assisting in surgery under Medicare Part B (Omnibus Budget Reconciliation Act PL 99-210).

Physicians Assistants: New Models of Utilization, edited by Zarbock and Harbert, is published.

1987 *The Physician Assistant in a Changing Health Care Environment*, by Schafft and Cawley, is published.

National PA Day, October 6, established, coinciding with the anniversary of the first graduating class of PAs from the Duke University PA Program 20 years earlier.

New AAPA National Headquarters at 950 North Washington Street, Alexandria, VA, is established.

AAPA contracts to publish *Journal of the American Academy of Physician Assistants (JAAPA)*. Editor selected is first PA hired as AAPA professional staff.

Additional Medicare coverage of PA services (in rural, underserved areas) approved by Congress.

1988 First edition of *JAAPA* published and distributed.

Duke University PA Program awards first Master's degree for PA education.

1991 AAPA assumes administrative responsibility of the Accreditation Review Committee on Education for Physician Assistants (formerly the JRC-PA).

Navy PAs commissioned.

1992 Army and Coast Guard PAs commissioned.

1993 *The Role of the Physician Assistant and Nurse Practitioner in Primary Care*, edited by Clawson and Osterwies, is published.

24,600 PAs are in active practice in 49 states, territories, and the District of Columbia.

1994 *Physician Assistant: A Guide to Clinical Practice*, edited by Ballweg, Stolberg, and Sullivan, is published.

1995 *The Physician Assistant Medical Handbook*, edited by Labus, is published.

Physician Assistants in the Health Workforce, 1994 (report of the Advisory Group on Physician Assistants and the Workforce [AGPAW]), is published.

1996 American Medical Association (AMA) grants observer status to AAPA in the AMA House of Delegates.

1997 *The Physician Assistant Emergency Medical Handbook*, by Salyer, is published.

28,500 PAs are in active practice; prescribing authorized in 40 states, the District of Columbia, and Guam.

Physician Assistants in American Medicine, by Hooker and Cawley, is published.

1

Overview of the Profession

THE PHYSICIAN ASSISTANT PROFESSION

The concept of the physician assistant (PA) in the United States emerged in the 1960s as a strategy to cope with a shortage of primary care physicians. The concept spawned a handful of graduates and a new profession, which struggled to survive, grow, and become recognized. Three decades later, this profession is a mature and capable component of the medical workforce, with over 30,000 members, a stable and strong set of educational programs, and a growing importance within the health care system.

In the decades following the origin of the profession, there have been debates about the need for additions to the health workforce and predictions of a surplus of both physicians and nurses by the end of the century. Why then has this new profession prospered, and will its success and growth continue into the next century? The answer to these and other questions about this profession are not yet clear, but they are part of the warp and woof of a rapidly evolving health care system in the United States, which evidence seems to point to continued growth and success for this young profession.

EVIDENCE REVIEWED: THE SUCCESS OF THE CONCEPT

The startling growth and success of the physician assistant concept from its origins in the 1960s could not have occurred in the absence of ferment and change in the health care system, which made it possible and even necessary. Consumers of health care, existing health care professions, government, bureaucratic hierarchies, educational institutions, and accrediting bodies are all involved and have, implicitly if not explicitly, aided in the process by creating a positive political climate.

The innovation was born after a 20-year period of scientific breakthroughs, development of new medical specialties and subspecialties, and overgrowth of hospitals and hospital services. Young physicians, exposed early to this exciting display of technical power, were flocking to hospital-based specialties. The education and training of the generalist physician, once the foundation of the medical workforce, had shrunk after the Korean War, and the new graduates of residencies were not replacing the general practitioners who were retiring. The consequences of this gap were not so obvious in cities with good hospitals and a strong cadre of the newly trained specialists, but in small towns and rural areas, the impact was devastating.

Thus, the stage was set for entry of a new alternative provider that promised improved access to health care for these areas. The country's leaders were well aware of inequities in the distribution of health care, and most were convinced that the problem was one of inadequate numbers of medical providers. A series of actions was undertaken, at both the federal and state level, aimed at correcting these problems.

With the advent of the PA profession, and the development of the nurse practitioner, the following actions were taken in the 1970s:

- Medical schools were rewarded for increasing class size
- New medical schools were created
- The generalist physician was "revived" in the form of a new general specialty—family medicine
- Special offices to promote medical practice in underserved areas were created in many states
- Dispersed medical educational systems (area health education programs) were created in many states

An added factor in the mix was the war in Southeast Asia, which was reaching its tragic conclusion at this same time in our history. Military medical care had been significantly improved by trained medical care teams operating in combat areas and by forward area battalion aid stations. Physicians, nurses, military personnel, and corpsmen were returning home with knowledge of these improvements and the key roles played by nonphysician members of these field teams.

Yet another factor was the social climate within the country. The "War on Poverty" had brought to public attention the poverty and deprivation of some within the bounds of the "richest country on earth." President Lyndon Johnson's "Great Society" program brought an optimism that solutions might be found for these chronic social ills.

It is easy to understand why this was a favorable time for the entry of physician assistants on the health workforce stage. Governments, both state and federal, were also willing to support some of the most far-reaching demonstration projects seen to that time to increase access to health care, and the public supported these demonstrations. The fact that this innovation tapped the newly available source of returning military corpsmen was an added boost.

Intertwined with these circumstances were events more directly related to the PA profession. In 1961, the president of the American Medical Association proposed the idea of utilizing military trained personnel as assistants to physicians. In the mid-1960s, Dr. Richard Smith, then a deputy director of the Office of Equal Health Opportunity, moved to a new role in which he proposed to create a new source of health providers for rural areas. A notable academic pediatrician, Dr. Henry Silver, with Dr. Loretta Ford, a nurse educator, began to develop at the University of Colorado a new pediatric practitioner model for underserved areas.

At Duke University, the first physician assistant program began with a small group of ex-Navy corpsmen, under the direction of Dr. Eugene A. Stead, an academic physician leader, who had been impressed by the need for new personnel, both in the medical center and in the rural areas of his state. His previous experience with military personnel convinced him that the training period for assistants in this new program could be much shorter than that for medical students, and that close supervision by their physician employers would ensure competence and further development of skills in practice.

The history of the Duke program will be discussed in more detail in a later chapter, but at this point, several unique features of Dr. Stead's conceptual model should be recognized. Two have already been mentioned: the relatively brief duration, and the role of the employing physician in continued supervision. The program was patterned after the familiar medical model, a period of basic science education, followed by clinical skill development under medical instructors. The assistant would be trained to take a medical history, elicit symptoms, develop diagnoses, examine the patient, and take over some medical management tasks. Complicated cases or procedures were to be referred to the supervising physician. Although it was expected that the new personnel might spend more time with patient education and preventive interventions, the activities and skills would be similar to those of the physician, with the assistant assuming some but not all of the physician's tasks.

Another feature of the Duke model was its clear intention to train a generalist assistant, whose training and skill development were adequate to serve as a platform for further education and further skill development by the physician employer. The generalist assistant could work with a rural practitioner, gaining further insights and skills with time, but could also work with a narrow specialist, who would add another layer of expertise to the general education of the PA.

As might have been predicted, state and federal governmental attention was quickly achieved by the new PA program at Duke. Among the interest of government was the regulation of this new category. The Department of Health, Education and Welfare sponsored a study and a series of conferences at Duke University on the regulation of practice of physician assistants. This activity, under the direction of Martha Ballenger, JD, and E. Harvey Estes, Jr, MD, resulted in model regulatory laws that were enacted by many states, and prepared the way for the 1971 Health Manpower Act. This legislation provided funds for medical schools to increase the number of students to meet the perceived shortage of medical personnel. It also included funding for physician assistant training programs. The availability of funding quickly increased the number of training sites, so that 50 such programs were active in 1974.

In 1971, the American Medical Association (AMA) recognized the new profession and lent its name and resources to the process of national certification and codification of educational programs and practice. This recognition did not ensure acceptance by all physicians, and occasional roadblocks to acceptance and permission to practice persisted within the jurisdiction of certain state medical components of the AMA until the 1990s.

The PA Today

In 1997, there were approximately 28,828 physician assistants in active clinical practice in the United States. The stability and dedication of this workforce to their profession are demonstrated by the fact that this represents about 83% of all of the 34,683 persons formally trained as PAs since the first class graduated in 1967.

The mean age of PAs is 40 years; 53% are men and 47% are women. The age reflects the relative youth of the profession. The early dominance of men in the profession, related to the male gender of the former military students of the early years, is changing rapidly, and women dominate in many current classes.

Thirty-three percent of PAs practice in communities with a population under 50,000, and 17% practice in communities under 10,000 (AAPA 1996).

PAs practice in all the types of clinical settings served by physicians. They serve as commissioned officers in all US military branches, including the US Public Health Service. In clinical practice, most spend their time in office or clinic settings, but some work in hospitals and divide their time among the wards and the operating and delivery rooms. In addition to primary care roles in all the primary care specialties, PAs can be found in all non-primary-care specialties. They are underrepresented in nursing home care and home health care, perhaps because of the difficulties in receiving reimbursement for care in these settings and restrictive practice acts in some states.

While all the health professions would like for their members to reflect the racial and ethnic composition of those they serve, this objective has not been achieved. The PA profession has 10% of its members from underrepresented groups. Of those in active clinical practice, 3.5% are African Americans, 3.3% Hispanic/Latinos,

1.9% Asian/Pacific Islanders, and 1% are American Indian/Alaskan Natives. The remaining 90% are Caucasian or do not choose to identify their racial/ethnic origin.

PA practice distribution in the early years of the profession reflected the federal and state initiatives and the interest of the medical profession in extending primary care into areas of need. The early recruits were individuals with experiences that enabled them to practice with minimal supervision, which probably enhanced this emphasis. As the capability of PAs to fit into specialties outside primary care has become known, and as their ability and productivity have been confirmed, physicians in these specialties have successfully "outbid" the primary care specialties for their services. This trend has been blunted or reversed in recent years. In comparison with physicians, PAs remain more likely to be found in primary care practice (45% of PAs, 32% of MDs) and more likely to be in rural and other medically underserved areas.

The Duke model of PA education has been confirmed by the adaptability of PAs to new roles in the medical and surgical specialties, but the price of this has been diverting them from their roles in primary care and underserved areas. In both the primary care and specialty roles of the PA, the relationship between the PA and the supervising physician remains constant. The physician and the physician assistant become a functional team. Eugene Schneller characterized this relationship as "negotiated performance autonomy," reflecting the continually evolving delegation of medical tasks from physician to PA based on a mutual understanding and trust in their respective professional roles. Schneller proposed that this mutual evolution was a major determinant of clinical practice effectiveness of the PA and was advantageous to both (Schneller 1978).

The recognition and acceptance of this beneficial relationship are key to understanding the relationship between the PA and physician, and in understanding the official stance of the profession that it does *not* desire autonomy from physician supervision. Dr. Eugene Stead's early recognition of this principle is reflected in his prediction that PAs would gain greater freedom and growth from delegation by wise physician supervisors, who share the benefits of this growth, than from legislated autonomy.

Delegation of tasks from physician to PA is also contained in the basis of legal and regulatory authority granted to PAs in most state laws. Model legislation proposed as a result of the Duke conferences on this topic in the late 1960s permitted PAs to work in the full range of clinical practice areas: office, clinic, hospital, nursing home, or patient's home. This wide latitude was considered essential for a full range of services and effectiveness. The model legislation recognized the authority of physicians to delegate medical tasks to qualified PAs while holding them legally responsible through the doctrine of "respondeat superior." North Carolina, Colorado, and Oklahoma were the first states to amend their medical practice acts in this manner in the late 1960s, and most states have followed in kind.

These practice regulations and the supervisory relationship have also contributed to the striking versatility among the practice roles of PAs, as they are permitted to assist the physician in any task or function within the scope of the physician's practice, but with the recognition that the responsibility and legal liability for this delegation remain with the physician. This delegation is not limited to the immediate presence of the physician, but in most states, it can be extended to locations from which the supervising physician can be readily contacted for consultation and assistance, such as by telephone.

While there has been a steadily increasing demand for PAs and steadily growing acceptance of and respect for their role as health care providers, added emphasis on cost-effectiveness under managed care has greatly augmented the importance of the profession in health care. Managed care organizations have found them to be capable of providing primary care at a lower cost than physicians and to be willing to move into areas in which it would not be cost effective to place a physician. The supervising physician role remains unchanged from that described previously. This development and the increasing demand for PAs in these settings have caused a reversal of the shift of PAs away from primary care. Additionally, PAs have been willing to move into a variety of other settings that have not been popular with physicians, such as correctional health systems, substance abuse clinics, occupational health clinics, and geriatric institutions.

In summary, there has been continual evolution and enlargement of the role of physician assistants, and the process will continue. The utility of a generalist assistant, capable of further growth and an ever enlarging role under responsible supervision of a physician partner, continues to be explored and confirmed. The original concept has been modified and enlarged so much that the American Academy of Physician Assistants (AAPA) felt the need to develop a new definition of the profession, which was adopted in 1995 by its House of Delegates. This definition addresses the versatility of the profession, its distribution in all geographic locations, and the various nonclinical roles that PAs might pursue.

Physician assistants are health professionals licensed to practice medicine with physician supervision. Physician assistants are qualified by graduation from an accredited physician assistant educational program and/or certification by the National Commission on the Certification of Physician Assistants. Within the physician/PA relationship, physician assistants exercise autonomy in medical decionmaking and provide a broad range of diagnostic and therapeutic services. The clinical role of physician assistants includes primary and specialty care in medical and surgical practice settings in rural and urban areas. Physician assistant practice is centered on patient care and may include educational, research and administrative activities (Fray 1996).

Some interpretation of this definition of PAs may be required. The following explanations are provided by the Professional Practices Council of the AAPA.

Physician assistants are health professionals.

This recognizes the scope of PA practice, advanced knowledge required to be a physician assistant, exercise of discretion and judgment, use of ethical standards, and orientation toward service.

… licensed to practice medicine with physician supervision.

This may be of concern to PAs accustomed to the terms *certified* and *registered*. Examination of accepted definitions of occupational regulation, however, reveals that PAs are subject to de facto licensure regardless of terminology used by the state.

Registration is the least restrictive form of regulation. It is the process of creating an official record or list of persons, for example, voter registration. Its main purpose is not to ensure the public of its quality but rather to serve as a record-keeping function.

Under a certification system, practice of an activity or occupation is not directly restricted, but limits are placed on the use of certain occupational titles. The label *certified* publicly identifies persons who have met certain standards, but does not prevent uncertified practitioners from engaging in the activity.

Under licensure, the most restrictive method of regulation, persons have no right to engage in a particular activity without permission to do so by the state. Such permission is generally conditioned upon stringent requirements, such as certain educational qualifications and passage of an examination.

Because PAs must meet such standards and may not practice without state approval, *licensed* is the most appropriate way to describe the control exercised by states over PA practice. PAs are qualified to practice by graduating from an accredited PA educational program and/or by certification by the National Commission of Physician Assistants. There are two major criteria for being a PA. The connector *and/or* is in accord with AAPA policy, which recognizes that informally trained, nationally certified PAs are an integral part of the profession.

Within the physician/PA relationship, physician assistants exercise autonomy in medical decisionmaking and provide a broad range of diagnostic and therapeutic services.

This reinforces the concept of team practice, yet emphasizes the ability of PAs to think independently when making diagnoses and clinical decisions. It also refers to the broad scope of services that PAs provide.

The clinical role of physician assistants includes primary and specialty care in medical and surgical practice settings in rural and urban areas. Physician assistant practice is centered on patient care and may include educational, research, and administrative activities.

This piece addresses the versatility of the PA profession, the distribution of the profession in all geographic regions, and the nonclinical roles that PAs may pursue.

PHYSICIAN ASSISTANT: THE NAME

The name, *physician assistant,* has a historical base; some of that history is outlined in Chapter 3. It is a name that has been used since the concept originated but has not always been universally embraced.

The original concept of the PA was an assistant who would be able to handle many aspects of a physician's work. The initial focus was on the education process and not on the name. It was not a copyright term such as *physical therapist* or *psychologist,* but it generally conveyed what everyone thought should be conveyed. Other names were proposed and continue to be proposed (Table 1-1).

It was evident that the PA role filled a health delivery need, but before long the movement was growing and taking on new dimensions. However, confusion arose about the label *physician assistant,* which, after coming to public attention, was misused to describe a variety of

Table 1-1 *Partial list of proposed names for assistants to physicians*

Physician assistant (PA)
Physician's assistant
Physicians' assistant
Physician associate
Physician's associate
Medex (Mx)
Child health associate (CHA)
Surgeon's assistant (SA)
Anesthesia assistant and associate
Clinical associate
Community health aide
Community health medic
Medical services assistant
Ophthalmic assistant
Orthopedic physician's assistant
Pathology assistant
Primex (Px)
Radiology physician's assistant
Synarist
Urologic physician's assistant
Flexner
Osler

Modified from the AAPA Professional Practice Council, 1994 (AAPA PPC 1994b).

individuals, including support personnel from physicians' offices (Fasser 1984).

The title *physician assistant* is not a legally recognized term nationally. However, National Physician Assistant Day (October 6) is observed on the state level in 49 states (Mississippi excepted), the District of Columbia, and some of the trust territories (Puerto Rico, Guam, American Samoa). It is up to the states to protect the public health, safety, and welfare by determining how the term *physician assistant* is used. Generally, this means setting minimum standards and regulations to practice using a certain health profession or occupation (AAPA PPC 1994). With a few exceptions, most state statutes or regulations define PAs as individuals who have graduated from an accredited program, and/or passed the NCCPA examination. While this has not prevented some imposters from occasionally emerging, the known incidences are rare, and the checks and safeguards in place in most states seem fairly sound (Fisher 1995).

From this historical review, we learned that members of the PA profession did not determine the title by which they would be known. The very first suggestions for a name were made by educators, physicians, regulators, and advocates of the concept. Later, PAs did exert some influence in the drive toward title uniformity when state laws were being enacted, accreditation and certification mechanisms were being established, and professional organizations were being founded. It was at this point that Eugene Stead of Duke University observed, "The time has come to consider a new name for the product produced by Duke and other similar programs." Although he favored the title *physician's associate*, Dr. Stead concluded that "agreeing on a name is the important step. What name is adopted is secondary" (Stead 1971). A number of names were advanced, including *Medex*, coined by Dr. R. Smith at the Medex Northwest Physician Assistant Program in Seattle.

Although *physician assistant* is the dominant title, some believe that the term assistant is demeaning. They argue that the term leaves the impression that PAs are mere helpers or auxiliary personnel who facilitate the work of their superior, or function in a subordinate position. Inclusion of the word assistant leads people to draw parallels with medical assistants and nurses' aides.

A second argument for changing the title is that it does not accurately describe what PAs do. The scope of medical services and the level of care that PAs provide go beyond assisting physicians. In many underserved areas, PAs are the sole or primary providers of health care. Even if the term at one time appropriately described PA practice, it is no longer accurate. The AAPA describes PAs as "practicing medicine with physician supervision."

Another point made by advocates for change is that the title is not readily understood. The word *assistant* implies entry-level knowledge, on-the-job training, or trade school education. It fails to reflect PAs' substantial clinical and didactic education and the fact that many have earned graduate degrees (Mastrangelo 1993). Patients may be confused and may sometimes ask when the PA plans to attend medical school. Other health care providers such as nurses resist taking orders from PAs because they do not understand the PA's role. The title is not universally recognized and understood, which leads to problems with insurers, employers, and others.

Proponents of name change tend to favor the term *physician associate* because they believe it more accurately reflects the PA-physician relationship, avoids comparison with medical assistants, and is less confusing to the public. In other parts of the world, *doctors' assistants* and *physician assistants* are well-defined terms for people who support general practitioners (Fischer 1995). Advocates point to the change from Medex to PA that occurred easily and could occur again, given the relative simplicity of changing the word from assistant to associate. Other suggestions include the terms *medical practitioner, physician practitioner, clinical practitioner, assistant physician, clinical associate,* and *associative physician.*

Defenders of the title *physician assistant* argue that replacing the term *assistant* with *associate* does not guarantee greater respect. Respect and self-esteem is to practice with excellence and skill and provide the best possible medical care to patients. These defenders find little or no dissatisfaction with the current title. For them, the title correctly conveys the dependent nature of the relationship with their supervising physician.

The issue is one of semantics. Clerks and telemarketers may be called sales associates, whereas high government officials hold the title special assistant to the president; in academics, assistant professors are still professors.

Supporters of the current name say that time and growth, not a new name, will produce more recognition. The lack of universal recognition occurs because the profession is small and has a relatively brief history. The profession has already made an enormous investment in educating the patients and public about the true meaning of the title physician assistant. State laws define the qualifications of those who use a particular title, and once the title physician assistant is abandoned by the profession, it could be awarded to another category of health provider, such as unlicensed medical graduates.

Another important observation is that the laws of 51 jurisdictions and the federal government could not be changed simultaneously. A period of years would pass during which many different individuals would reap the benefits achieved by the PA profession by assuming the name and calling themselves PAs. In addition to the changes required by the state legislatures, licensing boards, and the federal government, other agencies would be required to make changes. Educational institutions, state and national PA organizations, and the accrediting and certifying agencies would need to be persuaded to change. Many of these organizations would have to bear significant administrative and financial costs to make the change.

As the AAPA Professional Practice Council concluded (Tiger 1993), "the argument most strongly expressed by opponents of change is that this debate draws time and effort away from issues that demand urgent attention. The PA profession is at a crossroads and is faced with unprecedented opportunities to define and influence its future. The options are varied. One observer says 'it is time for PAs to dedicate themselves to achieving the greatest benefit for the greatest number of people by becoming advocates for health promotion and preventive medicine.' "

Certified Physician Assistants

PAs who have passed the Physician Assistant National Certification Examination (PANCE) have the option of putting the word *Certified* behind the title Physician Assistant. This title, *Physician Assistant—Certified*, is abbreviated PA-C. The intent of using PA-C is to distinguish formally trained PAs who are nationally certi-

fied from PAs who are informally trained and not eligible to sit for the PANCE. In the 1970s and 1980s, this was thought to be important since the percentage of non-certified PAs was small but significant, and formally trained PAs felt they should have some way to show the public the difference.

Many PA observers feel that the identification of PA-C is unnecessary and probably confuses more people than it reassures. It is simply an indication that one has passed a test, a fact known, for the most part, only by the profession. The accomplishment is debatable and pales in light of other more commonly recognized letters such as MPH, PhD, and MBA. Adding additional letters such as *R* for registered as in RPA-C, which is done in New York, confuses people even more. This letter stands for *registered*, which means that the PA has completed a form and sent a specified sum to an official New York address. Physicians must be licensed but do not place initials after MD or DO (e.g., MD-L). Nurses who have passed their boards do not put RN-B (Begley 1993).

Generic Terms for Nonphysician Providers

One of the more confusing evolutions of names has been the effort on the part of health services workers and medical sociologists to develop a generic term that encompasses both PAs and other workers that fill traditional physician roles such as nurse practitioners (NPs) and certified nurse midwives (CNMs). One early term used in the early 1970s was *new health professionals*. This was the term the most frequently used throughout the 1970s for both PAs and NPs. Other terms that came into vogue were *physician extenders* and *midlevel practitioners*. These terms were never defined and remain largely meaningless: midlevel between whom? What does it mean to extend a physician? Another term carelessly used is *allied health*. *Allied health providers* is a term used rather restrictively to indicate only those occupations that are allied with the medical profession through their cooperative scheme of accreditation and certification organizations. This term has a fairly precise definition and is usually reserved for those occupations that support physician services such as x-ray technicians, physical therapists, and laboratory personnel. Nurses are in an occupation that is not considered part of allied health personnel, so it is not appropriate to refer to advanced practice nurses such as NPs and CNMs as allied health, nor is it appropriate to refer to PAs as allied health.

One attempt to encompass both PAs and NPs has been the advancement of the term *affiliated clinician*. It was suggested that somehow the two professions, PAs and NPs, should merge under one title (Mittman 1995). Not unlike the *affiliated staff* term used at Group Health Cooperative in Seattle, this effort was to counter the otherwise seemingly negative-sounding term *nonphysician provider*. The response from readers to an editorial in *Clinician Reviews* on the term affiliate clinician was one of disapproval. The term *nonphysician provider* (NPP) was introduced in 1988 in the public health literature and seems to have been largely adopted and used by medical sociologists and the federal government. More recently, nonphysician clinician has emerged in some of the HMO literature. For now, the easiest practice seems to be to use the term *PAs* and *NPs* (PA/NP) and to leave the search for a generic term for another time.

THE EVOLVING ROLE

During the formative years of the PA profession, many arguments were put forth about why this new health occupation was not needed or would fail. Among these arguments was the idea that PAs would be frustrated in their role and leave the field for greener pastures. The sources of frustration envisioned by these critics was the stress and strain of being an "almost doctor," without the intrinsic or extrinsic rewards that our society provides for physicians. The intrinsic rewards of professional autonomy in clinical practice would not be available because of the need for close supervision by a physician (Perry 1989).

Over the last three decades, the PA occupation has helped to fill a health sector with highly skilled professionals. These professionals are capable of carrying out responsibilities that in the past had been within the physician's domain. Given the degree of formal training involved, the PA profession offers highly challenging and satisfying work.

The demand in the health sector for PAs exceeds the available supply (A. Simon 1996). The legal and bureaucratic obstacles preventing a broader scope of responsibilities in diagnosis and treatment have largely been overcome during the first two decades. The initial view held by some that physician assistants would be frustrated because of a narrow and limited professional role is now untenable. The intrinsic rewards are there.

A career as a PA is an attractive alternative to the years of competition, pressure, long hours, and expense required to enter and to complete medical school and to finish residency training. "The career as a physician assistant is also an alternative to the narrower scope of work and lower pay available to the nursing profession" (Perry 1989).

PAs, by and large, have all the responsibility and independence most could reasonably expect. Role frustration, while certainly present, does not appear to be a dominant problem (Freeborn 1995). Although salary levels and career advancement opportunities may be less than optimal, they are certainly not problematic enough to cause a significant exodus from the PA profession. There is a greater demand for graduates of PA programs than there are applicants entering the PA training programs (A. Simon 1996).

In the first decade of the PA movement (1965 to 1975), there was considerable interest in exploring the characteristics of this new health profession. As the profession begins its fourth decade, we expect to see renewed vigor for research that will shed new light on our understanding of this group of highly motivated, well-trained, compassionate health care providers. Such research should help the PA profession to become an even more dynamic force in the improvement of the quality and availability of health care in the United States.

Qualification for Practice/Legal Parameters

State medical practice statutes and regulations define the scope of practice activities, delineate the range of diagnostic and patient management tasks permitted, and set standards for professional conduct. Qualification for entry to practice as a PA in nearly all states requires that individuals possess either a certificate of completion verifying graduation from a PA educational program accredited by the Accreditation Review Committee-Physician Assistants (ARC-PA), and/or proof of having sat for and obtained a passing score on the Physician Assistant National Certifying Examination (PANCE). The PANCE is a standardized test of competence in primary care medicine administered annually by the National Commission on Certification of Physician Assistants (NCCPA) and is assembled and scored through the National Board of Medical Examiners. Presently, certification by the NCCPA is a qualification for practice as a PA in 46 states, and more than 92% of all PAs in active practice hold current NCCPA certification. To maintain certification, the NCCPA mandates that PAs fulfill annual continuing medical education requirements, and to recertify by formal examination every 6 years. PA practice is recognized by licensing boards for health occupations in 49 states and the District of Columbia; 39 states, the District of Columbia, and Guam allow PAs to legally prescribe.

The clinical professional activities and scope of practice of PAs are regulated by state licensing boards, which are often boards of medicine, but in some instances comprise a separate PA licensing board. The PA profession appears to be very comfortable with its dependent practice role and, since its inception, has not wavered in that stance. In contrast, nurse practitioners have articulated a position of practice independent from physicians. Statements by professional nursing organizations have stirred debate on the national level, with physician groups regarding the turf of primary care and related legal practice barriers and regulations. While NPs are professionally autonomous in the performance of nursing care functions, most state medical and nursing practice regulations require that NPs work in collaboration with a physician practice, recognizing the fact that their extended roles encompass medical diagnostic and therapeutic tasks. Thus, in providing medical care tasks, most NPs work closely with physicians in a majority of clinical settings.

In contrast, the legal basis of PA practice is centered on physician supervision. Doctors are ultimately responsible for the actions of the PAs, and state laws often require that physicians clearly delineate the practice scope and supervisory arrangements of employed PAs. However, wide latitude exists within the physician's practice for the PA to exercise levels of judgment and professional autonomy in medical care decisions.

It has been noted that the level of acceptance and integration of PAs in American medicine is related to its continued adherence to this position and to the PA's willingness to practice in settings, locations, and clinical care areas that physicians deem to be less preferable. Observers believe that PA utilization will continue as long as it extends the medical care services of physicians without competing for or challenging physician authority and autonomy. How these providers compare to other providers is profiled in Tables 1-2 to 1-4.

Table 1-2 *First-year enrollments in selected health professions schools, selected academic years, 1970–1971 through 1995–1996*

HEALTH OCCUPATION	NUMBER OF STUDENTS					
	1970–1971	1975–1976	1980–1981	1985–1986	1991–1992	1995–1996
Medicine						
Allopathic (MD)	11,348	15,295	17,186	16,963	17,071	17,058
Osteopathic (DO)	623	1,038	1,496	1,737	1,974	2,274
Podiatric medicine (DPM)	351	641	695	811	725	
Dentistry (DDS/DMD)	4,565	5,763	6,030	4,843	4,047	
Optometry (OD)	884	1,057	1,258	1,251	1,355	
Pharmacy (RPh)	5,694	8,710	7,551	7,084	8,343	
Veterinary medicine (DVM)	1,430	1,712	2,239	2,282	2,225	
Nursing (RN)	78,524	112,174	110,201	100,791	113,526	
Physician assistants (PA)						2,400
Nurse practitioner (NP)						5,000

(Data from American Association of Medical Colleges. AAMC Data Book, Statistical Information Related to Medical Education, January, 1992; American Association of Colleges of Osteopathic Medicine. 1992 Annual Statistical Report; American Association of Colleges of Podiatric Medicine. Unpublished data; American Dental Association, council on Dental Education. Annual report on Dental Education, 1991/93. Also prior annual reports; American Schools and Colleges of Optometry. Unpublished data; American Association of Colleges of Pharmacy. Profile of Pharmacy Students, 1992, Also unpublished data; Association of American Veterinary Medical Colleges. Unpublished data; National League for Nursing. Nursing Datasource, 1992: Vol 1; Oliver 1993; Morgan 1993.)

Table 1-3 *Estimated supply of selected health personnel and practitioner-to-population ratios, selected years, 1970–1995*

HEALTH OCCUPATION	NUMBER					
	1970	1975	1980	1985	1990	1995
Physicians (active)	326,900	384,500	457,500	534,700	602,300	643,720
Allopathic (MD)[a]	314,200	370,400	440,400	512,800	574,200	618,000
Osteopathic (DO)[b]	12,700	14,100	17,100	21,900	28,100	35,720
Podiatrists	7,100	7,300	8,900	10,500	12,000	10,300
Dentists[c]	102,200	112,00	126,200	140,700	162,300	155,000
Optometrists[d]	18,400	19,900	21,900	24,000	26,000	28,000
Pharmacists[e]	112,600	121,800	142,400	153,500	161,900	170,000
Veterinarians[e]	25,900	31,100	36,500	42,100	51,000	59,000
Registered nurses[e]	750,000	961,000	1,272,900	1,538,100	1,715,600	1,977,000
Physician assistants						32,470
Nurse practitioners						36,000
	PRACTITIONERS PER 100,000 POPULATION					
Physicians	157.1	175.4	197.8	220.1	237.1	248.6
Allopathic (MD)	151.0	168.9	190.4	211.1	226.1	236.0
Osteopathic (DO)	6.2	6.5	7.5	9.1	11.2	12.6
Podiatrists	3.4	3.4	3.9	4.4	4.8	
Dentists	49.5	51.6	55.4	59.0	64.9	
Optometrists	8.9	9.2	9.6	10.0	10.3	
Pharmacists	54.5	56.1	62.2	64.0	64.4	
Veterinarians	12.5	14.3	15.9	17.6	20.3	
Registered nurses	366.0	449.0	560.0	644.0	690.0	
Physician assistants						8.6
Nurse practitioners						Unknown

[a] The numbers of active MDs are adjusted to include approximately 90 percent of those MDs either with unknown addresses or not classified as to activity status by the American Medical Association.

[b] American Osteopathic Association, 1996, estimated number of active DOs.

[c] Methodology changed in 1990

[d] American Optometric Association, 1996.

[e] U.S. Department of Labor, Bureau of Labor Statistics, Current Population Survey.

(From data estimated by Health Resources and Services Administration, Bureau of Health Professions, American Academy Physician Assistants, and Morgan 1993.)

Table 1-4 *Estimated percent distribution of practicing physician assistants by specialty: selected years, 1984–1996[a]*

SPECIALTY	1984	1989	1990	1991	1992	1994	1996
Primary care[a]	55.8	49.3	45.9	43.6	42.8	45.2	50.8
Family medicine	42.5	37.9	33.0	31.3	31.4	33.7	39.8
General internal medicine	9.2	7.8	9.0	9.9	8.9	9.2	8.3
Pediatrics	4.1	3.6	3.0	2.4	2.5	2.3	2.7
Non-primary care	44.2	50.7	55.0	56.4	57.2	48.5	49.2
Obstetrics/gynecology	3.1	4.6	4.0	3.4	3.3	2.9	3.0
Surgical subspecialties	9.0	7.5	9.0	9.0	9.8	10.5	8.8
General surgery	9.2	7.9	8.0	9.2	8.0	7.7	3.1
Internal medicine subspecialities	4.8	3.8	6.0	5.9	7.1	6.3	5.8
Pediatric subspecialties	0.0	1.0	2.0	1.0	1.2	1.2	2.1
Emergency medicine	6.4	6.2	7.0	7.9	8.0	8.7	7.0
Orthopedics	4.1	5.6	6.0	7.1	7.6	7.8	6.9
Occupational medicine	4.1	3.8	5.0	4.0	3.9	3.4	3.0
Other specialties[d]	3.5	10.3	8.0	8.9	8.3	6.3	9.5

[a] Practicing Physician Assistants are figured at 85% of the total graduates.

[b] Primary care includes Internal Medicine, Family/General Practice, Pediatrics

[c] Includes General Medicine

[d] Includes Correctional Medicine, Neurology, Geriatric Medicine, Psychiatry, and Industrial Medicine.

(Unpublished data from American Academy of Physician Assistants.)

2

Development of the Profession

FACTORS INVOLVED IN THE CREATION OF A NEW HEALTH PROFESSION

The introduction and development of new types of health care professionals are recurring phenomena in societies observed in the health systems of a number of countries over several time periods. While physicians are typically regarded as the "captain of the ship" in the systems of most countries, and their status may be thought of as the "gold standard" of health care professionals, numerous other workers assume roles in clinical practice similar to those of physicians. The practice roles of these health professionals often overlap considerably with those of physicians. In several countries, particularly after times of societal/cultural turmoil such as war and revolution when doctors are in short supply, new professionals were introduced who often initially assumed roles as generalist physician substitutes. Some were later incorporated into health systems where their utilization and status became institutionalized, their clinical roles evolving to include a broad range of clinical practice activities. Generally, these nonphysician providers have fewer years of formal training than physicians, have a regulated, dependent status, and in some cases a largely technical scope of practice. In nearly all instances, the major rationale for the introduction of such providers is to supplement and extend the delivery of medical care services to the population. The clinical roles of some nonphysicians blend medical care tasks with skills imported from other health care paradigms and disciplines. In such instances, practice is not merely substitutive of physician functions, but is expanded to encompass services that may be termed *physician-complementary*, e.g., health and medical services not performed by physicians.

The notion of using health practitioners who are not physicians to provide medical services is not new. Physicians have trained and employed many types of assistants throughout the history of medicine. In many countries during the last two centuries, a number of nonphysician health providers who were not physicians have played important roles in meeting nations' medical services needs (Roemer 1977). Sometimes, the emergence of health professionals comes about after a cultural upheaval, which led to a physician shortage in a country. The introduction of various types of nonphysician health professionals has been shown to be an effective health workforce stopgap measure in several countries' health systems (Rousselot 1971; Storey 1972; Roemer 1977).

Based in part on the developmental experience of the physician assistant (PA), and in part on natural history models in other health systems, some of the more notable recent experiences with nonphysician providers is reviewed below. In describing the creation and natural history of new types of health care professionals, using the US PA as a model, we propose at least five somewhat overlapping stages in the evolution of new health professionals (Table 2-1).

CREATION OF THE PHYSICIAN ASSISTANT

PAs were created with a public and medical establishment mandate to assume clinical roles that extend the capabilities of a generalist physician to deliver primary care to medically

---

Table 2-1 *Stages in the development of new health professionals*

Stage I — Ideology

The existence of an appropriate social, medical, and political climate; medical personnel factors; and educational influences that lead to a coherent rationale and expected role necessitating the creation of a new category of health personnel. This rationale must gain the acceptance of critical existing stakeholders in the health system, e.g., physicians and nurses, government health policy makers, educational institutions, medical regulators, state legislators, and health administrators. The climate in which the conceptualization of new health occupations develop helps set the stage. Stakeholders must perceive a benefit. Public policy makers must be convinced that introduction of a new health profession will benefit society in improving health services, and not directly threaten existing professions.

Stage II — Implementation

Key health policy, medical education, and organizational collaboration to implement the conceptual framework, educational preparation, and professional regulation of the new profession. A variety of critical areas must be determined: length and level of training, curriculum content, scope of practice, legal status and mechanisms of regulation, sponsorship and funding, and credentialing. Academic institutions begin to develop educational programs. Organization of levels of state recognition (licensure, regulation, or certification) of practice activities for new practitioners entering medical practices. Establishment of systems of educational sponsorship, academic recognition and accreditation, professional credentialing, occupational regulation, definition of practice scope.

Stage III — Evaluation

Conduct and evaluation of organized health services research and public policy analysis designed to measure the levels of clinical performance effectiveness and practice characteristics of the new professional: measurement of levels of acceptance by patients, physicians, and other professionals; content and quality of care; cost-effectiveness; practice deployment; and role satisfaction. Also, studies begin to examine longitudinal trends of provider utilization patterns and professional demographics in the health system.

Stage IV — Incorporation

Steady growth and acceptance of the new professionals. Utilization extends from original generalist/primary care roles to include specialty areas. Clinical practice settings include private solo and group medical offices; hospitals, health facilities, and organizations; academic centers; managed care systems; long-term care facilities; and public health clinics. Legislation is promulgated in states authorizing in statute for medical licensing boards to regulate the new health professional; regulations adopted permitting new professionals to be eligible for fractional reimbursement for professional services (payment to the employing practice). Inclusion of new professionals in health workforce supply and requirements planning; publication of summary policy reports on impact and practice experiences.

Stage V — Maturation

Acceptance and institutionalization of the profession among the health occupations. The acceptance of educational institutions in the form of faculty appointments for PA educators. Professional utilization patterns are characterized by steady, ongoing demand for practitioners' services by both patients and physicians, and continuing utilization in a variety of medical care settings.

underserved populations. Now a quarter of a century later not only is there widespread recognition of the competence and effectiveness of PAs in medical care delivery, but their utilization has been shown to enhance access to health care and to expand the capacity of physician practices.

Roots of the PA Profession

When PAs were introduced into medical practice in the United States in the 1960s, the principal hope of the creators of the concept was to improve primary health care delivery due to generalist physician shortages brought about by the fading of the general practitioner. PAs were envisioned as a new type of medical generalist—one whose role could build on prior medical experiences, one who could be trained in a reasonably short period of time and rapidly deployed to practice locations in medically needy areas.

The concept of new types of health personnel to extend physician services in the United States was first suggested by Charles L. Hudson, then President of the National Board of Medical Examiners, in a speech to the House of Delegates of the American Medical Association (AMA) in 1961. In this address and a subsequent article in *JAMA*, he articulated the rationale for new health personnel based on changing medical labor/hospital staffing personnel demands and advancing technology (Hudson 1961).

Stead and Estes noted the short supply of primary care physicians at that time, and that physicians were becoming more specialized. This led them to propose a new category of personnel to augment physician capacity to deliver needed generalist/primary care services (Carter 1982).

THE PREDECESSORS OF PAs

For centuries, all over the world, individuals who are not fully trained doctors have been involved in health care delivery. Known by a variety of names, given differing clinical prerogatives by societies, and discharging vastly different functions, these types of health providers play important roles in delivery systems, often, but not exclusively, in primary care. In the main, nonphysician health providers and the way they function are a product of the systems and nations that have fostered their development and incorporated their roles.

While the role of "doctor" as chief minister to and advocate for the person who is ill has existed since time immemorial, the role of the physician is a more recent incarnation. In the United States, a wide variety of health providers were in practice in Colonial times, some of whom were better trained than others. By the mid 1800s, the establishment of the US medical profession was based on a profound European influence in training and role, the incorporation of newly developing scientific advancements, and a propensity to exert political and economic strength to define and protect professional prerogatives (Starr 1982). There were a number of rivals popular with patients, but allopathic medicine prevailed based largely on adherence to a philosophical and scientific approach.

Nonphysician Providers

At one time or another, many countries have utilized a variety of health care workers, which we broadly define as nonphysician providers. Implicit in our definition is the notion that these health providers perform medical tasks that in some societies have been the domain of physicians. Such tasks could include skills in physical examination, diagnosis of common illnesses, minor surgical skills, knowledge of basic medications, and so forth. Countries in Africa, Asia, and South and Central America continue to employ these types of providers mainly to increase primary care delivery to poorly served regions.

A number of industrial nations, curiously sometimes after periods of social upheaval, have turned to nonphysicians to provide needed health services. At times, this approach has taken advantage of existing resources and circumstances on which to build a new cadre of health providers. Various objectives underlie strategies to incorporate nonphysicians into health systems: the need for primary care, medical assistance in times of doctor shortages, and the need for trained personnel to staff developing technology (Fulop & Roemer 1987). Sometimes the incorporation of nonphysicians into a nation's health system appears to be connected to social strife, and a type of health provider emerges to fill specific health manpower policies (Table 2-2) (Cawley 1983b).

FRANCE: THE OFFICIER DE SANTÉ

In 1803, shortly after the French Revolution, the eminent scientist and educator Fourcroy submitted a report to the legislature outlining plans for a major reorganization of the French medical care system. Among his proposals was the creation of a new, independent grade of health officers who would help alleviate health personnel shortages in the military and the civilian sector, particularly in rural areas. These providers were called *Officiers de Santé* (Health Officers).

Qualifications for the grade of Officier de Santé in the French health system required either a 6-year apprenticeship with a physician, a 5-year period in a hospital, or 3 years in medical school; to fully qualify as a physician required 6 years in medical school. The scope of practice of the Officier de Santé was limited. For example, this professional could not perform major operations, but could suture and do minor surgical removal of lesions. Under certain conditions Officiers de Santé were legally liable for malpractice (Bonner 1976).

Despite the good intentions of Fourcroy, as might be expected, this personnel policy stirred substantial opposition from physicians. Officiers came under attack from the medical profession soon after their inception and remained so almost constantly until their abolition in 1892. As French social and economic conditions changed and improved over the years, the clamor from physicians to reestablish

---

Table 2-2 *Types of nonphysician health providers in different countries* [a]

NAME	COUNTRY	TIME
Officier de Santé	France	1803–1892
Feldsher	Russia, Eastern Europe	1600s–Present
Midwife	Universal	>10,000 to present
Nurse midwife	United States, Europe, others	1900–present
Village health worker	Developing countries, Alaska	1940–present
Barefoot doctor	China	1966–present
Physician assistant	United States	1965–present
Nurse practitioner	United States, Canada	1966–present
Community health technician	Colombia, Mexico, Peru, Guyana	1970s

[a] A wide variety of names denote health care workers who were modeled after the Barefoot Doctor. These nonphysician providers were introduced and promoted by WHO in many developing countries: Dresser, medical auxiliary, health assistant, paramedic, medical aide, assistant medical officer, Medicin Africain, and rural health technicians.

(Data from Cawley 1996a.)

a single qualifying degree in medicine became increasingly insistent. The argument of the entrenched physicians to the French legislature was bolstered by the reluctance of Officiers to practice in rural areas. The grade of Officier was attacked by physicians as sustaining "second-class practitioners" and after 1850 was considered by medicine to have outlived its usefulness. After several legislative measures had reduced their practice privileges, Officiers were abolished in 1892. Although judged to be an asset to health care delivery during the immediate post-revolutionary years, the Officier de Santé eventually became a personnel anachronism as medical opposition grew and the French physician population reached adequate numbers (Heller 1978).

RUSSIA: FELDSHERS

Originally, feldshers (from the German *Feldscherer*) were German military assistants to the "barber-surgeons" of the seventeenth century. These feldshers were introduced into the Russian armies by Peter the Great in the 1860s. Following military service, early feldshers were often the only available providers for the rural peasant population. Typically, they were apprenticed to physicians for some time and provided low-cost health care for much of the Russian countryside (Sidel 1968).

For many years, feldshers were widely used by the armies of several East European countries, but eventually, in most instances, they were replaced by more highly trained personnel. In Russia, during several periods, feldshers were extensively used as primary care providers, mainly in rural areas. In these settings, they were often the only type of trained medical personnel available and typically functioned in an independent manner (Storey 1972; Knaus 1981).

After the Bolshevik Revolution, it was decided that each Soviet citizen deserved to be treated by his or her own physician, and feldsherism was considered to be second-class rural medicine without a place in a society that was committed to the "equality" of its citizens. For a while, younger feldshers were sent to medical school, and older ones were allowed to continue their service. However, an abundance of physicians did not change the distribution of medical care, and the rural areas continued to suffer limited access to health care. In 1936, the Soviet government reinstituted formal training for feldshers. By the mid-1970s, the Soviets were training approximately 30,000 feldshers annually (Condit 1977, Condit 1984).

Feldshers receive between 1 and 3 years of medical education following graduation from secondary school. Length of training depends on the specialty the feldsher elects: general feldsher 2½ years, midwife 2½ years, feldsher-laborant 2 years, and sanitarian feldsher 1 to 1½ years. Candidates usually enter directly from secondary school. Instruction is given by physicians only, although feldshers serve on the faculty. Tuition is free, stipends and living expenses are provided, and positions are guaranteed at the completion of training.

The upper 10% of graduate feldshers are encouraged to go on to medical school. Otherwise, they can take evening study at medical school after 3 years of clinical service. Once admitted, these students are eligible for advanced placement. It is now estimated that as many as 25% to 30% of physicians in the former Soviet Union were initially trained as feldshers.

The role of the feldsher in present day Russia is basically twofold: (1) in the urban areas as side-by-side assistants to physicians (similar to PAs and nurse practitioners [NPs] in the United States) and (2) as alternatives to physicians in underserved regions. Like contemporary PAs, they are responsible to a particular physician in their clinical activities. Up until the late 1980s, about 30,000 new feldshers entered practice each year; over a million are in current practice (Kenyon 1985). The latest reports are that feldshers are on the wane with the breakup of the Soviet Union and restructuring of health care in Russia. There seems to be an oversupply of physicians in Russia, with similar maldistribution patterns as in the United States.

Feldshers have had a checkered history in Russia as political and medical forces changed. For many years following the 1917 Soviet Revolution, feldshers were labeled as second-class doctors and considered to be an expedient solution to health personnel problems. As the years went by, feldshers retained their role as the enormity of the health care needs of the newly formed Soviet Union, then the largest country in the world, became apparent. At first, feldshers practiced in the rural and underserved regions of Russia and entrenched themselves as an important personnel link in the health care system: the delivery of primary care. More recently, as the supply of physicians began to grow in Russia, feldshers were perceived as expendable practitioners. Policy makers, on one hand, regarded feldshers practicing in rural areas as necessary, but only to the degree that they can be replaced by physicians (Terris 1977; Knaus 1981). The trend toward replacing rural feldshers with physicians has occurred, until recently, in most of the other Eastern European countries where feldshers are employed.

It is reported that feldshers have adapted to shifts in the patterns of Russian health care and assume a role in technical and specialized areas. Although regarded by Western standards to be less technically advanced, Russian medicine has become specialized in various areas, and specific roles for them have developed. Feldshers are employed as assistants to specialist physicians, advanced clinical technologists, industrial health specialists, school health workers, emergency room assistants, laboratory technicians, and midwives. Some are trained additionally in public health and industrial hygiene and function in those roles in diverse settings. Reportedly, feldshers are not extensively utilized in Russian polyclinics or the tertiary centers in urban areas that deliver specialty care.

Despite forces seeking to reduce the numbers of feldshers and the attempt to replace them in rural areas with physician-staffed centralized health centers, Russia's 1.5 million feldshers remain an important health manpower contingent in the health system. They have become key health personnel in the nation's health systems, playing an intermediary role in medical labor, with capacities in primary medical care and the ability to assume technical and specialized roles. While the early developers of the PA concept did not have the feldsher in mind, there is a remarkable parallel between the feldsher and the American PA today.

It is difficult to determine the future of feldshers. In Russia, the physician ratio to population is 350:100,000, which suggests that feldshers are likely to continue in their present role. Training as a feldsher is a necessary step in the preparation of many physicians. Application to training programs is competitive, and the top 10% of each year's graduating class of feldshers goes on to medical school. Russia appears to be comfortable with the role of an adaptable mid-level health care provider that can fill multiple roles in health care delivery and despite aristocratic claims that medical care by feldshers perpetuates second-class care. For those already relegated to second-class care, the population appears to accept the notion that it is not necessary to have a fully-trained physician present for every illness.

CHINA: BAREFOOT DOCTORS

The Chinese barefoot doctor is a health care worker initially described as a "poor cousin of the Russian feldsher," overly romanticized in many quarters in the 1970s (Terris 1977). A type of nonphysician health care provider, they are not comparable to feldshers or American PAs and NPs in that their training and level of function are on lower levels. Armed with only 3 to 6 months of medical education, the aim was to increase the basic level of primary care delivered to China's enormous and expanding population.

Barefoot doctors emerged from the social cataclysm that marked the 1966 Cultural Revolution in China. During that period, drastic reductions in medical education took place under a campaign against medical and professional elitism. This profoundly anti-intellectual thrust lead to a massive reorganization of the system of medical education. Many medical schools were closed, with a reduction in the length of physician training and a dispersal of faculty to the rural villages. Chinese leader Mao Ze-dong attacked the medical status quo with a vengeance and called for the formation of a legion of primary health care workers based in the village of China who, when not providing health care, would tend the rice fields (Wen & Hays 1975). Barefoot doctors received only 3 months on-the-job training in the villages, which they would serve and their roles were oriented to prevention of common diseases.

In the ensuing years, several million barefoot doctors were trained and deployed in China. As the fervor of the Cultural Revolution waned, the system of medical education was restored, and China worked steadily to rebuild its system of medical education and increase its supply of physicians (Blendon 1979). Policy assessments of the introduction of barefoot doctors note that "the program has not been a panacea; the usefulness of the barefoot doctor lies in there being a stop gap measure rather than a long-term solution to the shortage of physicians" (Hsu 1974).

Barefoot doctors comprise the first tier of Chinese medicine and are the entry point to the system for peasants seeking curative services. Their numbers have declined somewhat from a high of over 2 million in the late 1970s to about 1.2 million in 1984. This reduction coincided with economic reforms in China, resulting in a decline in the cooperative medical system, the last vestige of the Cultural Revolution ideology. Hsiao observed that the extent of health services coverage, specifically for primary care and basic sanitation, was falling in the mid-1980s as the health system shifted in economic emphasis. China's change from a collective agricultural production system to one that rewards peasants according to their individual output has altered the once-strong rural system of primary care in China (Hsiao 1984). Current health care system conditions are very different from those of the 1960s. A deserved triumph of

the cooperative medical system, due in part to the contribution of the barefoot doctor, has been the dramatic reductions in rates of infectious diseases and the establishment of basic standards of public health and sanitation throughout China. The policy shift of the 1960s has resulted in higher life expectancy and lower infant mortality rates than those of New York City. The Chinese health system is in transformation, more recently feeling the pressures of high technology and privatization. Yet its commitment to primary care and demonstrable success in raising the fundamental health level of the population serve as a model for developing countries worldwide (Kristof 1991).

Developing Countries

The incorporation of nonphysician health providers into the health system depends fundamentally on the extent of the needs of that country for medical services. In many developing countries, where the supply of physicians is lacking, various types of practitioners are employed to ensure delivery of essential primary care services such as prenatal care, immunization, and disease screening. In the later half of this century, many countries have successfully utilized nonphysicians, propelled by the increasing demand for health services, the emphasis on primary care, and the World Health Organization policy of "Health for All by the Year 2000" (Fulop 1982; WHO 1980; WHO 1987a; WHO 1987b).

Throughout many countries in Africa (Algeria, Sudan), Asia (Burma), South America (Venezuela), and Oceania (Micronesia, Melanesia, and Polynesia), health workers are known by many different titles (health officers, community health aides, medical auxiliaries, health assistants, village health workers, Algerian adjoint medicaux de lasante, the Burmese health assistant, the Sudanese medical assistant, and the Venezuelan auxiliar de enfermeria) (WHO 1968). They provide primary health care in small communities and in rural areas.

These health providers vary greatly in their backgrounds and level of clinical function (Smith 1978).

The World Health Organization (WHO) has been involved in providing leadership in health personnel, activities in developing countries with the aim of improving primary care and other basic health services such as sanitation and public health. In the 1980s, the major WHO objective in health personnel was total population coverage for health care services. Only by a rapid expansion of programs incorporating use of multipurpose auxiliary health personnel would developing countries achieve this goal (Storms 1979; WHO 1980; Fulop 1982; WHO 1987b).

Through support by the Pan American Health Organization, several programs also exist that lend themselves more closely to comparison with the PA in the United States.

Peru trains and approves health providers with professional status; this training is provided by a specialized high school education leading to the title "Bachelor in Health" (Acuna 1977).

Colombia and Mexico started several experimental training programs in the 1970s for Community Health Technicians—with components of clinical and preventive medicine, public health, and community practice—that involve postsecondary education. The modalities may vary, but the principle of incorporating the PA in the health team is gaining acceptance (Acuna 1977).

In the 1970s, Guyana took a further step by approving the training of a full-fleged PA with the characteristics and functions similar to those of the American version. Experience there has attracted the interest of neighboring countries (Acuna 1977).

Developed Countries

A number of developed countries, faced with the trends of increasing physician specialization and demand for primary care services,

have adopted different approaches in medical education to encourage primary care deployment. A major policy thrust in some industrialized countries has been to place limitations on the numbers of physicians who can become specialists. This fundamental determination in personnel ensures a country's health system of an adequate supply of primary care providers and precludes the need for a nonphysician provider in this role. In most countries, such as Europe, the use of nonphysicians to provide primary care in rural areas or similar types of health providers in urban tertiary-center roles is unheard of. Fully trained physicians deliver primary care and medical generalist service to most, if not all, of the population. To be sure, roles exist for advanced nursing practitioners and nurse midwives in several countries, England being the most noted. In the health systems of most developed countries such as Denmark, however, health personnel and primary care staffing are well established and planned by governments and key groups. In addition, the homogeneity of individual European countries' societies, the common belief that health care is a fundamental right, the smaller geographic areas of these nations, and the less entrepreneurial approach to health services delivery systems are major reasons why most European countries have not adopted the nonphysician health personnel concept. In Latin American countries, the health systems do not include the utilization of nonphysicians of any type; some countries in Latin America, as in Europe, have an oversupply of physicians, particularly in urban areas. For a time, Canada followed the US model by promoting the development of the NP concept, but steady pressure from physicians over time eroded their effectiveness in the system; at present, their numbers are dwindling (Morgan & Cohen 1992).

The Alaska program trains local residents to provide emergency and primary care services in villages that are often hundreds of miles away from the nearest physician. Most Alaska Natives live in small villages isolated by mountain ranges, glaciers, stretches of tundra, impassable river systems, and vast distances. These individuals, called Community Health Aids (CHAs), use procedures set forth in an easy-to-read manual and consult daily by telephone or radio with a hospital-based physician. The foundation for the CHA program was laid in the 1940s and 1950s when the federal government, in response to tuberculosis epidemics, used village volunteers to dispense medicine in remote villages. These volunteers, mostly women, generally act as intermediaries between patients and hospital-based physicians. The title Community Health Aid was chosen to show the position's link to the community and to emphasize that the person in this role did not practice independently of a physician. In 1991, CHAs served about 45,000 Alaska Natives and handled more than 253,000 patient encounters. While the program's effects have not been measured by rigorous study, available data indicate that the program has achieved substantial acceptance among the population it serves and has played a major role in improving the health status of Alaska Natives. The federal government assumes responsibility for medical malpractice claims against services provided by CHAs (GAO 1993).

Feldsherism: Policy Implication

The term *feldsherism* has been used to denote the policy of using nonphysicians to provide primary care health services (Sidel 1968). As a personnel strategy, it has been used by many countries, particularly when health care needs are great and physicians are in short supply. The acceptance of the policy of feldsherism depends in large part on the system of health manpower organization and the needs of the population. In developing countries, increasing the numbers of primary care workers is essential (Roemer 1977; Orubuloye 1982; WHO Study Group 1987); their level of skill in high technology areas is irrelevant. What is needed are providers skilled in the delivery of basic health services referent to the acute needs of the populations of these countries. Specifically, clinicians with knowledge of infectious diseases and their treatment, immunization, fluid replacement therapy, prenatal care, screening for cancer, surgical and orthopedic procedures, and health education to avoid environmental health hazards are essential in providing health services to populations. The advanced skills of the physician are not required in health roles such as these (WHO 1987a; WHO 1987b).

In developed countries, generalist physicians, rather than nonphysicians, are the principal providers of primary care. Roemer notes that this has been the explicit personnel policy in countries such as Belgium, Norway, Canada, and Australia where directions have focused on increasing the proportion of generalist physicians, limiting physician specialization, and giving priority to primary care. Roemer suggests that the US policy, coming on the worldwide trend of experimentation in health manpower in the 1960s, was a hasty expedient to shortages in primary care in America. Roemer (1977) states:

> In the world's most affluent nation, there would hardly seem to be economic justification for the use of physician extenders for primary care. Current American policies can only be attributed to an unwillingness to impose social obligations on the physician (e.g., location in areas of need) and to train adequate numbers of primary care doctors. Such policies are an unfortunate acknowledgment of failure by medicine to fulfill its social mission.

Feldsherism is often thought of as an interim health personnel approach. In Russia, for many years, feldshers were viewed as expedient providers, necessary only until the physician supply became adequate. This view, however, implies that primary care is best delivered by a fully-trained physician, a notion that clearly is an open question. It is unnecessary and a misuse of medical talent to suggest that a physician need be present to deal with every human infirmity. American medical pundit

Daniel Greenberg likens the Western system of medical education to putting all bus drivers through astronaut training, the point being that most physicians are overtrained for the role of the primary generalist.

In a number of countries where nonphysicians have been used over long periods of time, roles have changed with advances in health care delivery and policy shifts. In Russia, feldshers were employed for many years on the front lines of primary care in much of the countryside. As the health system in the country became more sophisticated, and as the supply of physicians came into balance with the medical needs of the population, policy makers and citizens criticized feldsherism as sustaining second class care to those already relegated to second class health care in the system. As indicated, in none of Western Europe, the countries of the Pacific Basin, or in Central or South America is there any movement to incorporate nonphysician health providers as the primary source of health personnel for the future (Nakatani 1987).

Feldsherism is at times championed as an attack on medical elitism and the professional establishment. Others view it as imposing a second tier of medical care. As an expedient policy solution to primary health personnel needs, it has strong advantages. Yet the perpetuation of feldsherism as the best way of providing primary care to a population runs the risk of institutionalizing a lower level of care for the poor, those in medically underserved areas, and other disadvantaged members of society. The employment of nonphysicians in a variety of roles, spanning some primary care functions as well as technical and perhaps even public health duties, appears to be the most appropriate niche for them in the systems of those countries who have elected to use them.

THE AMERICAN EXPERIENCE

In 1960, Dr. Charles L. Hudson spoke before the AMA about an idea he had for a new health practitioner (Hudson 1961). He proposed to "extend the usefulness" and experience of Army and Navy corpsmen as efficient assistants who "could not be expected to exercise medical judgment, but he might well develop considerable technical skill which could be a source of satisfaction." He believed "a curriculum could be devised, consisting of 2 or 3 years of college work with certain prescribed courses" that paralleled medical school, and that these new health providers should be called "externes" in a broader sense than just "medical students."

Hudson writes that reaction to this proposal was generally favorable, but there were some dissenting opinions. Little seems to have come from this proposal, and it was largely believed to have died in some AMA committee. People who spoke with Dr. Hudson in the early 1980s say that he was amazed at how the PA concept exceeded his imagination.

Eugene Stead was Chairman of Medicine at Duke University in the 1960s and recognized changing medical service and personnel needs in and around Duke Medical Center. Stead was a highly respected figure in academic medicine at that time and became interested in developing training programs for new health care personnel. Before coming to Duke, he had been a professor of medicine at Emory University during World War II and worked with very capable third- and fourth-year medical students at a time when the intern staff went from 15 to zero. In spite of their limited training, they gave "superb medical care" (Stead 1979). Knowing what could be accomplished with minimal training, he envisioned a new type of "mid-level" generalist (between the level of a doctor and a nurse), a medical clinician who could be trained in a relatively short time period to assist physicians in a broad range of practice settings. Stead believed that such providers should work closely with the physician and established the role in a configuration that would not directly threaten physicians. He was first approached by Thelma Ingles, RN, at Duke who wanted to develop an advanced medical educational program for nurses. Together, Stead and Ingles' concept was to expand nursing roles in generalist care delivery. The nurses "... were very intelligent and they learned quickly, and at the end of a year we had produced a superb product, capable of doing more than any nurse I had ever met" (Stead 1979). This program could have initiated the NP movement, but was opposed by the National League of Nursing and never continued due to lack of award of national accreditation. The attempt failed because on three occasions, the National League of Nursing, the accrediting agency for degree-granting nursing programs, denied accreditation on the basis that delegating medical tasks to nurses was inappropriate (Fisher 1977). This early foray into an advance practice nursing program was eventually phased out. Ingles left Duke for the Rockefeller Foundation, and Stead was left with a conviction that people with varied backgrounds can deliver high quality patient care.

During this time, Stead developed and Duke University sponsored a continuing medical education (CME) program for physicians living in the region. The CME program failed because of lack of attendance. Stead sought the reasons for the failure and found that many physicians were interested in such a program, but could not attend because of their patient load and because the intensity of their practices was too demanding. He reasoned that if the physicians had well-trained assistants, they would be able to leave their practices for a day or two to attend the seminar programs (Howard 1969).

The idea of an assistant may have been suggested to him by Amos H. Johnson, a solo general practitioner in Garland, a small rural town in the piedmont region of North Carolina. Dr. Johnson was able to attend the CME programs, as well as accept professional appointments such as the president of the American Academy of General Practice (1965–66) because he had an assistant. In fact, the assistant, Henry "Buddy" Treadwell, had been trained by Johnson for his practice needs and functioned in many ways like a contemporary PA, assuming many tasks such as diagnosing and treating (Gifford 1987a; Gifford 1987b).

Because organized nursing was not interested in an expanded role for nurses, Stead conceived of an entirely new category of health professional to assist physicians. He next turned to former military corpsmen. The idea was not entirely without precedent. Duke physicians had been in the military, and many were in the Reserves or were consultants in the major military hospitals in the area. In those hospitals, they had observed corpsmen and medics working with physicians in direct patient care, as well as in technical areas of diagnosis and treatment. Former military corpsmen also worked in special clinical units at the Duke Medical Center Hospital and other hospitals in the region (Carter 1982). The technologic advances in medicine had put pressure on hospitals for well-trained technicians. Many of these veterans were able to assume a large portion of these tasks with little or no additional training.

In the spring of 1965, the Vice Provost for Medical Affairs at Duke University appointed an ad hoc committee to evaluate the existing programs and personnel needs at Duke's hospital. The committee concluded that two types of medical personnel were needed: one, a very highly skilled technician limited to a specific medical discipline or specific area; the other, a more advanced specialist with a broad and basic knowledge of medicine (Stead 1966, 1967; Estes 1968c; Estes 1968e; Estes & Howard 1970b; Howard 1972).

Dr. Herbert Saltzman, of the Duke faculty, had applied for a grant from the National Health Institute seeking support for training chamber operators in hyperbaric medicine citing a need for paramedical technicians "to provide the doctors with support needed in their clinical and research endeavors." Saltzman's concept of the type of personnel needed was consistent with Stead's concept for the PA. Before 1965, the National Heart Institute had not funded "nonprofessional" training programs, but Stead had recently served on the Institute's study section, and its members were aware of this thinking. When the grant was approved in April 1965, the successful piggy-backing of the PA concept, with a source of funding, permitted plans for the first training program to proceed (Carter 1982).

With limited funding by the National Heart Institute, the first Physician Assistant Program was formed at Duke University. On October 4, 1965, four former Navy corpsmen became the first students to begin a 2-year training program. Almost by accident, the new concept received nationwide publicity. *Reader's Digest* produced a series of articles entitled "Where the Jobs Are" (Velie 1965). Even before the curriculum for the first class was planned, the *Digest* announced to its readers that the Duke faculty hoped the program would help to make up for the dwindling number of rural doctors. Halfway through the training program, the students were portrayed in a September 6, 1966 article in *LOOK* magazine. This article, "More Than A Nurse, Less Than A Doctor," was the first airing of the concept to the general public. The article began with a paragraph implying that the social change taking place in providing the public increased access to health services would be accomplished through "the use of mid-level providers" (Berg 1966):

> There is a shortage of doctors, and it's getting worse. With the demand for medical care swelling and treatment itself growing more complex daily, the supply of physicians cannot keep up with the need for their skills. Although plans are under way to build more medical schools and expand existing ones, the experts figure it takes almost ten years from the time a medical student drops into one end of the funnel and a practicing physician emerges from the other. Sick people can't wait that long.

Three of the four students graduated a year later. For 2 years they had utilized the house staff's television lounge in the medical center hospital as their classroom. Their graduation ceremony was held in a small Durham barbecue restaurant. Within such inauspicious environments, these prototype PAs began formulating a new role, a role as yet uncharted.

The Duke program began to expand. In September 1967, just before the first class graduated, the training program moved from the Department of Medicine to the Department of Community Health Sciences under the direction of Dr. E. Harvey Estes, Jr. In that year, Stead retired from active professional duties and Dr. D. Robert Howard was appointed the first full-time director of the program. Under Howard's leadership, the program continued to grow, increasing its number of students and its physical facilities. From the house staff television lounge, the program moved to a small white trailer purchased by the newly formed *American Association of Physician's Assistants.*

From a historical standpoint, it is noteworthy that initially Stead and his colleagues were insistent that the PA, being in a dependent role, could not and would not enter into the medical problem-solving process. The PA would enter the process before and after the stages of diagnosis and prescription. The original intent was that the diagnosis and prescription would be reserved for the physician (Schneller 1978). E. Harvey Estes, chair of the Duke University Department of Community Health Sciences Department in 1968, explained (Estes 1968b):

> Practicing medicine is basically diagnosis and prescribing treatment. The new assistant will take no part in traditional doctor functions. -

During the same year, D. Robert Howard, MD, Duke PA Program Director, wrote (Howard 1969):

> ... the physician's assistant will not be able to make diagnosis or prescribe management for patients, but they can learn to do just about anything else. The diagnostic and prescriptive functions obviously belong to the physicians.
>
> These functions belong to them now and should always stay with them.

In fact, one of the innovative features of the original concept was to avoid seeking licensure for the PA to perform any specific task yet developing some autonomy. The features of physician dependency and being excluded from the diagnostic and prescriptive process were believed to be compatible and did not require licensure (Ballenger 1971). An even more interesting fact is that physician assistants have come to assume diagnostic and therapeutic management responsibilities in their clinical roles. The level of PA clinical function subsumes diagnostic and patient management tasks.

If the idea of a PA movement was in the eye of its creators, it also rested squarely on the shoulders of its first students. One of the first students recalls thinking then that if any of them did poorly, it could be the early demise of such a movement. The idea of a PA was generally cooly received by the physicians, and only a few were willing to engage in the novel experiment of an improved assistant for doctors. Ken Ferrell, from the first Duke class, recalls that some of the physicians who would have benefited most from assistants were quite resistant to the idea. They were reluctant to relinquish any of their responsibilities, even though they were overworked (Mastrangelo 1993).

The idea of the PA persisted, and the notion of training of a new category of health professionals to assist the physician spread to other institutions. In 1968 a program began at Bowman-Gray School of Medicine in Winston-Salem, North Carolina, similar to the Duke program. In the same year, Alderson-Broaddus College, a small private school in Phillippi, West Virginia, admitted its first class to a 4-year degree program for educating physician assistants (Fasser 1992a). Unlike the Duke program, students enrolled in the Alderson-Broaddus College directly from high school with the intent of majoring in medical sciences and receiving a bachelor degree at the end of 4 years. The director of the program, Hu C. Meyers, was a local general practice physician. He was promoted to professor and chairman of the Department of Medical Science to oversee this program. The development of the Alderson-Broaddus College program was supported by grants from The Commonwealth Fund, The Robert Wood Johnson Foundation, and the Department of Health, Education and Welfare (Meyers 1978).

At the University of Washington in Seattle, Richard Smith, MD, MPH, Professor of Health Sciences, began a 1-year program (later increased to 15 months, and now 24 months) to augment the training of former military medical corpsmen. This was called the MEDEX program, a contraction of the two words MEDicine and EXtension. Graduates would refer to themselves as Medex, and put Mx after their name. The program, which began in 1969, relied heavily on its students receiving most of their training through "on-the-job" preceptorships with selected physicians in rural areas of the Pacific Northwest.

While credit is rightfully given to Stead, Howard, and Estes at Duke for pioneering PA education, the Medex model developed by Smith deserves a special place in PA history. It has remained a viable model of PA education and is often referred to as the collaborative model because the curriculum was built to augment a specific group of individuals with enriched medical backgrounds. Dick Smith was a physician with a wealth of experience in medical care in the Third World as well as in the United States. Having worked in Cambodia and Laos in the 1960s where he was exposed to the *Officier Medicine Indochinoise*, the Asian version of the French African Medical Officer, he had also been in the Peace Corps, and was part of the US delegation to the World Health Organization in the mid 1960s. Even a brief time with Albert Schwetzer in Africa helped shape what he envisioned would be an assistant to the primary care physician. Smith returned to the United States in the mid-1960s as Planning Director for Surgeon General William Stewart. In this position, he continued to nurture the idea of the creation of a new category of health care professional, one who could assume the majority of care that a physician provided. During this time, Smith also met the same Amos Johnson from Garland, North Carolina, who helped influence Eugene Stead in his PA concept. Johnson, a country doctor, was a dominant figure in North Carolina medical politics at that time. He was president of the American Association of Family Practice and an influence in the AMA. He had heard of Smith's ideas, knew of Stead's work, and introduced Smith to the leadership in the AMA who provided encouragement in developing the PA concept that Smith envisioned. He often mentioned the relationship he had with Buddy Treadwell and wanted Smith to develop a similar type of assistant (R. Smith, personal communication, 1996).

Dick Smith wanted his program to be more than a demonstration project that was typically underwritten by the federal government and then forgotten a few years later. To succeed, he chose a state with a conservative legislature. Thinking that if he could sell his concept to physicians in a conservative state, it would have a better than usual chance of success elsewhere. He chose the University of Washington in Seattle for a site with some familiarity since he had completed his MPH at this institution and understood some of the politics there. This program differed from the Duke model in that entering students needed to have a sponsoring physician who agreed to be their mentor for the preceptorship. Often these physicians became their employers as well (R. Smith, personal communication, 1996).

Within a few years, eight Medex programs evolved, mostly consisting of 3 months of intensive didactic work in basic and clinical sciences at the university medical center, followed by a preceptorship with a practicing primary care physician for 9 to 12 months. These programs were widely distributed from the inner city of the Watts district of Los Angeles, to rural areas such as Alabama, Dartmouth, North Dakota, and Hershey, Pennsylvania. Not all were bootstrap programs. One program was started at Drew University and another in Salt Lake City at the University of Utah. Upon completion of the preceptorship, the student received a certificate (Smith 1969).

The third prototype of PA education was at the University of Colorado Child Health Associate program and also began in 1968. Under Henry Silver, a well-respected professor of pediatrics, and Loretta Ford, RN, this program recruited nurses and other applicants with diverse backgrounds for a 5-year (later reduced to 3 years) training program to assist pediatric physicians (AMA 1970). Originally, the mission was to supply preventive and routine care to children and began as an NP program. This was later expanded to almost all areas of pediatric primary care and enrolled non-nurses (Fisher 1977). Even though graduates of this program put CHA after their names, they usually take the Physician Assistant National Certifying Examination (PANCE), and many are certified as pediatric PAs.

Other movements in specialization took place in the late 1960s as well. There was a surge of new programs to train nonphysician providers in very specific areas of care. Some of these programs include the Orthopedic Assistant and the Urologic Physician's Assistant, which were 2-year programs designed to train personnel to work directly for specialists. The only requirement for entry into a 4-month "health assistants" training progam sponsored by Project Hope in Laredo, Texas, in 1970 was that the student had to be 18 years old. Eight of the eleven students who entered the first class lacked high school equivalence and were able to earn their General Equivalency Diploma Certificate upon completion of the program (Sadler 1972). Programs sprung up of various duration in length of training were developed in gastroenterology, allergy, dermatology, and radiology. By 1971, more than 125 programs in 35 states announced they were training "physician support personnel" (Bureau of Health Manpower Education 1971). Few nonprimary care programs survived past 1975, with the exception of the surgical assistant, the pathology assistant, and child health associate programs.

While not all programs flourished, most primary care-based ones did. By 1972, 31 programs were in operation: 21 of the programs were federally supported by agencies such as the Office of Economic Opportunity, the Model Cities Program, the Veterans Administration, the Public Health Service, the Department of Defense, and the Department of Labor, while the remainder were financed by private foundations and institutional sources (Fisher 1977).

In 1970, the National Congress on Health Manpower (sponsored by the AMA's Council on Health Manpower) sought to develop uniform terminology for the many emerging PA programs. Congress concluded that *physician's assistant* was too general to be adopted as the single generic term because PAs were receiving varied levels of training. They decided that *associate* would be a preferred term for health workers who assume a direct and responsible role in patient care and act as colleagues to physicians, rather than as their technical assistants. Congress noted that the PA terminology is often confused and used interchangeably with the established *medical assistant*, the title for the nonprofessional office helper who functions in a clerical and technical fashion (Curran 1972). The AMA's House of Delegates rejected the *associate* terminology in the belief that *associate* should be applied only to physicians working in collaboration with other physicians (this criticism ignores the apostrophe "s," which denotes that the *associate* is not another physician). Thus no consistent position emerged from organized medicine (Sadler 1972).

In 1970, the Board on Medicine of the National Academy of Sciences classified physician's assistants according to the degree of specialization and level of judgment. The Board on Medicine Report states:

> The Type A assistant is capable of approaching the patient, collecting historical and physical data, organizing the data, and presenting them in such a way that the physician can visualize the medical problem and determine appropriate diagnostic or therapeutic steps. He is also capable of assisting the physician by performing diagnostic and therapeutic procedures and coordinating the roles of other more technical assistants. While functioning under the general supervision and responsibility of the physician, he might under special circumstances and under defined rules, perform without the immediate surveillance of the physician. He is, thus, distinguished by his ability to integrate and interpret findings on the basis of general medical knowledge to exercise a degree of independent judgment.

> The Type B assistant, while not equipped with general knowledge and skills relative to the whole range of medical care, possesses exceptional skill in one clinical specialty or, more commonly, in certain procedures within such a specialty. In his area of specialty, he has a degree of skill beyond that normally possessed by a Type A assistant and perhaps that normally possessed by physicians who are not engaged in the specialty. Because his knowledge and skill are limited to a particular specialty, he is less qualified for independent action. An example of this type of assistant might be one who is associated with a renal dialysis unit and who is capable of performing these functions as required.

> The Type C assistant is capable of performing a variety of tasks over the whole range of medical care under the supervision of a physician, although he does not possess the level of medical knowledge necessary to integrate and interpret findings. He is similar to a Type A assistant in the number of areas in which he can perform, but he cannot exercise the degree of independent synthesis and judgement of which Type A is capable. This type of assistant would be to medicine what the practical nurse is to nursing.

On the surface, the new classification seemed to be helpful but quickly created some confusion in hierarchy and uniform nomenclature. When Medex graduates were assigned a Type C rating and Duke graduates were assigned a Type A rating, resentment by Medex leaders was raised and this was later changed (Estes 1970a).

In June 1972, the Bureau of Health Manpower, Health Resources Administration, Department of Health, Education, and Welfare, mandated by Section 774a of The Public Health

Service Act as amended by PL 93-157 was initiated. This was "The Comprehensive Health Manpower Training Act of 1971," and under this important act the responsibility for 24 of the 31 programs was assumed and contracts with 16 developing programs were initiated. This federal support represented an investment in experimental programs to test the hypothesis that nonphysician health professionals could provide many physician-equivalent services in primary and continuing care. The Bureau's programs were designed to carry out the intent of Congress to relieve problems of geographic and specialty maldistribution of physicians and the US health care workforce. This intent was reflected in the contract process, which required each PA program to emphasize three major objectives in its demonstration:

1. Training for delivery of primary care in ambulatory settings
2. Placing graduates in medically underserved areas
3. Recruiting residents of medically underserved areas, minority groups, and women as students for these programs

Each program was free to devise various curricula and methods of instruction, but the preceding three requirements were held constant to carry out the intent of Congress (Fisher 1977). This brought about the demise of most of the Type C and B programs. They either folded up in a few years for lack of funding support or converted into primary care programs. The only survivors are the Surgeon's Assistant and the Pathology Assistant programs.

There was also a brief experimentation with a more appropriate name since the title physician's assistant was not always widely accepted. Silver suggested a new term *syniatrist* from the Greek *syn* signifying "along with" or "association" and *-iatric*, which means "relating to medicine" or a "physician" (Silver 1971a). He proposed the syniatrist terminology by a prefix relating to each medical specialty; for example, general practice would be a General Practice Syniatrist Associate or a General Practice Syniatrist Aide (Salder 1972). Smith opted for Medex and saw his graduates placing the letters Mx after their names as the appropriate title. Other proposed titles in lieu of PA included *Osler, Flexner*, and *Cruzer* in honor of famous people in American medical history (Smith 1971). The intent of these new names would be neutral and less demeaning than PA. Little interest in these names developed and the title PA remained.

Support of Organized Medicine

The PA concept would not have germinated and become successful had it not been for the overt support and active involvement of major physician groups. The AMA, in particular, contributed substantially to confirming legitimacy and acceptance of the concept and had a strong role in the establishment of standards of PA educational program accreditation and professional credentialing organizations. Support for the development of the PA profession also came from the American College of Surgeons, the American Academy of Family Physicians, the American Academy of Pediatrics, and other medical groups in shaping the infrastructure of the PA profession.

During the formative stages of the PA profession, a notable feature was the impressive degree of collaboration among organized physician groups, PA educators and professional leaders, public policy agencies, and national medical regulatory bodies. These groups worked to build the critical components of the professions' structure, particularly legal and regulatory components. A good example of physician group collaboration was the 1973 creation of the National Commission on Certification of Physician Assistants (NCCPA). The NCCPA is an independent health credentialing agency that administers the Physician Assistant National Certifying Examination (PANCE). Physician groups worked with government agencies, the National Board of Medical Examiners, the Federation of State Medical

Licensing Boards, and members of the general public. PA practice certification mechanisms were patterned to a large degree on their counterparts in the medical profession.

EVOLUTIONARY DEVELOPMENT OF THE PA PROFESSION

To understand the evolution of the PA profession, it is helpful to examine the history by important milestones or segments. The transition from an idea in 1960 to the mature profession that exists in 1997 and beyond has a number of elements. We have identified these as ideology, implementation, evaluation, incorporation, and consolidation.

Period of Ideology (1961–1965)

When PAs were introduced into medical practice in the United States in the 1960s, the principal hope of their creators was to improve primary health care delivery, which was suffering due to generalist physician shortages brought about by the demise of the general practitioner. PAs were envisioned as a new type of medical generalist, one whose role would build on prior medical experiences, who would be trained in a reasonably short time and be rapidly deployed to practice locations in medically needy areas. The concept of new types of health personnel to extend physician services in the United States was first suggested by Charles L. Hudson, then President of the National Board of Medical Examiners, in a speech to the House of Delegates of the AMA in 1961. In this address and in a subsequent article in JAMA, he articulated the rationale for new health personnel based on changing medical labor/hospital staffing personnel demands and advancing technology (Hudson 1961). Later, Stead and Estes noted the short supply of primary care physicians and that physicians were becoming more specialized. (Stead 1967b; Estes 1971).

Period of Implementation (1966–1972)

The federal government provided strong support for the creation and development of PAs in the health system. Domestic policy in the early 1970s sought to improve citizen access to health services by increasing health care personnel. Most believed there was a shortage of physicians overall and a decreasing proportion in general practice. Because organized medicine had not adequately addressed these issues in the past, this new federal workforce approach was composed of two major elements: (1) expansion of physician supply by expanding medical education and (2) promoting the introduction of new practitioners whose roles would focus on primary care. The PA concept began as one model among a number of new health practitioner models (e.g., nurse practitioners, health assistants, Medex, and many others). Shortly after Stead introduced the PA model at Duke in 1965, other versions of the concept of the PA emerged with the Child Health Associate Program, developed by Henry Silver in 1966 at the University of Colorado, and the Medex program founded by Richard Smith at the University of Washington in 1969 (Smith 1971).

LEGAL/REGULATORY CHALLENGES

The introduction of the PA into the American health system brought with it the necessity to consider appropriate legal and regulatory approaches to enable these and other emerging health practitioners to enter clinical practice. Important decision points were the determination of the professional scope of practice of these new professionals, appropriate levels of state board recognition (licensure, registration, certification), and stipulations for supervision and prescribing activities (Estes 1971; Ballenger 1971).

To support the entry of PAs into clinical practice, the House of Delegates of the AMA in 1970 passed a resolution urging state medical licensing boards to amend health occupations statutes and regulations to permit PAs to qualify as medical practitioners.

Among the first states to amend medical acts allowing PAs to practice were Colorado, North Carolina, California, and New York. On the federal level, important leadership in the early nurturing of the PA concept was provided by the federal government in the form of grant support for PA educational programs. Initial legislative initiatives included the Allied Health Professions Personnel Act of 1966 and the Health Manpower Act of 1968. PA programs quickly sprang up in medical centers, hospitals, and colleges; programs were also supported by state legislatures and private foundations.

The Comprehensive Health Manpower Act of 1973 was an important milestone, which marked the inclusion of PA program funding support programs under Title VII of the Public Health Service Act. Since then, federal awards have totaled $140 million supporting PA educational programs; in FY-96, programs received a total of $5.7 million (AGPAW 1995).

STATE REGULATION

The legal basis of PA practice is codified in state medical practice statutes granting authorization to licensed physicians to delegate a range of medical diagnostic and therapeutic tasks to individuals who meet educational standards and practice requirements. Authority for medical task delegation is based on the legal doctrine of *respondeat superior*, which holds that it is the physician who is ultimately liable for PA practice activities, and mandates that doctors who employ PAs appropriately define and supervise their clinical actions. State acts exempt PAs from the unlicensed practice of medicine with the stipulation that they function with physician supervision.

Professional activities and the scope of practice of PAs are regulated by state licensing boards, which are often boards of medicine, boards of health occupations or, in a few instances, separate PA licensing boards. Laws define PA qualification requirements, practice scope and professional conduct standards, and the actions of the PAs. State laws often require physicians to clearly delineate the practice scope and supervisory arrangements of PAs.

State medical practice acts defining the boundaries of PA practice activities tend to vary considerably by state, particularly with regard to scope of practice, supervisory requirements, and prescribing authority. This variability leads to barriers to PA practice effectiveness in a number of states (Sekscenski 1994).

As originally envisioned, the role of the PA encompassed working with physicians in the full range of clinical practice areas: office, clinic, hospital, nursing home, surgical suite, or in the patient's home. Laws in many states were written to give PAs a practice scope, allowing the physician to delegate a broad range of medical tasks to PAs. This latitude allows PAs to exercise a degree of clinical judgment and autonomic decision making within the parameters of state scope of practice regulations and the supervisory relationship. This is considered essential for PAs to be fully effective in practice. Geographic practice isolation in rural and frontier settings may, by necessity, result in varying degrees of off-site physician supervision and require the PA to exercise some autonomy in clinical judgment, particularly when the PA is the only available on-site provider. Regulatory reluctance to support such MD-PA relationships in satellite and remote clinical settings restricts the PA in extending and/or providing services that might otherwise be unavailable.

PA practice regulation has progressed from a delegatory model achieved by amending medical practice acts to a regulatory/authority model wherein health licensing boards are explicitly authorized to govern PA practice. Typical state regulatory acts establish PAs as agents of their supervising physicians; PAs maintain direct liability for the services they render to patients. Supervising physicians who define the standard to which PA services are held are vicariously liable for services performed by the PAs under the doctrine of *respondeat superior*.

PRACTICE QUALIFICATION

Qualification to practice as a PA in nearly all states requires that individuals be graduates of a CAAHEP-accredited PA educational program

(Committee on Accreditation of Allied Health Education Programs), CAAHEP, and/or pass the Physician Assistant National Certifying Examination (PANCE). The PANCE is a nationally standardized examination in primary care medicine that is administered annually by the National Commission on Certification of Physician Assistants (NCCPA). The PANCE comprises both written and practical components, and its content and standards were developed in cooperation with the National Board of Medical Examiners (NBME). At present, initial successful completion of the NCCPA is a required qualification for PA practice in 47 states (over 92% of all PAs in active practice hold current certification). To maintain certification, the NCCPA requires PAs to obtain continuing medical education hours annually and to recertify by formal examination every six years.

PA EDUCATION

Formal standards for PA educational programs were initially established by CAAHEP's predecessor in the AMA in 1971. These standards were established with the publication of *Essentials of an Approved Educational Program for the Assistant to the Primary Care Physician* (AAPA 1979). Compliance with the *Essentials* is the basis for awarding accreditation to PA educational programs. It defines the core components of PA educational programs: level of institutional sponsorship support, curriculum content, clinical training affiliations, basic and clinical science course offerings, faculty qualifications, and admission and selection guidelines, which must be fully met before the award of accreditation. It has also allowed PA educational programs a degree of latitude in which to create curricular configurations based on a structure awarding several types of academic degrees. Reflecting the multiple changes affecting educational preparation occurring within a rapidly developing field, the *Essentials* were revised and updated in 1978, 1985, and 1990. Accreditation is necessary for PA programs to receive federal Title VII grant funding and, in a large majority of states, for program graduates to qualify for entry to practice.

Period of Evaluation (1973–1980)

A great deal of health services research was performed during the 1970s examining the impact of the introduction of PAs into medical practice. Early results showed that PAs were safe and competent practitioners in primary care, that there was a high degree of patient acceptance of the PA role, and that most were in primary care practices in medically needy areas (OTA 1986).

With regard to cost, studies have clearly shown that within their spheres of practice competency, PAs can lower health care costs while providing physician-equivalent quality of care (Record 1980). Despite the fact that PA cost effectiveness has not been conclusively demonstrated (or even studied) in all clinical practice settings, substantial empirical and health services research supports this finding. The present increasing utilization and market demand for PAs in clinical practices would be unlikely if they were not, to some degree, cost effective.

Evidence indicates that the organizational setting is closely related to the productivity and possible cost benefits of PA utilization. Scheffler and colleagues documented that PAs employed in institutional settings are more productive than those in private practice in that they see more patients in the same period of time (Scheffler 1979).

Initial PA practice distribution tended to reflect the federal and medical sector intent that PAs assume primary care roles in areas of need. Early recruits to the PA profession were often individuals with extensive levels of prior health care experience (i.e., military medical corpsmen, registered nurses), factors contributing to their ability to function effectively with a minimal level of physician supervision. Selection of precepting physicians in rural areas remains a goal of many of the programs. Upon graduation, most of these individuals tended to select practices working with primary care physicians typically located in a rural or medically underserved community (Willis 1990c).

Many of the clinical performance aspects of PA utilization were performed in ambulatory practice and in HMO settings. In such settings, PA clinical performance has been impressive. Their productivity (number of patient visits) has been shown to approach levels of primary care physicians (Sox 1973; Hooker 1993). Record carefully documented PA productivity rates in a large group model HMO. She determined that the physician PA substitutability ratio, a measure of overall clinical efficiency, was 76%. This assumed a practice environment where PAs were utilized to their maximum capacity to perform medical services (consistent with educational competency and legal scope/supervision), and that they worked the same number of hours per week as physicians (Record 1978; Record 1980).

By the end of the first decade of practice for PAs, experience and empirical research indicated that American medicine's adoption of the PA had been generally positive (Sox 1973; Scheffler 1979). PAs were responsive to the public and the medical mandate to work in generalist/primary care roles in medically underserved areas. As their numbers crested at 10,000 in 1980, PAs were gaining recognition as being competent, effective, and clinically versatile health providers (Nelson 1975).

Period of Incorporation (1981–1990)

Conclusions from the first 15 years of health services research and practical experience with PAs (as well as NPs) were positive with regard to critical factors such as patient and professional acceptance, quality of care, cost effectiveness, productivity, and versatility (Carter 1984a; Schafft 1987a).

The PA role broadened during the 1980s when utilization extended beyond primary care into inpatient hospital settings and specialty areas. The trend toward specialization by PAs was due in part to their clinical versatility and also to health workforce demand. PA utilization increased, despite the prediction by the Graduate Medical Education National Advisory Council (GMENAC) of a rising number of physicians

in the workforce. However, not all demand arose from within primary care. More PAs were entering specialty and/or inpatient practices; the numbers in primary care began to fall. In 1981, the percentage of PAs working in the primary care specialties, defined as family practice, general internal medicine, and general pediatrics, was 62%; by 1994, that percentage had fallen to 45%. Over the same period, the percentage working in surgery, and the surgical subspecialties rose from 19% to 28% in 1994; PAs in emergency departments rose from 1.3% to 8.5% (Hooker 1992; Jones 1994a).

This period also marked the milestones indicating increasing recognition of PAs in the workforce: approval of reimbursement for services in certain settings under Medicare Part B (OBRA, 1986) commissioned officer status in US uniformed services and the passage and/or updating of medical practice acts in many states.

Period of Consolidation (1990–present)

The changes taking place in the PA profession are consolidation and stabilization. The most marked change during this period is the way PAs are incorporated into health policy projections and debate. Instead of enlarging the breadth and scope of practice, the PA movement is consolidating gains. Longevity is adding depth to PA roles and status. On the federal level, they are considered significant players in health care reform under various proposals. States continue to modify their legislation to enable PAs to practice with few barriers. With over 30 years of experience, many institutions such as HMOs, the Veterans Administration, and the military have fading memories of what it was like to have medical staffs without PAs.

CONCLUSION

The history of the PA profession is a remarkable one from a number of standpoints. Some give credit to Charles Hudson, president of the AMA for the idea. Others give credit to visionaries such as Stead and Estes at Duke University, to Silver and Ford at Colorado, and to Smith at the University of Washington. Still others believe that unmet demands for health care was the impetus for a nonphysician provider (Stanhope 1992). There are precedents in a number of countries and going back to the French Revolution (Cawley 1996a). In all instances, the product seems to have exceeded even the boldest imagination of its creators. Many ideas are born out of well-meaning intent, but few have succeeded like the PA movement. Why did the PA movement survive when other labor movements have failed? Perhaps because there is a long tradition of nonphysicians filling the roles of physicians when there were shortages of physicians to meet the demand. Perhaps there was a niche in health care delivery that demanded a different kind of provider to meet the diverse needs of Americans. Some believe the incorporation of the profession with a national certifying examination helped solidify the profession in the eyes of physicians gaining legitimation. Others believe that had family

practice developed 10 years earlier, the PA profession would not have gained enough momentum. Certainly the policy of federal support for such an enterprise helped make it possible (Table 2-3). Perhaps all of these ideas contributed to making the PA in American medicine what it is today. These contributions also makes it probable that the utilization of PAs in the US health system will continue as long as they remain flexible and extend the medical services in physician practices without challenging ultimate physician authority.

Table 2-3 *Federal health policy that affected PA development*

LEGISLATION	DATE
Allied Health Professions Act	1966
Health Manpower Act	1968
Health Manpower Training Act	1972
Health Educational Assistance Act	1976
Rural Health Clinics Act	1977
OBRA (PL 99–509)	1986

3

Current Status:
A Profile of the Profession

To understand the current status of physician assistants (PAs), one must understand where they are dispersed in American society and why. There is virtually little unemployment among PAs. Some believe that a shortage of PAs exists based on the job opportunities for recent graduates. This observation has not been missed by many educational institutions as they gear up to either expand or start new programs. The choices appear to be particularly wide for formally trained PAs with 2 or more years experience.

INFORMATION ON PAS

Information that makes up most of what is known about PAs comes from a limited number of sources. The General Census Database of the American Academy of Physician Assistants (AAPA) is a survey effort that provides detailed and timely information on socioeconomic aspects of the PA profession. It collects continuous information from annual membership renewal in the AAPA. Although initially this database was used for membership and mailing purposes, it now contains current and historical data on a large proportion of the PA population, including members and nonmembers of The Academy. The AAPA membership was originally composed of the first few graduates of the Duke University PA Program. Formed in 1968, as other PA programs were developing (Stanhope 1992), it now serves as the national register for all PA graduates.

Today, the census database is considered to be a source of PA-related information and provides much information of the current status and trends in the profession. Each PA student, on entry into a PA program, is registered in the AAPA database. This information links the program name, year of graduation, gender, birthdate, and AAPA membership status to the student. These data become particularly useful in medical labor force planning and research. Creating this information requires a commitment from PA members and their professional society to provide accurate and complete information.

Another source of information the profession relies on is the Annual Report on Physician Assistant Educational Programs. This report is organized by the Association of Physician Assistant Programs (APAP). While the AAPA Census database relies on individual responses from Academy members, the *Annual Report* is data gathered by the individual programs.

A third source of information is the National Commission on the Certification of Physician Assistants (NCCPA). One of the roles of the NCCPA is to register all PA graduates who have sat for the Physician Assistant National Certifying Examination, and to log their medical education time for maintaining certification (see section on NCCPA).

Together, these three databases provide a remarkable breadth and depth of information about the profession. The APAP database provides information on students and new graduates. The NCCPA details where certified PAs are distributed, and the AAPA database collects information about what they are doing, and in what type of setting. The data contained here are primarily from information collected in the membership renewal survey.

Other sources of national data on PA are obtained from time to time. Historically, this has included the National Ambulatory Medical Care Survey by the National Centers for Health Statistics and the American Medical Association. Smaller samples of national data can be found in various surveys of managed care and other health industry reports (Hooker 1994a).

DISTRIBUTION

As of January 1997, 34,683 PAs have graduated from an approved physician assistant program (Table 3-1). This number is expected to exceed 45,000 by the year 2000 based on estimates of new and expanding PA program capacity. Table 3-1 depicts the growth of PAs based on new graduates and the total number of graduates. This demonstrates that there is a fairly steep increase of new graduate PAs with some fluctuations in certain years due to closure of certain programs and expansion of others. The exact number of PA programs in the first few years is not known because of different types of specialty PA programs that were in existence that were counted in different ways by different organizations.

The distribution patterns of practicing PAs by state roughly parallels that of the population, with the highest percentages located in New York (11.4%), followed by California (10.7%), Texas (5.8%), Pennsylvania (5%), and Florida (5%). Marked differences have been noted among practicing PAs with regard to their patterns of specialty and geographic location of clinical practice setting. In the western states, PAs are utilized mainly in office-based, ambulatory, and rural practice settings, with a concentration within primary care practice specialties (internal medicine, family practice,

and general pediatrics). Such patterns differ markedly from those observed in the eastern states, where it is far more common for PAs to

Table 3-1 *PA graduates*

YEAR	NEW GRADUATES	CUMULATIVE GRADUATES	PA PROGRAMS
1967	3	3	1
1968	a	a	2
1969	a	a	4
1970	195	237	NA
1971	75	312	NA
1972	278	590	NA
1973	667	1,257	NA
1974	1,090	2,347	NA
1975	1,357	3,704	NA
1976	1,573	5,277	NA
1977	1,587	6,864	NA
1978	1,345	8,209	NA
1979	1,334	9,543	NA
1980	1,489	11,032	NA
1981	1,519	12,551	NA
1982	1,376	13,927	NA
1983	1,362	15,289	NA
1984	1,236	16,525	NA
1985	1,178	17,703	53
1986	1,187	18,890	51
1987	1,081	19,971	49
1988	1,081	21,052	50
1989	1,162	22,214	51
1990	1,195	23,409	51
1991	1,383	24,792	55
1992	1,595	26,387	54
1993	1,737	28,124	56
1994	1,952	30,076	63
1995	2,139	32,215	63
1996	2,500[b]	34,683[b]	68
1997	2,600[b]	37,315[b]	84
1998	2,700[b]	40,015[b]	94[b]
1999	2,850[b]	42,865[b]	98[b]
2000	3,000[b]	45,865[b]	100[b]

Abbreviation: NA, not available.

[a] Unknown

[b] Estimate based on expanding PA program trend.

(Data from American Academy of Physician Assistants, Research Division, 1996.)

be employed in clinical practice roles in acute care hospital settings, or in inpatient-related clinical practice specialties. Over 40% of PAs in the northeast region of the country are employed by a hospital or perform some of their duties in a hospital setting.

In recent data obtained from a cohort of over 11,000 practicing PAs, the percentage of those working in primary care specialties in the western US states was 77%, versus 48% in eastern states. When percentages of PA employment levels in hospital and institutional settings were compared, only 13.9% of PAs in western states were working in such settings, compared to 45.5% in eastern states (Oliver 1993b). These practice differences appear to stem from the multiple, sometimes competing, medical marketplace demands in different geographic regions and are influenced by state licensing regulations that affect the scope of practice and prescribing authority. The preponderance of primary care PAs in western states and locations in medically underserved regions reflects one of the major policy objectives of the Title VII PA training grant program. Those PA educational programs located in the western states, which tend to have practice statutes with less physician supervisory requirements than those in eastern states, have successful track records in the deployment of PA educational graduates and have developed effective mechanisms to disperse primary health care providers among medically underserved communities (Shi 1993).

PRACTICE SETTINGS

Patterns of choice of practice setting have been stable over the last decade, with almost 40% of all PAs working in either solo or group private practices, 28% in hospitals, and the remaining in settings such as public and private ambulatory clinics, health maintenance organizations (HMOs), geriatric facilities, corporate/occupational health settings, correctional systems, and other health care practices and institutions (Table 3-2).

PRACTICE SPECIALTY

As the physician workforce becomes increasingly specialty oriented, the specialty orientation of PAs seems to follow as well. After a decade in which PAs were largely deployed in primary care, more recent patterns reveal a trend toward PA practice in nonprimary care specialties and location in urban and inpatient settings. The number of PAs in primary care specialties has fallen steadily since the early 1980s (Table 3-3).

Among currently practicing PAs, 50.8% work in the primary care clinical practice specialties, which are defined by the federal Department of Health and Human Services as the specialties of family practice, general internal medicine, and general pediatrics. This pro-

Table 3-2 PA employment setting

SETTING	NUMBER	PERCENT
Clinic	1,193	9.7
Group practice	3,667	29.7
Solo physician practice	1,265	10.2
HMO	850	6.9
Other managed care organization	150	1.2
Home health agency	6	0.0
University hospital	841	6.8
Hospital (nonuniversity)	2,024	16.4
Inner city clinic	84	0.7
Military facility	527	4.3
Corrections facility	147	1.2
Nursing home	27	0.2
Rural clinic	297	2.4
Self-employed	132	1.1
Veterans Administration facility	366	3.0
Industrial facility	91	0.7
Academic faculty	130	1.1
PA program	68	0.6
Public Health facility	115	0.9
Other government	165	1.3
Other clinic setting	198	1.6
Total	12,343	100.0

(Data from Annual Census Data, American Academy of Physician Assistants. American Academy of Physician Assistants, Alexandria, VA, 1995.)

Table 3-3 *Percentage specialty distribution trends of PAs, 1974-1996*

	YEAR (NUMBER)						
SPECIALTY	1974 (939)	1978 (3,416)	1981 (4,312)	1984 (6,552)	1987 (10,692)	1995 (12,281)	1996 (12,701)
Family practice	43.6	52.0	49.1	42.5	38.7	37.2	39.8
General internal medicine	20.0	12.0	8.9	9.2	9.5	7.7	8.3
General pediatrics	6.2	3.3	3.4	4.1	4.0	2.5	2.7
General surgery	12.1	5.5	4.6	5.1	8.8	2.8	3.1
Surgical specialties	6.8	6.2	7.7	12.5	13.8	19.1	8.3
Medical specialties	3.9	6.3	2.7	4.8	7.1	7.4	5.8
Emergency medicine	1.3	4.9	4.5	6.4	6.5	8.4	7.0
Occupational medicine	1.8	2.7	3.1	4.1	4.1	3.1	3.0
Other specialty	4.3	7.1	16.0	11.3	7.5	7.0	9.5

(Data from the 1981 National Survey of Physician Assistants, Association of Physician Assistant Programs, 1984; The 1984 and 1987 Masterfile Surveys of Physician Assistants, American Academy of Physician Assistants. 1985, 1987; Oliver, DR. Eighth Annual Report on Physician Assistant Educational Programs in the United States, 1991-1992. Alexandria, VA: Association of Physician Assistant Programs. American Academy of Physician Assistants, General Census Data on Physician Assistants, 1996.)

portion is down from the 57% reported in 1980 who practiced in the primary care specialties. In 1996, 39.8% of all PAs were working in family practice, 8.3% in general internal medicine, and 2.7% in general pediatrics (AAPA Census 1996). Over the last decade, the percentages of PAs who work in the primary care specialties have substantially declined with a corresponding increase in proportions employed in hospital-based and specialty care practices. Fluctations in numbers may be due to shifting trends as well as variations in assigning specialty categories.

In the last 15 years, the percentage of PAs employed by hospitals has remained fairly constant, after rising from 14% in 1974. As the proportion of PAs in primary care practice declined, the rates of PAs working in acute care settings in medical and surgical specialties and subspecialties rose correspondingly. Key factors in expanding the role of the PA and their numbers in positions in inpatient care were hospital cutbacks in physician residency programs, curtailed availability of international medical graduates (IMGs), and cost effectiveness in inpatient roles.

It may be argued that trends in PA utilization patterns over the last decade have closely mirrored those of physicians. With the physician workforce becoming increasingly specialized, and with changes in physician-determined patterns in the division of medical labor, PA utilization has moved toward specialty areas, a process to be expected of any developing occupation. While primary care remains the major practice thrust of the PA profession, recent trends emphasizing specialty practice in the PA profession continue. What is not known is how much primary care is provided by PAs working within specialty practices.

DEMOGRAPHIC DATA

The median age at graduation has generally declined, with the current age at approximately 33. The average age, as well as the median of all practicing PAs, is 40. Since 1974 the trend in age of practicing PAs has risen from 30.6 (Perry 1976), to 38 in 1991, to 40 and is expected to hover around this age for a few years (AAPA 1995).

By the beginning of 1997, there were approximately 34,683 PA graduates, of which approximately 28,828 were in active clinical practice in the United States. Thus, about 83% of all persons trained as PAs are still practicing (Table 3-4). The AAPA membership survey reports that the mean years in clinical practice for PAs is 9.5 years, and a median of 9.0 years. A sizable proportion of those in the profession have been in clinical practice for less than 3 years (22%), and 15% have been in clinical practice less than 6 years.

The attained educational degree is the highest degree reported. Over 84% of graduates have at least a Bachelor's degree. This percentage is increasing each year for two reasons. First, more PA programs are shifting from a certificate to a Bachelor or Master's program each year. This is due in part to the desire to remain competitive with other programs and also to the pressure of a competitive job market that demands at least a baccalaureate degree for professional legitimacy. The second reason is that more and more students already have degrees when entering programs. More than 73% of the 1992–93 students possessed at least an undergraduate degree before entering training programs (Oliver 1993). The trend toward degree-granting programs and applicants with degrees already in hand is expected to continue.

Certification, the last portion of Table 3-4, refers to the percentage of PAs who are nationally certified. While certification is not a requirement everywhere, more and more states, federal government agencies, and private employers are requiring it as a condition of employment. Currently, approximately 93% of

Table 3-4 *Full-time practicing PAs, 1996*

	PERCENT	NUMBER
Total PA graduates		34,683
Total practicing PAs	83	28,828
Total graduate PAs not practicing	17	5,855
Gender		
Female	49.4	
Male	50.6	
Ethnicity		
Asian/Pacific Islander	1.9	
Black/African American	2.9	
Hispanic/Latino	3.1	
Native American/Alaskan Indian	0.8	
White (not Hispanic)	91.3	
Highest attained degree		
Certificate	26.1	
Associate	12.2	
Bachelor	55.4	
Master	6.2	
Doctorate	0.7	
Current certified		
Yes	92.7	
No	7.3	

Information is self-reported at time of membership enrollment/renewal.

(Data from American Academy of Physician Assistants, 1996a.)

PAs are certified. The issue of certification is discussed in Chapter 4.

DISTRIBUTION

The PA profession was asked by its early proponents to prove that it could provide quality care to the underserved, reduce the perceived personnel shortage in health care, and make the lives of physicians less harried. In the first 10 years, all of these goals were achieved within the confines of the limited number of personnel being trained in relatively small programs. However, the criteria by which effectiveness is judged have changed, and the health care context has also shifted radically, raising new questions about the role of PAs.

The supply of working PAs varies considerably from state to state (Table 3-5). California and New York account for one-sixth of the graduates. At the other end of the scale, low population states such as Arkansas and Wyoming have the fewest number of PAs.

Barriers to practice such as legislation also influence the distribution of PAs. Mississippi, with a population of 5 million, has only a handful of nonfederal PAs, reflecting the fact that, as of 1997, there is no law on the books that allows PAs to practice there (White 1994).

Marked differences have been noted among practicing PAs with regard to patterns of specialty practice and geographic location of clinical practice setting. Practice patterns of PA utilization in the western states tend to be set in office-based, ambulatory, and rural practice settings, with a concentration within primary care practice specialties. Such patterns differ markedly from those observed in the eastern states, where it is far more common for PAs to be employed in clinical practice specialties.

While the majority of PAs are spread throughout the United States, approximately 2% also report residencies overseas. These locations are in the US territories (Guam, Virgin Islands, American Somoa, etc.), in the US military (Germany, Japan, Turkey, etc.), in private agencies that have medical facilities outside the United States (Central America, Southeast Asia, Saudi Arabia, etc.), in the State Department, in the Central Intelligence Agency, and in the Peace Corps (Tonga, New Guinea, Africa, etc.).

About 35% of all PAs are in communities of less than 50,000, and 18% are practicing in communities of less than 10,000 people (Table 3-6). The community size in which PAs practice varies from the largest metopolitan areas to the most rural.

Population alone cannot account for all state variations. Mississippi, for example, is thirty-first in population and is tied with Guam for the lowest number of PAs and the highest population to

Table 3-5 *Distribution by state and territory in which PAs practice (N = 13,111)*

STATE	PERCENT	STATE	PERCENT
Alabama	0.6	Mississippi	0.1
Alaska	0.8	Montana	0.5
Arkansas	0.2	Nebraska	1.4
Arizona	1.7	Nevada	0.5
California	8.3	New Hampshire	0.7
Colorado	2.6	New Jersey	0.6
Connecticut	2.2	New Mexico	1.2
District of Columbia	0.6	New York	11.2
Delaware	0.2	North Carolina	5.5
Florida	5.3	North Dakota	0.7
Georgia	3.2	Ohio	2.3
Guam	.0	Oklahoma	1.5
Hawaii	0.3	Oregon	1.3
Idaho	0.5	Pennsylvania	5.7
Illinois	1.6	Rhode Island	0.5
Indiana	0.7	South Carolina	0.6
Iowa	1.7	South Dakota	0.9
Kansas	1.3	Tennessee	1.3
Kentucky	1.2	Texas	6.4
Louisiana	0.6	Utah	0.9
Massachusetts	2.4	Vermont	0.4
Maryland	3.1	Virginia	1.6
Maine	1.3	Washington	2.8
Michigan	4.6	West Virginia	0.9
Minnesota	1.6	Wisconsin	3.0
Missouri	0.9	Wyoming	0.3

(Data from American Academy of Physician Assistants, 1996a.)

PA ratio in the country. Lack of enabling legislation for PAs to practice in this state and a strong nursing society that is reluctant to accept PAs are believed to be the reasons for this disparity (White 1994). Another important reason for the concentration of PAs in states such as New York, Texas, and California is that they also have the greatest number of PA training programs. Implicit in the location of state-supported PA programs is that many of the graduates of a program will remain in the state.

The geographic distribution of PAs in the health work force is responsive to a number of factors:

Table 3-6 *Practice setting, population base, years as a PA, years in current position, 1994*

SETTING/LOCATION OF PRACTICE	PERCENT
Clinic	9.8
Group practice	29.5
Solo physician practice	10.2
HMO	6.8
Other managed care organizations	1.2
Home health agency	0.0
University hospital	7.0
Hospital (nonuniversity)	16.5
Inner city clinic	0.7
Military facility	4.3
Corrections facility	1.2
Nursing home	0.2
Rural clinic	2.4
Self-employed	1.1
VA facility	3.0
Industrial facility	0.7
Academic facility	1.0
PA program	0.5
Public health facility	1.0
Other government	1.4
Other clinical setting	1.6

POPULATION BASE	
<5,000	9.6
5,000–10,000	7.0
10,000–50,000	15.8
50,000–250,000	22.0
250,000–500,000	12.0
500,000–1,000,000	12.7
1,000,000–5,000,000	13.7
>5,000,000	7.1

NUMBER OF YEARS AS A PA		NUMBER OF YEARS IN CURRENT POSITION
<1 year	3.6	10.5
1-3 years	22.0	49.8
4-6 years	15.3	18.7
7-9 years	11.9	7.6
10-12 years	14.3	5.6
13-15 years	12.3	3.8
16-18 years	10.5	2.4
>19 years	9.6	1.7
Mean	9.2 years	4.2 years
Median	9.0 years	2.0 years

(Data from American Academy of Physician Assistants, 1996a)

- Market demand and wages
- Enabling state legislation (ability to practice and prescribe)
- Location of PA training programs (Hooker 1992)

Some caution should be taken in accepting this hypothesis since the data are limited and the variables untested. A longitudinal study of the education, work history, and changing place of residence of several classes of PA graduates is needed to understand how and why PAs are distributed the way they are.

SPECIALTY

One of the more remarkable aspects of the evolution of the PA profession has been its incorporation into specialty medical practice. Although the initial mandate for PAs was to serve as primary care practitioners, a rather large proportion have entered specialty and subspecialty practice with equal success (Schafft & Cawley 1987a; Hooker 1992). Table 3-7 illustrates the specialty distribution of practicing PAs for 1996. This exhibit reveals that the primary care specialties of family practice, general internal medicine, and general pediatrics have the largest groups of PAs (51%).

The next largest group of PAs is composed of general surgery and the surgical subspecialties (13%). When this group is combined with orthpedics (8%), the surgical subspecialties make up over one fifth of the PA workforce. The activities of surgical PAs and surgeon assistants (SAs) has been fairly well described in the literature (Mauney 1972; Faircloth 1976; Maxfield 1976; Sonntag 1977; Miller 1978a; Miller 1978b; Perry 1983; Beinfield 1991.)

Many specialties do not differ substantially from primary care. For example, much of gynecology, occupational medicine, and emergency medicine are largely composed of primary care activities, but are not counted as primary care disciplines because they do not generally follow the patient longitudinally.

Productivity Features of PA Practices

PA utilization refers to the quantity of services PAs provide to their patients. The number of patient visits or patients seen in the hospital is a measure that captures a large proportion of overall PA utilization in most specialties. The time spent in practice by PAs is measured in hours per week and patients per day. On average, PAs spend 37.6 hours a week in an outpatient setting and see 19.3 patients a day (Table 3-8).

In Table 3-9, an inpatient practice is considered (although undefined in the survey) to exist when a PA makes hospital and/or surgical service patient visits (hospital rounds). The table is an approximate measure of inpatient practices. Hospital utilization refers to the number of patients seen per day on average.

Many PAs who have an outpatient practice primarily may provide some of their work in a hospital. Likewise, many PAs working in hospitals may see only ambulatory patients.

The PA labor market is not dominated by any one type of employer, although close to 28% work in the hospital. Conversely, the other 72% are outpatient based. The greatest concentration of PAs outside the hospital are in group practices (22.1%), followed by solo practices (10.6%). The high proportion of PAs in outpatient settings is consistent with the high demand for this type of medical labor. It is in this area of outpatient medicine that the greatest shortage of PAs is believed to exist.

Although formally trained PAs are employed by a variety of industries, agencies, and firms, the dominant employer is a physician or a group of physicians who provide outpatient primary care.

In recent years, a number of changes in the PA labor market have had a profound effect on the supply:

- Rising incomes for PAs
- A higher proportion of women than men entering the profession
- Enabling state legislation that improve the use of PAs

Table 3-7 *Distribution of PAs by specialty, 1996*

SPECIALTY	PERCENT	SPECIALTY	PERCENT
Allergy	0.3	Pediatric general	2.7
Anesthesiology	0.2	Pediatric subspecialty	
Dermatology	0.5	Cardiology	0.1
Emergency medicine	10.3	Endocrinology	0.0
Family/general medicine	39.8	Heme/oncology	0.2
Geriatrics	0.9	Nephrology	<0.1
Indus/occupational medicine	3.1	Neurology	<0.1
Orthopedics	7.8	Pulmonary	<0.1
Internal medicine, general	8.3	Other	0.1
Internal medicine subspecialty		Physical medicine/rehab	0.8
Cardiology	2.2	Psychiatry	0.8
Critical care	0.3	Public health/	
Endocrinology	0.2	preventive med	0.4
Gastroenterology	0.2	Radiology	0.1
Hematology/immune	0.1	Surgery, general	3.1
Infectious disease	0.6	Surgery, subspecialty	
Nephrology	0.5	Cardiovascular	4.5
Oncology	0.9	Colon/rectal	<0.1
Pulmonology	0.2	Hand	0.1
Rheumatology	0.1	Neurosurgery	1.4
Other subspecialties	0.2	Pediatric	<0.1
Neurology	0.3	Plastic	0.6
Obstetrics/gynecology	3.0	Thoracic	0.1
Ophthalmology	0.2	Trauma	0.2
Otolaryngology	0.4	Urology	0.8
Pathology	<0.1	Vascular	0.4
Other medical specialty	1.5	Other	0.2
		Transplant	0.2
		Other surgical specialty	1.5

Total Primary Care = 50.8%; Total Surgery = 13.1%.

(Data from American Academy of Physician Assistants, 1996a.)

Table 3-8 *Full-time outpatient practice of PAs, 1995*

HOURS/WEEK	PERCENT	PATIENTS/DAY	PERCENT
1–20	2.5	1–10	10.5
21–30	3.1	11–20	47.6
31–40	63.7	21–30	32.9
41–50	26.1	31–40	6.7
51–60	4.2	41–50	2.3
>60	0.4		
Mean = 37.6		Mean = 19.3	

(Data from American Academy of Physician Assistants, 1996a.)

Table 3-9 *Full-time inpatient PA practices, 1995*

HOURS/WEEK	PERCENT	PATIENTS/DAY	PERCENT
1–20	3.8	1–10	40.5
21–30	1.7	11–20	40.0
31–40	39.9	21–30	13.9
41–50	37.3	31–40	4.1
51–60	14.7	41–50	1.5
>60	2.6		
Mean = 41.3		Mean = 13.6	

(Data from American Academy of Physician Assistants, 1996a.)

- The increasing popularity of the profession with managed care organizations

- Decreasing opportunity costs (tuition plus lost wages) of PA education and increasing future benefits (higher salaries)

- The development of a critical mass of PAs so that most people now know what a PA is

- Increasing enrollment in PA programs

Along with concern about the adequacy of the total supply of employed PAs in the United States is the problem of an unequal regional distribution.

PAs PRACTICING PART-TIME

When all occupations (not just health care workers) are investigated, it appears that women make up the bulk of part-time workers (72.2%). In the aggregate, they are often married (with the husband present) and can be considered as secondary wage earners. While an age-participation profile is not available at this time, we believe that part-time PAs fall into this category as well since the majority of part-time workers are female. However, apart from the fact that only 9% of PAs practice less than full-time, the distinction between full-time and part-time employment from the data presented here does not differ significantly. Part-time PAs are more likely to be in primary care (71% versus 56%) but with the exception of the gender differences, the type of setting, ethnicity, and number of years in current position are only marginally different between full-time and part-time PAs (Table 3-10).

Ideally, the data needed to better understand part-time work would include total family income, excluding the earnings of the part-time PA spouse. In studies that rely on data obtained from individual families, it is sometimes possible to estimate such variables.

Table 3-10 *PAs practicing part-time, 1993*

GENDER	PERCENT	
Female	72.2	
Male	27.8	

NUMBER OF YEARS AS A PA	PERCENT	YEARS IN CURRENT POSITION (%)
<1 year	3.1	19.8
1–3 years	9.7	40.7
4–6 years	20.2	19.0
7–9 years	21.8	9.5
10–12 years	22.9	5.9
13–15 years	14.0	3.4
16–18 years	6.9	1.4
>18 years	1.4	0.3

(Data from American Academy of Physician Assistants 1993 General Census Data, 1994a.)

COMPENSATION

Income generated by an occupation, considered either at a point in time or as a stream received over the working lifetime of an individual, strongly influences the choice of that occupation and is the most frequently mentioned attribute of an occupation.

Although the time structure of earnings is the key determinant in measuring occupational models, the annual earnings at a point in time can give a rough idea of the relative income ranking of different occupations (Fig. 3-1).

The term *compensation* includes the combination of salaries and benefits. It is the amount the employer foregoes to retain the services of the employee. While salary is fairly easy to figure, benefits are more nebulous. Some benefits have a definable amount, such as the cost of dental insurance for an employee and his or her family. Other benefits are really perquisites of the job such as an automobile or medical liability insurance.

The AAPA conducts a national census of its members. The survey provides information on demographics of PAs, current practice patterns, and trends in the profession. It also provides salary and benefits information because this is the most frequently requested information from the Research Division.

Salary

The mean income for PAs at the end of 1996 was $65,125. Between the years 1991 and 1996, the salary increased on average $5,000 (Table 3-11). This increase was slightly more than inflation.

Although what accounts for this modest increase is not clear, many factors can influence the amount of money a PA earns. Practice specialty, years of experience, employment setting, city size, and the region of the country or state in which a PA works all have an effect on salary. The first variable to consider for PA salary analysis is practice specialty.

Viewing income distribution as a probability density, the data show a right-sided kurtosis. This shape curve is classic for salary distribu-

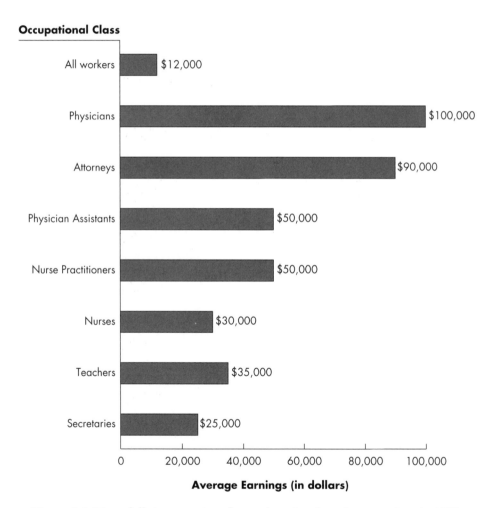

Occupational Class

Figure 3-1 Mean full-time earnings for workers in selected occupations in 1992. (Data from Handbook of Occupations, 1992.)

tions and predictable because income increases until some peak density is attained and then decreases, declining exponentially at higher levels of income. The ever-diminishing tail represents the very few, who, for whatever entrepreneurial reasons, have incomes two to four times greater than their cohorts.

Geography influences the average salary for PAs. The geographic location of the PAs not only affects their salary, but also may help explain why PAs locate in some areas more densely than in others. For example, salaries are high in the West, and there is a high prevalence of PAs in that region. Conversely, PA income is the lowest in the Southeast where some states have few employed PAs. Salary also tends to increase along with the size of the city. Large metropolitan cities tend to pay PAs more than small towns. However, in some different parts of the country (i.e., the Southeast and North-central regions), PAs in rural areas are paid better if the region has difficulty recruiting workers.

Not surprisingly, PAs with more experience are commanding higher salaries. Table 3-12 shows the progression of wages from entry level to the most senior level (19 years or more). However, PAs with 13 years of experience are paid almost as much as PAs with more than 18 years of experience. That is not to say that these PAs aren't receiving annual raises; each group averaged $3,000 to $4,000 more than they received in the previous year.

The types of compensation arrangements being negotiated are also changing. Bonuses were reported for 20.8% in 1996, an increase of 1.8% over the previous year. Other arrangements including partnerships and percentages of revenues are presented in Table 3-13. Details of these partnerships have not been collected.

Benefits

In 1993, the AAPA conducted a survey to determine the types of benefits that employers commonly offer to PAs. A total of 2,372 practicing PAs completed the survey (56% response rate).

Table 3-11 Distribution of average salary, 1995

| | PERCENT | |
SALARY	OVERALL	1994 GRADUATES
<$20,000	0.5	0.3
20,000–24,999	0.1	0.2
25,000–29,999	0.2	0.3
30,000–34,999	0.8	1.7
35,000–39,999	3.1	6.5
40,000–44,999	9.6	22.1
45,000–49,999	13.3	23.7
50,000–54,999	17.5	19.8
55,000–59,999	12.7	10.8
60,000–64,999	12.0	7.4
65,000–69,999	7.3	2.8
70,000–74,999	6.4	1.3
75,000–79,999	4.0	0.5
80,000–84,999	3.7	1.0
85,000–89,999	2.2	0.2
90,000–94,999	1.6	0.6
95,000–99,999	1.3	0.0
100–104,999	1.3	0.3
105–109,999	.6	0.0
110–114,999	.4	0.2
115–119,999	.3	0.0
120–150,000	.9	0.0
Over 150,000	.4	0.1

| | SALARY | |
PERCENTILE	OVERALL	1994 GRADUATES
Mean salary	$61,010	$50,770
10th percentile	43,066	40,371
25th percentile	49,176	43,721
50th (median)	57,077	48,982
75th percentile	68,593	55,208
90th percentile	83,395	63,506

Full-time, nongovernment PAs only. The data are collected throughout the year, only one time per respondent. The final data are reported at the end of the year by the AAPA. 11,016 surveyed.

(Data from 1995 Membership Census Report, American Academy of Physician Assistants, 1996b.)

The demographic distribution was reported as representative of the practicing PA population by specialty, setting, population base, and gender.

Table 3-12 *PA income by years of experience, 1993*

YEARS AS A PA	AVERAGE SALARY	CHANGE IN SALARY
<1	$43,200	
1–3	47,700	+$4,500
4–6	52,100	+4,400
7–9	54,600	+2,500
10–12	56,600	+2,000
13–15	58,500	+1,900
16–18	59,700	+1,200
19 or >	59,700	+0

Total annual income from all PA-related work.

(Data from AAPA News October 1993.)

Table 3-14 *Breakdown of PA benefits, 1993*

BENEFIT	FULLY FUNDED (%)	PARTIALLY FUNDED (%)
Medical insurance (individual)	62	26
Medical insurance (family)	39	38
Malpractice insurance	94	1
Profit sharing	21	11
Retirement fund	39	38

BENEFIT	AVERAGE/YEAR
Maternity leave	5.6 weeks
Paid vacation	17.2 days
Sick leave	7.4 days
Medical education leave	5.9 days
Earnings over base	$6,018
Medical education funds available	$1,075

(Data from AAPA News October 1993.)

Aside from the base salary information, questions included areas such as insurance benefits, paid leave (vacation, continuing medical education [CME], ill time and maternity leave), and other earnings through bonuses (Table 3-14).

The mean bonus earning is $9,000, although this is a bit misleading since two-thirds earned a bonus less than $5,000 per year in additional revenue. More than 15% of the PAs report additional earnings ranging from $10,000 to more than $20,000.

Table 3-15 describes the findings for insurance benefits, benefits other than insurance, and the mean number of days available for various leave categories. It should be noted that the average amount of funding for CME is $875 per

year, although 33% report recurring $1,200 to more than $3,000.

The benefit structure of government workers, both state and federal, tend to be more encompassing than that for those in the private sector. For example, in the federal system, vacation is 30 days a year. Sick leave is generous; Medical, dental, and malpractice and life insurance is automatically covered. The retirement benefits of federal employment make this sector particularly attractive.

TURNOVER AND MOBILITY

PAs are fairly mobile, which means they tend to change jobs from time to time. This is sometimes expressed as turnover. One method of determining the turnover rate is the number of PA clinical positions held divided by the total number of years in practice as a clinical PA. For all respondents to the 1995 membership census who practice full or part-time, the rate is 0.47 (K. Kraditor, personal communication 1996). On the whole, more than 60% of the profession has spent less than 3 years in their current positions, and for the past 5 years, the percentage of

Table 3-13 *Income type, 1995*

TYPE OF SALARY	PERCENT
Salary	82.5
Salary and revenue sharing	3.8
Salary and bonus	20.8
Partnership	.6
Self-employed	2.3

Active duty military PAs excluded.

(Data from American Academy of Physician Assistants Membership Census Report, 1996b.)

Table 3-15 *Types of benefits provider by employer*

BENEFIT TYPE	FULL COVERAGE (%)	PARTIAL COVERAGE (%)	NOT A BENEFIT (%)
Individual medical	63	26	11
Family medical	39	38	23
Dental	28	41	30
Disability	47	28	25
Vision	15	57	28
Term Life	48	19	33
Full Life	16	8	76
Malpractice	94	1	5

OTHER BENEFITS PROVIDED BY EMPLOYERS	FULL SUPPORT(%)	PARTIAL SUPPORT(%)	NOT A BENEFIT(%)
Profit sharing	21	11	68
Retirement	39	38	23
Annuity	6	18	76
License fees	64	4	32
NCCPA annual registration	57	3	40
NCCPA recertification exam fee	60	5	35
AAPA dues	66	3	31

LEAVE TYPE	MEAN NUMBER OF DAYS
Vacation	13
Sick/administrative	9 or more
CME	9 or more
Maternity	6 weeks

(Data from AAPA News June 1993.)

PAs who have remained in the same position more than 10 years has averaged around 8% (Table 3-16). Even PAs with more than 15 years of experience report that they have been with their current employer, on average, less than 3 years. This suggests PAs negotiate contracts frequently. Little is understood about this phenomenon other than the observation that PA graduates tend to take the first job as an entree to the workforce, which may not be the most attractive, and then tend to look around for a way to raise compensation by switching employers. Anecdotal reports suggest that few positions are filled by a PA that haven't been occupied by a PA previously.

Table 3-16 *PA mobility, 1993*

NO. OF YEARS	YEARS AS A PA (%)	YEARS IN CURRENT POSITION (%)
<1	8.1	23.3
1–3	16.9	34.0
4–6	16.5	17.6
7–9	13.1	7.8
10–12	16.5	7.9
13–15	12.2	4.4
16–18	10.8	2.7
>19	5.9	2.2
Mean	8.8	4.5

(Data from American Academy of Physician Assistants, 1994a.)

AGE

Figure 3-2 indicates that in 1995, the majority of PAs were younger than 40 years of age (52%). The 41- to 45-age interval accounted for the highest (23%). Relatively few PAs have reached traditional retirement age (1%), but this number is expected to triple over the next 5 years.

DISTRIBUTION BY SPECIALTY

Specialty data are reported on the membership renewal questionnaire and are detailed in Chapter 6 and in Table 3-7. Forty-six specialties are listed by the AAPA. In contrast, 117 specialties are listed by the American Medical Association (Roback 1993).

THE CHANGING COMPOSITION OF PAs

The profile of the PA has changed relatively fast, compared to those in other professions. In contrast to a group of three male veterans in 1967 (Condit 1993), the average PA graduate in the 1990s is female, approximately 33 years of age, and has a nonmilitary medical background.

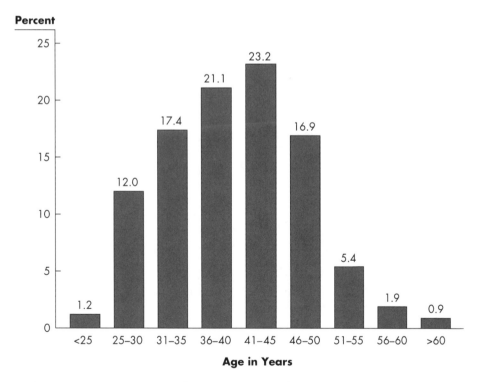

Figure 3-2 1995 Census on physician assistants by age. (Data from American Academy of Physician Assistants 1996b.)

As the national complexion of PAs changes, we can make some predictions about what the professsion will look like in the future. First, the gender distribution of PAs will probably remain generally even over the next decade because the PA profession is popular and the pool of applicants is basically equal. Programs seem to be naturally inclined to enroll their classes in roughly even numbers of men and women. Second, the average age of PAs in the workforce will slowly increase to approximately 42 years and then plateau because the aging PA is raising the age, while the average age of entrants to PA programs is relatively stable. While little is known about the life cycle of a PA and what the average age of retirement will be, we believe that at least three-fourths of all PAs will remain in their careers until retirement. This is evident anecdotally, although little data exist about the career trends of older PAs. PAs tend to be satisfied with their career which suggests some profession stability (Freeborn 1995). Historically, physicians have unusually long work lives; the average 35-years-old physician can expect to practice almost to the age of 70 (Kletke 1987). Whether this holds true for PAs is not clear, but our observation is that some PAs are working beyond age 65.

MILITARY/FEDERAL AND STATE PUBLIC SERVICE

Presently, about 15% of all PAs are employed in positions within the public sector. Among all PAs reported in the AAPA Annual Census, 11.6% are employed in the federal government, with 3% working for the state, and 2% in local government agencies. The federal government is the single largest employer of all health care providers. Currently, about 1,350 of PAs serve in uniformed services branches, including 2% each in the Army and Air Force, 1.4% in the Navy, 0.1% in the Coast Guard (Department of Transportation), 3.8% in the Department of Veterans Affairs health system, 0.5% in the Department of Justice in the Bureau of Prisons medical system,

and 0.4% in the Indian Health Service (IHS) and other agencies in the US Public Health Service.

The overall number of PAs employed by the Department of Veterans Affairs system was 1,100 in 1996. PAs in the US military hold commissioned officer status, and in 1996 there was a vacancy rate of over 300 PA positions. PAs are avidly recruited by agencies in the US Public Health Service and the Bureau of Prisons (BOP), where the existing limitations in the available supply of PAs continue to cause ongoing vacancies in medical staffing. For example, the Indian Health Service (IHS) at present employs 98 full-time equivalents (FTE) PAs (about one-third are Native Americans) and reports 60 unfilled positions. Both the IHS and other federal agencies, such as BOP, anticipate that medical staffing requirements for PA personnel will increase substantially in the coming years. In 1996, BOP had 1,100 positions for PAs in its health system and projected that requirements for PAs would increase over the next 5 years. This is the fastest growing federal department, and the demands for PAs and other health workers is high. The distribution of PAs in the different types of government agencies is shown in Table 3-17.

Table 3-17 *Type of government employer*

EMPLOYER	PERCENT
Not government employed	84.5
Air Force	1.7
Bureau of prisons	0.3
Navy	0.9
Veterans Affairs	3.5
Public Health Service	1.0
Army	1.8
Coast Guard	0.1
National Guard	0.1
Other federal government	1.1
State government	3.5
Local government	2.0

(Data from American Academy of Physician Assistants, 1996a.)

Variations in PA practice patterns over the years may be best seen when data on practice patterns and characteristics derived from reports of state PA cohorts are compared. Table 3-18 shows comparisons of results obtained from surveys of practicing PAs conducted by professional organizations in three states (California, Connecticut, North Carolina) (Kohlhepp 1984; Fowkes 1990; Von Seggen 1993).

PAs IN UNDERSERVED SETTINGS

The major objective in the development of training programs for PAs was to increase the availability of health care in areas with physician shortages. These underserved areas include small communities in rural areas. The federal government defines rural as a county with less than 100,000 people and a town with less than 50,000 individuals.

Some of the first studies on PAs examined how PAs were employed in rural practices (Nelson 1975; Miles 1976; Ekwo 1979). Basically they filled vacant physician practices, and seemed to be well accepted by rural residents (Conant 1971; Litman 1972).

In 1996, about 14% of PAs were in practice in communities of less than 10,000 people, with an additional 14% working in communities of between 10,000 to 50,000. More PAs (29%) were working in practices in communities of less than 50,000 than either allopathic physicians (12%) or osteopathic physicians (15%) (COGME 1992; AMA Socioeconomic Survey 1992; 1996 AAPA Census 1996). The reasons for the distribution of PAs in underserved communities are multifactorial, but one of the leading reasons is the federal initiative to fund programs that serve small communities. Since the late 1970s, federal statute has required that PA programs receiving grants support curricula emphasizing primary care. Programs that demonstrate successful outcomes in deployment of graduates in primary care practices and in medically underserved areas have promoted

PA practice in rural communities (Lohrenz 1976; Oliver 1977). Until recently, a downward trend in the percentages of PAs practicing in small communities (less than 10,000 population) had been observed. Between 1981 and 1996, the percentage of PAs working in smaller communities has declined from 27% to 14%. Major factors responsible for this decline include a changing medical market and the changing demography of the PA profession. Some responsible factors overlap. Nearly all rural PAs (defined as those practicing in communities of less than 10,000) are employed by primary care practices (86%). The factors influencing PA employment trends away from both primary care and rural practice include the retirement of older male PAs (who are more likely than women to enter practices in underserved areas), the increasing proportion of women now in the profession, and the increasingly strong demand and consequently higher remuneration levels offered in urban settings and hospital-based practices. The same negative factors that discourage physicians from working in rural areas also affect physician assistants (i.e., large patient care load, long hours, professional and social isolation, fewer academic centers, and lower income). However, since the 1996 low of 14%, the percentages of PAs working in communities under 10,000 has somewhat improved. In 1992, the figure rose to 16.5%, in 1993 to 18% (Willis 1993) and in 1996 to 14%. The effect of federal PA funding preferences on grants for PA educational programs is believed to have offset to some degree the national trend among health professionals drifting away from rural practice (Table 3-19) (Willis 1990c; Willis 1993b).

Although PAs are supervised by physicians, many are in practices in isolated rural areas where they often function with considerable independence. Many rural communities are dependent on a PA staffed clinic to provide local medical care for residents. Physicians in rural communities rely on PAs to help balance patient care duties, on-call responsibilities, leisure time, and to help avoid problems of

Table 3-18 *Selected professional characteristics of PAs by state cohort, as reported in published surveys*

	CALIFORNIA	NORTH CAROLINA	CONNECTICUT
Date of report	1990[a]	1992[b]	1984[c]
Estimated number of PAs in state	1782	860	200
Number responding to survey	641	440	118
Response rate	36%	51%	59%
Gender			
Male	43%	52%	53%
Female	57%	48%	47%
Mean age (years)	38	39	32
Race/ethnic			
White	70%	95%	NR
African-American	11%	3%	NR
Hispanic	12%	1%	NR
Other	7%	2%	NR
Practice setting			
Office	56%	43%	19%
Hospital	17%	18%	68%
Clinic	27%	25%	13%
Community size			
50,000 population	NR	32%[a]	2%
Mean years in current position	3.7 years	NR	5 years
Degree achieved			
Bachelors or higher degree upon entry to PA program	58%	69%	68%
NCCPA Certified	NR	91%	NR
Practice Specialty			
Primary care (includes family practice, internal medicine, and general pediatrics)	73%	59%	49%
Surgery (includes general and subspecialties)	NR	25%	23%
Emergency medicine	4%	8%	20%
Other specialties	NR	18%	11%
Satisfied with PA career choice	NR	92%	NR

Abbreviation: NR, not reported.

[a] Data from Fowkes, VK. A Profile of California's Physician Assistants [correspondence]. *West J Med* 1990; 153: 328–329

[b] Data from VonSeggen, W., Hinds, A. Physician Assistants in North Carolina, 1992. *North Carolina Med J* 1993; 54: 276–280; VonSeggen, *North Carolina Med J* 1984; 45: 304–308

[c] Data from Kohlhepp, W., Fichandler, BC, Stasiulewicz, C., Barese, S., Beinfield, M. in 1982; Connecticut Physician Assistants. *Connecticut Med* 1984; 48: 657–660

social and professional isolation. PAs are cost effective to employing rural practices because their salaries are about one-third of physicians' salaries. Anecdotal reports suggest that most perform at productivity rates similar to that of physicians in these settings as well.

COMMUNITY AND MIGRANT HEALTH CENTERS

PAs are filling important roles in service to medically needy populations in rural communities. Shi and colleagues (1994) from the University of North Carolina examined the patterns and determinants of utilization of PAs and other nonphysician health care providers practicing in rural community and migrant health centers in all US geographic regions. The primary objective of the analytic methods of the study was to compare centers that employed PAs and other nonphysician health providers in 1991 with those not employing such providers. Data from the 243 responses received from rural and migrant health clinics gave findings related to the utilization of PAs, NPs, and certified nurse midwives (CNMs). Three quarters (77%) indicated that PA/NP/CNM health professionals were on their medical staffs. Also, 85% indicated that they were seeking to employ additional PA and NP health providers. The report projects that to meet anticipated demand for

Table 3-19 *PA specialty and practice settings in underserved areas (%)*

PRACTICE TYPE	TOTAL	HIGH POVERTY	TOTAL HPSA	URBAN HPSA	RURAL HPSA
Specialty					
Primary care[a]	42.4	36.8	66.0	41.2	87.0
Medical specialty[b]	25.4	29.8	18.9	29.2	10.2
Surgical specialty[c]	25.4	26.1	11.0	21.9	1.8
Obstetrician-gynecologist	4.4	4.8	3.4	6.8	0.5
Other[d]	2.5	2.5	0.7	0.9	0.5
Practice Setting					
Group office	25.7	15.6	17.8	21.2	15.0
Clinic medical office	23.5	31.8	48.8	32.1	62.6
Private hospital	15.1	17.1	10.0	19.6	2.1
Public hospital	14.1	20.9	9.5	14.3	5.4
Solo office	12.6	7.2	11.1	7.5	14.2
HMO	8.4	7.1	2.4	5.0	0.3
Other	0.7	0.4	0.4	0.3	0.5

Abbreviations: HPSA, Health Professional Service Area; HMO, health maintenance organizations.

[a] Family/general practice, general internal medicine, and general pediatrics.

[b] Allergy, dermatology, emergency medicine, geriatrics, internal medicine subspecialty, neurology, occupational medicine, pediatric subspecialty, psychiatry, and rehabilitation.

[c] Gereral surgery, surgery, ophthalmology, orthopedics, and otolaryngology.

[d] Anesthesiology, pathology, and radiology.

(Data from Physician Payment Review Commission 1994. Based on analysis of the AAPA 1992 General Census Data on Physician Assistants.)

primary care providers, community and migrant health centers would need to hire 726 physicians, 315 NPs, 218 PAs, 145 CNMs, and 169 other staff members (Samuels 1992). A major factor in the utilization of PAs and other nonphysician health care providers in rural and migrant health clinics is whether these facilities hold an affiliation with an educational program involved in the training of these providers. High proportions (77% for PAs, 67% for NPs, and 93% for CNMs) of the rural community and migrant health centers surveyed nationally are involved in training activities of these health professionals. Findings also suggest that the centers who actively seek to employ PAs and other nonphysician providers are more likely to establish training and employment channels with educational programs.

Working in primary care in rural community and migrant health clinics, PAs, NPs, and CNMs tend to function in roles that are largely substitutive of the physician. This study found a significant and inverse relationship between the number of physicians and the number of nonphysicians employed in these settings. Other factors shown to have an effect on patterns of utilization of nonphysician health providers in these clinical settings included (1) a significant positive relationship between the number of total staff and the number of nonphysician providers employed, (2) geographic region, (3) educational program linkage, and, (4) center clinical staffing policies (Shi 1993).

PAs IN MEDICALLY UNDER-SERVED URBAN SETTINGS

Recent studies suggest that working with the impoverished is appealing to some providers. For PAs and other health care providers who work in urban underserved areas, there seems to be a value placed on service to humanity and a strong sense of pride in making a difference. Focus groups of primary care providers in inner city areas reveal that they thrive on the challenge of creatively dealing with their patients' complex human needs with limited health care

resources. Factors critical to survival in an underserved urban setting include a hardy personality style, a flexible but controllable work schedule, and multidisciplinary practice teams. The camaraderie and synergy of teams generate personal support and opportunities for continuing professional development (Li 1995).

HMO/MANAGED CARE

PAs, as well as primary care physicians, will be in stronger demand in health maintenance organizations (HMOs) and managed health care systems. At present, however, figures from the Annual Census Data on Physician Assistants show that only 7% of all PAs nationwide report they are working in an HMO setting. Some believe that this may be an underestimate of the true number of PAs utilized in managed care systems, as reporting does not include categories for independent practice associations (IPAs), preferred provider organizations (PPOs), and similar organizational practice arrangements. While PA utilization has been slow to catch on in some HMO systems, the clinical staffs of many other organizations have a large mix of physician and nonphysician health care providers. Using findings from a survey of 10 HMOs nationwide, as well as data from several other HMO studies, Weiner (1994) estimated that there are approximately 18 nonphysician health providers (either PA or NP) per 100,000 HMO enrollees, with a range from zero to 67 PA/NPs. A Group Health Association of America study found that the mean number of full-time physicians per 100,000 enrollees is 142.3. The number of primary care physicians was 68.7 per 100,000 enrollees. When PAs/NPs were factored in, there was an inverse relationship (Dial 1995). Our interpretation of this observation suggests that PAs and NPs are substituting for primary care physicians in these settings in under appreciated levels (Hooker 1995b).

Other observations from this study find PAs and NPs providing direct patient care to all categories of patients (Table 3-20). NPs and CNMs tend to provide more obstetric and gynecology care than PAs, but both PAs and advance practice nurses are used extensively in primary care.

An example of the extensive integration of PAs into HMOs can be seen at Kaiser Permanente in Portland, Oregon. This is a well-established HMO with an enrollment of over 400,000 members, staffed by 550 FTE physicians and 150 FTE PAs and NPs within 29 clinical departments. PAs practice in both primary care areas and in specialty care roles and are fully integrated as members of the health provider team. Through the Kaiser Permanente Center for Health Research, it has been possible for investigators to measure longitudinally the clinical productivity, costs, and practice characteristics of both PAs and NPs in the HMO/managed care setting (Hooker 1993).

PAs are also utilized extensively in other major HMO systems as well: (The Southern California Kaiser Plan employs roughly 500 PAs and NPs; Pilgrim/Harvard Community Health Plan in Boston; Health Insurance Plan of Greater New York; Group Health Association and The George Washington University Health Plan in metropolitan Washington, DC; the Mayo Clinic in Rochester, Minnesota; Group Health Cooperative

of Puget Sound in Seattle; and the Family Health Plan Systems in Utah, California, and other western states. Over two-thirds of all group- and staff-model HMOs report that they employ PAs and/or NPs (Table 3-21) (Dial 1995).

Performance in Managed Care Systems

Major factors receiving increased attention in managed health systems relate to the clinical capabilities and cost effectiveness of PAs in such settings. In the HMO setting PAs and NPs have long played important roles in the clinical staffing patterns of these health facilities. PAs and NPs have proven themselves capable of delivering a majority of the health care services required at physician-equivalent levels of quality of care and at lower costs than physicians (Hooker 1993). When clinical productivity of PAs, as measured by the number of outpatient care visits per day, was compared to the patient visit rates of primary care physicians and NPs, PA clinical productivity was equal to and in some settings greater than those of these other primary care providers. In studies conducted at Kaiser Permanente Northwest, Record and colleagues (1981a) compared the clinical performance of PAs with primary care physicians in a large HMO in handling episodes of four specific morbidities: strep throat, upper respiratory infection (URI), bursitis, and bronchitis. Outcome criteria included patient safety as measured by the rate of adverse side effects from antibiotics and other drugs used in patient management. Over 1 year, no differences in the rates between PAs and physicians were observed.

QUALITY OF CARE

The spread of PA utilization in medical practices observed since the mid 1970s has been partly a function of practice efficiency and economic advantages, as well as a high degree of patient satisfaction with care provided by these providers. A number of health services research

Table 3-20 *Clinical responsibilities of PAs and NPs in HMOs*

	PERCENTAGE OF HMO[a]	
	PAS	NPS
Prescriptive authority	59.5	73.3
Primary provider	70.3	68.4
Included on provider list	35.1	36.8
Provide direct access to		
Obstetrics/gynecology patients	51.5	94.7
Well adults	97.2	91.7
Chronically ill patients	91.7	91.4
Other adults	73.9	63.6
Pediatric patients	71.4	89.2
Psychiatric patients	48.4	48.4

[a] N = 34, NPs includes CNMs.

(Data from Dial 1995; Group Health Association of America Survey of Clinical Staffing in HMOs.)

Table 3-21 *Characteristics of PAs in HMOs and group practices*

	ALL PAs (%)	PAs EMPLOYED BY HMO (%)	PAs EMPLOYED BY GROUP PRACTICES (%)
Years in clinical practice (median)	10	12	9
Years in current position (median)	3	4	3
Median age	40	42	39
Median years in current position	3	4	3
Median on-call hours per week	24	12	24
Median outpatient visits	20	20	20
Median outpatient hours	40	40	40
Median annual income	$57,500	$57,500	$57,000

(Data from American Academy of Physician Assistants, 1996a.)

studies conducted shortly after introducing a PA into practice concluded that PAs provide physician-equivalent levels of quality of patient care. Sox (1979) summarized data from more than a dozen well-conducted studies examining the clinical performance of PAs. He found that the quality of patient care delivered by PAs was at a level "indistinguishable" from that of physician care.

Although patient satisfaction is a related but imperfect measure of health provider quality of care, it is a partial determinant of utilization of health personnel. A high level of patient acceptance of PA services has been a consistently observed finding in many of the health services research reports published in the years after PAs were introduced into clinical practice (OTA 1986). In several of these studies, the proportion of patients reporting acceptable to high levels of satisfaction with health care services delivered by PAs averaged between 80% and 90% among individuals not previously exposed to PA care. This figure subsequently rose over 95% among patients surveyed after having received care from a PA (Nelson 1974b; Hooker 1993).

Public acceptance and familiarity with PA health providers have grown substantially, particularly over the last decade. Data from a recent report based on findings from a random sample of 687 adults surveyed by telephone in the Kentucky Health Survey indicated that 1 in 4 (25%) had received medical advice or treatment from a PA within the last 2 years. More than 90% of these subjects reported satisfaction with the care they received. Recipients of care from PAs did not differ from recipients of care from physicians with respect to income, education, insurance status, self-assessment of health status, or rural versus urban location (Mainous 1992).

The quality of care provided by PAs was assessed in primary care clinics of the US Air Force in which PAs delivered a considerable portion of primary care formerly provided by physicians. Quality of clinical care determinations were made on the basis of responses to predetermined diagnostic, therapeutic, and referral/disposition criteria. Therapeutic criteria included desirable actions on the part of the health care provider (i.e., prescribing the appropriate class of antibiotic for infectious otitis media at the first visit) and undesirable actions (e.g., prescribing an antibiotic for viral syndrome with gastroenteritis). On five of six such criteria, PAs performed as well as or better than physicians in identifying desirable therapeutic actions (Goldberg 1981).

Kane reported a study comparing the quality of clinical care performance of Medex-trained PAs to that provided by their employing/supervising physicians. Findings revealed that PAs were less likely than supervising physicians to use antibiotics in a manner judged to be inappropriate (i.e, prescribed for fevers of undetermined origin or viral URIs and to be somewhat less likely to use systemic steroids for conditions such as contact dermatitis or asthma). This suggests that the patient care management decisions for these morbidities made by PAs were as good as or better than those of physicians (Kane 1978a). In another study, Wright and colleagues (1977) compared the clinical performance of several types of providers of primary care services by recording decision patterns and outcome aspects of treatment by family practice residents, faculty, and PAs in two clinics staffed by health care professionals in a university family practice residency program. Activities measured in the study included patient functional outcomes, patient satisfaction, and mean cost per episode of care. Findings revealed that PAs performed as well as or better than other primary care providers in delivery of services in each of the end point measures (Wright 1977). Dutera and Harlan (1978) evaluated the appropriateness of patient care provided by PAs in 14 rural primary care settings. They concluded that PAs were clinically competent, in both diagnostic and therapeutic skills, as judged by performances observed in three specific practice circumstances: (1) when all patients were initially seen by the PA and then by a physician, (2) when undifferentiated patients were managed concurrently by physicians and PAs, and (3) when patients with specific problems were assigned to PAs. We conclude that quality care, based on the literature, does not seem to be an issue when PAs are the providers of care.

CLINICAL PREVENTIVE SERVICES/PHYSICIAN COMPLEMENTARY SERVICES

In addition to their proven abilities to safely and effectively handle a wide range of commonly encountered medical problems in ambu-latory practice, PAs are also capable, within a conducive practice setting, to provide health services that are complementary to those provided by the physician. In fact, PAs may extend the types of patient care services offered by employing practices. PAs, as well as other non-physician health care providers, have been shown to be better suited than physicians to perform certain types of clinical tasks, most of which are preventive in nature such as health education, behavioral counseling, management of patients with certain chronic diseases, and being attentive to including clinical preventive services in their patient encounters (OTA 1986).

COMPARING PAs TO OTHER HEALTH CARE WORKERS

Comparing what PAs do and how well they do it with other health workers is not easy. The level of responsibility and salary and benefit structure are two of the most important variables to hold constant when performing these type of comparisons. Other variables include the different types of settings and institutions that employ PAs. Fee-for-practice settings can differ markedly from health departments and Veterans Affairs clinics. Salaries differ widely depending on the region of the country and enabling legislation.

HMOs offer a number of advantages for comparative studies because they are primarily involved in health care delivery, tend to do this as economically as possible, and employ large numbers of health care workers. They also tend to have more reliable administrative data on employees than can be obtained by self-reporting. The following comparison of salaries in Table 3-22 is from an industrial survey of 475 HMOs around the country in the fall of 1995. All salaries listed are national averages and are based on full-time 40-hour-per-week salaries as reported by human resource personnel within participating plans. Salaries do not include bonuses/incentive payments or fringe benefits. These salaries differ widely depending on the region of the country.

MEDICAL-LEGAL CONSIDERATIONS

PAs typically protect their medical-legal risk, as well as their supervising physicians' malpractice liability risk, in one of two ways: by obtaining their own malpractice insurance (this varies by state and averages from $1,500 to $3,000 a year), or by attaching a rider to the physician's policy covering the activities of the PA. The rate of malpractice suits filed involving PAs has been quite low across a wide spectrum of practice settings and specialties (Borden 1990). One plausible interpretation is that because PA practice is known to be associated with improved patient communication and proper documentation (two leading categories of breeches prompting malpractice lawsuits) utilization of a PA can mitigate a practice's medical liability risk (see Chapter 11).

FEMALE PAs

In 1965, the first class of PAs were all men. Women entered the third Duke University class and have been part of the PA movement ever since. Stead (1966, 1967a) conceived of the PA as being composed predominantly of men because he thought they would have a greater commitment to a career and a greater willingness to meet the demands of their work. This attitude was short lived, and by 1974 the percentage of female PAs had increased to 16% (Perry 1976). This trend did not level off, and in 1996 more than 60% of the entering class were women (A. Simon 1996). Currently, the composition of the PA workforce is almost evenly divided between men and women. This is not as surprising as it may seem at first. Women have been moving into formerly male-dominated jobs in large numbers in recent years. For example, the percentage of female lawyers and judges rose from 4% in 1972 to 15% in 1982. Over the same period, the percentage of female accountants rose from 22% to 38% of the total. For economists, the increase has been from

Table 3-22 *Comparison of HMO employees average salary, 1995*

PROFESSION	AVERAGE SALARY
Phlebotomist	$18,654
Medical assistant	19,255
Staff LPN	24,432
Medical technician	24,654
X-Ray technician	27,815
Staff RN	34,915
Triage nurse	35,120
Substance abuse counselor	37,385
Psychologist (MA)	42,734
Physical therapist	46,846
Nurse practitioner	51,867
Physician Assistant	**52,881**
Staff pharmacist	56,087
Psychologist-PhD	58,144
Nurse midwife	62,000
Staff optometrist	62,262
Nurse anesthetist	75,623
General practitioner	106,554
Pediatrician	111,136
Family practitioner	114,451
Internist	115,289
Emergency medicine	126,756
Pulmonologist	140,052
Dermatologist	142,282
Pathologist	145,267
Oncologist	148,030
Radiologist	171,101
General surgeon	172,350
Urologist	173,939
Obstetrician-Gynecologist	181,162
Anesthesiologist	181,538
Cardiologist	182,271
Orthopedist	231,775

(Data from Warren Surveys. The HMO Executive Salary Survey, Fall 1995.)

12% to 25%. These changes reflect the different educational choices made by young women in recent years. For example, in 1968, women received only 8% of all medical degrees and 4% of law degrees. The percentages were 31% and 39% respectively, in 1986 (Browning 1992).

Nationally, women are 11 times more likely than men to voluntarily quit a job. On average, they work 8 months in each job, while men work 3 years, and they are more likely to be part-time workers. Sustained work experience has an important effect on earnings, so these differences between men and women are relevant. Marriage also seems to affect women and men differently. Married men earn more than single men, but single women earn more than married women. This result may occur because, historically, marriage freed men of household duties and permitted more single-minded attention to jobs, but has had the opposite effect for women. Actually, women in their thirties who have worked without interruption since high school earn slightly more than men with the same background. Unmarried female faculty members at colleges and universities earn slightly more than unmarried male academics with similar credentials (Sowell 1980; Ehrenberg 1988).

In trying to determine whether wage differences are due to discrimination, we must compare groups of workers who are equally capable, experienced, and motivated. This comparison is not easy to make given the numerous factors that affect the current earnings of any worker. Using statistical techniques, economists have tried to take into account easily measured factors such as age, years of schooling, region, and hours of work. They have generally found that from one-half to three-fourths of the gross differences in earnings between men and women can be explained by these factors (Ehrenberg 1988). Whether the remaining differences are due to discrimination or to as yet unquantified productivity differences is, and probably will continue to be, a controversial issue.

Female PAs earn less than male PAs even when influencing factors such as on-call hours, years as a practicing PA, years in current practice, setting, and community size are controlled in the analysis (Carter 1983; Willis 1989, Oliver 1993a). Analysis by specialty also reveals that salary differences remain for family/general practice, pediatrics, obstetrics and gynecology, emergency medicine, and orthopedics. However,

no statistical differences emerge in the specialties of surgery, internal medicine, or occupational/industrial medicine (Willis 1990b). Other studies have found that female and male PAs that were hired at the same salary level did not have significant salary differences a few years later (Parnes 1991).

The reasons for salary differences are not easily explained. Shortcomings of some studies have been in ignoring hourly wage, productivity (patient visits per hour), and total revenues generated by the PA. Other considerations to explain the differences may relate to initial starting salaries, the ability to negotiate for raises, participation in profit sharing, and the development of partnerships when private practices are examined.

Future studies should address whether there are different expectations between women and men in specific settings and if employers are satisfied with the job performance between men and women. Do male PAs ask for more frequent and larger raises than women? Are there changes in the way women and men are perceived in their roles and in how they are reimbursed? What experiences discourage or block female PAs from obtaining jobs with greater potential for productivity, income, and advancement? Finally, what can women do to alter discriminatory practices (Parnes 1990)?

MINORITIES

Racial and ethnic diversity is the cornerstone of American culture, and adequate representation of all races and ethnic groups is essential to the viability of the PA profession. Without a heterogeneous mix of Americans adequately representing the profession, meeting the cross-sectional needs of Americans will fall short. The proportion of survey respondents with an underrepresented ethnic or racial group is rising within the profession. Groups showing the largest increases are Hispanics in the South Central region and African Americans in the Southeast (AAPA 1996b). Trend data suggest that African Ameri-

Table 3-23 *Ethnicity of PA trends*

	1991 (%)	1993 (%)	1995 (%)
Asian/Pacific Islander	3.3	3.8	3.8
Black/African American	4.3	4.9	4.0
Hispanic/Latino	5.5	6.1	6.1
Native American/ Alaskan Indian	0.9	1.6	1.8
White (not Hispanic)	86.0	83.5	84.3

(Data from American Academy of Physician Assistants, 1996a.)

cans, Native Americans, and other distinct ethnic groups are participating more than ever before in the profession, as less than 85% of all PAs are white (Table 3-23).

Historically there have been many efforts to improve the configuration of the profession. Three PA training programs actively recruit minority PAs, predominantly African Americans. A program for Native Americans functioned for a few years in New Mexico but closed in the late 1980s. Both the Health Professions Educational Assistance Act and the Health Professions Scholarship Program are designed to attract minorities to the health professions. Other efforts are underway such as programs to promote the sciences to minorities where they are also underrepresented.

The Minority Affairs committee survey on a cross section of PAs in 1992 found a higher percentage of graduate degrees among minority PAs than among the PA population overall. More minority PAs worked in inner-city clinics, military facilities, prisons, and nursing homes than nonminority PAs (Valentine 1992).

ATTRITION

If career mobility is one side of the PA professional coin, then attrition is the other side. Attrition, in this regard, is the gradual and natural reduction of membership or personnel from the profession. Surveys of PAs, both on a nationwide basis and selected populations from training programs, indicate that about 85% of all PA graduates are working in patient care positions. This level of professional retention is higher than for most health professionals, although not quite as high as the level of physician retention. Little is known about those who are no longer practicing as PAs. Men, former military medical corpsmen, and graduates of military PA programs have the lowest attrition rate (Perry 1984).

Clearly, a number of these individuals drop out because of health, retirement, death, parenting responsibilities, burnout, etc. and some have used their PA background and experience to branch into related fields. Still others have acquired further formal education. Employment experience and training have led many PAs into more complex and advanced roles. Some have shown the ability and interest to expand their horizons in the health care field by creating their own new roles and opportunities. Program alumni surveys estimate that approximately 4% of all PAs have gone on to medical, osteopathic, dental, chiropractic, or podiatric school. A considerably larger number have sought graduate education, for example, a Master's degree in public health or administration, medical education, health planning, occupational health/industrial medicine, or other sectors of the health care industry. One study conducted in 1993 identified 213 PAs who had a doctorate degree other than medical (e.g., PhD, DrPH, EdD). Most of these individuals acquired their terminal degrees after graduating from a PA program (P. Eugene Jones, personal communication, 1993). However, program directors report that applicants with doctorate degrees are also applying for PA training. In 1992, 1% of applicants had a doctorate degree (Oliver 1993b).

Employment patterns for PAs are extremely varied, depending on the interests, capabilities, and personalities of the individuals. Some have relied solely on an advanced degree to achieve or enhance positions in medical fields, whereas others have used the combination of clinical background and advanced degree to move to other positions.

The PA credential is increasingly recognized in the health care field as representing a valuable background that permits individuals to move into many types of expanded clinical and non-clinical roles. Attrition seems inevitable but does not appear to be a major problem for the PA profession. One can argue that, in any profession, a number of people would be expected to explore new and expanding areas of opportunity, and the PA profession seems like a reasonable spring-board for this. Because a large number of PAs sought this profession after making one or more career changes, it seems only natural that they be afforded this view as well if they seek career latitude or an alternative role.

PA BELIEFS AND PRACTICE ATTITUDES

Understanding some of the unique characteristics of PAs is important if we are to better understand the occupation. This section lists some of the health beliefs and behaviors of PAs that have been reported over the last decade.

Assisted suicide continues to be a topic of debate among health care professionals, and PAs are no exception. In a Michigan survey conducted in 1994, 48% of responding PAs tended to support provider-assisted suicide, and 40% were opposed (Hayden 1995). One state's cross-sectional survey, a state where physician-assisted suicide has been very controversial, cannot be generalized to PAs at large, nor can it suggest that these attitudes are static.

Recommendations by authorities seem to be important motivators for PA and medical students equally. At the University of Iowa College of Medicine, PA and medical students responded to recommendations to receive the hepatitis B immunization series at a higher rate than residents and staff physicians (Diekman 1955a).

Impaired providers is an important topic for state medical boards who have the charge to protect their constituents' health and exposure to unhealthy conditions. The majority of PAs in one study were either nondrinkers or ex-drinkers. An overwhelming number are non-smokers as well. A substantial majority of PAs, 87%, reported that they rarely or never relied on drugs or medication to affect mood or to relax. Most respondents in this study reported either occasional physical activity (47%) or regular physical activity at least three times a week (47%). Interestingly, this same study also found that PAs were oriented more strongly toward general health matters and prevention than toward illness or sick role-related beliefs (Glazer-Waldman 1989).

A 1991 national survey of PAs reported that 60% thought that treating patients with human immunodeficiency virus (HIV) placed them at risk for acquired immune deficiency syndrome (AIDS). About one-third thought that health care workers had a right to refuse care to patients with AIDS. However, more than 80% indicated they were willing to provide health care to patients with HIV, as well as those considered to be in high-risk groups (Currey 1992).

SOCIAL STATUS OF PAs

Social class or status is one of the most important variables in social research. The socioeconomic position of a person affects his or her chances for education, income, occupation, marriage, health, friends, and even life expectancy. This variable, however, has proved difficult to measure in a pluralistic, egalitarian, and fluid society such as exists in the United States. Nevertheless, many researchers have tried to identify the social strata and to measure variables associated with them. Occupation has been shown to be the best single predictor of social status, and overall occupational prestige ratings have been found to be highly stable. A number of factors act in close relationship between occupation and social status. Both individual income and educational attainment are known to be correlated with occupational rank. Education is a basis for entry into many occupations and for most persons, income is derived from occupation. House type and dwelling area constitute other highly correlated factors (Miller 1991).

Several scales are available to determine social status, and each has its proponents and detractors. They vary in length and number of factors included in the scale. The standard Duncan Socioeconomic Index (SEI) is the most widely used and is generally considered to be superior for most survey and large-sample situations. It takes into account income, education, and occupational prestige. Another scale is the Siegel Prestige Score. This score is based on subjective rankings to establish the standing of respondents' in a wide variety of occupations and represents an effort to secure a "pure" prestige rating.

The third scale is the Nam-Powers, which is based on the 1970 US Census. It has been used as a socioeconomic status score for most occupations. Scores are based on average levels of education and income for US workers in 1970. Researchers have the option of choosing the Nam-Powers Socioeconomic Scores if they wish to employ a measurement without prestige weights. A correlation of .97 is reported between the Duncan Socioeconomic Index and Nam-Powers Socioeconomic Status Scores.

In Table 3-24, the three social status scores are shown for the medical occupational group developed for the 1980 census. The Duncan and Nam-Powers SEI scores can take values approximately between 0 and 100 on both indexes, but because they are constructed somewhat differently, it is not appropriate to make direct comparisons. The Siegel Prestige Scores have a much smaller range, with bootblacks at the lowest (09.3) and college/university teachers at the highest (78.3).

Little is known about the social or occupational standing of PAs. The Census Bureau only started listing PAs as an occupation in 1980 as *Health practitioner n.e.c.* (not elsewhere classified) but gave it a score of 96.

Of the 12 health occupations listed in Table 3-24, PAs rank behind physicians, the same as marine scientists, and ahead of pharmacists, university professors, and economists.

To date, neither the Duncan SEI nor the Siegel Prestige Scores have rated PAs or nurse practitioners, although they may be considered "kindred workers" from a sociologic viewpoint. With increased examination of the profession, we expect that social scientists will modify these occupational classifications for PAs to be consistent with increased understanding of their income, status, mobility, and prestige of PAs across the spectrum of social situations.

CONCLUSION

Data on the current status of PAs indicate that PAs are improving the specialty and geographic maldistribution of the medical workforce in the United States. They are more likely to be working in primary care fields and in smaller communities, as well as moving into areas of medical subspecialty in all the states and territories of the America. The potential for making major contributions in this area is increasing. Their composition is reflective of the gender and ethnic makeup of Americans and efforts to improve this picture seems to be working as well.

The average age of the employed PA is 40 and employed for approximately 9 years. The age range of most PA students is between early 20s and late 40s, with the average around 33. One of the problems with the work-related rewards received by PAs appears to be that they will reach an early peak in the first several years after entry into the profession, and then plateau. This may be a problem for an individual who enters the PA profession early in his vocational career and who has relatively high career aspirations. An older individual who has been employed for some time and then makes a career move to become a PA may see this as a major career advancement. As the workforce changes, the PA profession will need to adjust to these changes as well.

Table 3-24 *Occupational classification system of three social status scores for health care workers, 1980*

CODE	OCCUPATION	1970 DUNCAN SEI SCORE	1970 SIEGEL PRESTIGE SCORE	1980 NAM-POWERS (US CENSUS SCORE)
	Health professional, technical, and kindred workers			
061	Chiropractors	75.0	60.0	96
062	Dentists	96.0	73.6	100
063	Optometrists	79.0	62.0	99
064	Pharmacists	81.3	60.3	95
065	Physicians (MD, DO)	92.1	81.2	100
071	Podiatrists	58.0	36.7	99
072	Veterinarians	78.0	59.7	99
073	**Physician Assistants**			96
073	Nurse Practitioners			96
074	Dieticians	39.0	52.1	64
075	Registered Nurses	44.3	60.1	73
076	Therapists (PT, OT)	59.9	40.5	73
	Other			
086	Clergymen	52.0	69.0	70
052	Marine Scientists			96
091	Economists	74.4	53.6	95
100	Social Workers	64.0	52.4	75
104	Biology Teachers	84.0	78.3	85
113	Health Specialties Teachers	84.0	78.3	85
124	Coaches, Physical Ed Teachers	64.0	53.2	74
140	College/University Teachers	84.0	78.3	91
161	Surveyors	48.4	53.1	64
163	Airline Pilots	79.0	70.1	93
175	Actors	60.0	55.0	76
211	Funeral Directors	59.0	52.2	81
265	Insurance agents, brokers, underwriters	66.0	46.8	81
364	Receptionists	44.0	37.1	38
461	Machinists	32.9	47.7	57
802	Farm managers	36.0	43.7	54
941	Bootblack	8.0	9.3	2
964	Police officers and detectives	40.5	47.7	79

(Data from Miller DC. Handbook of Research Design and Social Measurement, 15th Ed. Sage Publication, Newbury Park, CA, 1991; 327-429.)

4

Physician Assistant Education

Physician assistant (PA) educational programs were created more than 30 years ago, most within institutions preparing traditional health care professionals. Educational curricula designed to prepare these health care providers were based on the existing medical educational model. PA programs have kept pace with advancing concepts in health professions education and represent health professions curricula that have maintained a socially responsive, practically focused, and multidisciplinary educational approach. These programs have been innovations in the development of strategies proven effective in medical generalist/primary care preparation. PA programs have earned a distinct identity within medical education (Sadler 1972; Golden 1981; Carter 1984a; Schafft 1987a; Fasser 1992a).

CURRENT STATUS

There are currently 85 accredited educational programs for PAs (Table 4-1). These programs are accredited by the Accreditation Review Committee-Physician Assistant (ARC-PA), formally the Committee on Accreditation for Allied Health Educational Programs (CAAHEP). At least 10 other programs are expected to be on line by the end of 1997. PA educational programs exist in 30 states and the District of Columbia. Of these programs, all but two pre-

pare PAs for roles as primary care providers; two programs prepare surgeon's assistants (SAs). As of 1997, more than 34,000 individuals have completed PA education programs, with 85% in active clinical practice (AAPA 1996a).

PA education programs are sponsored by universities, academic health centers, schools of medicine, osteopathy, health-related professions, and 4-year colleges. The remainder are sponsored by teaching hospitals, community colleges, and the US military (see Appendix 3) (A. Simon 1996). The Association of Physician Assistant Programs (APAP) estimates that at least 19 new PA educational programs are preparing for entry to the ARC-PA accreditation process, with an additional 30 institutions expressing interest in sponsoring PA educational programs (AAPA 1996b).

Traditionally, PA education has relied on the philosophy that student performance is based on demonstration of a standard level of clinical competency and has tended to avoid assignment of a specific academic degree for what may be termed "standard" PA educational preparation. The competency-based PA educational philosophy holds that proficiency in the clinical skills identified as being necessary for future competence in primary care/generalist practice should be the "gold standard" of PA educational preparation, rather than necessitating adherence to institutional requirements for a specific academic

Table 4-1 *Number of students and graduates from PA programs, academic years, 1984–1996*

ACADEMIC YEAR	NUMBER OF PROGRAMS	ENROLLED STUDENTS	ANNUAL GRADUATES
1984–1985	53	2549	1176
1985–1986	51	2498	1148
1986–1987	49	2461	1094
1987–1988	50	2386	1141
1988–1989	51	2514	1204
1989–1990	51	2526	1227
1990–1991	55	3086	1499
1991–1992	54	3408	1594
1992–1993	58	3800	1710
1993–1994	58	4200	1850
1994–1995	60	5109	2500
1995–1996	64	5520	2600
1996–1997	78	6000[a]	3200[a]

[a] Estimate.

degree. Allowing for variability among PA programs regarding the terminal degree and/or certificate awarded has proven to be an effective approach in preparing PA health care professionals to assume a wide range of roles in clinical practice settings and specialities. This approach has also facilitated the recruitment of individuals from diverse ethnic, cultural, and educational backgrounds into PA educational programs and represents those graduates most likely to work in primary care roles in medically needy areas (Leiken 1985; AGPAW 1995). The competency-based orientation of PA education has proven to be effective in preparing health care professionals to qualify for the national certifying examination and to meet state licensing board requirements. The generalist philosophy of PA education produces graduates who have assumed clinical practice roles in a wide range of health care settings and specialties.

Of all institutions sponsoring PA programs, 26% are classified as Research I Universities as defined by the Carnegie Foundation for the Advancement of Teaching (Jones 1994a). At present, 80% of PA educational programs award either a Bachelor's or Master's degree. The remainder award either an Associate degree or a certificate of completion (Table 4-2).

A recent trend among sponsoring institutions has been to award the Master's degree for PA education. This is not without some contention, as some educators believe that the Bachelor's degree should be the minimum degree for PAs (Sadler-Sparks & Stein 1988). Since 1987, a number of PA programs have restructured their curricula for standard PA educational preparation, with approximately one-fourth of the programs now offering a graduate degree (typically either the Master of Health Science [MHS] or Master of Science [MS] degrees) or a Master's degree option. The PA programs of Duke University, Emory University, Baylor University, the George Washington University, the University of Iowa, the University of Nebraska, the University of Texas, and the University of Colorado now award the Master's degree for completion of PA professional education. Most PA programs continue to award the Bachelor's degree, but also

Table 4-2 *Characteristics of PA educational programs, 1996*

TYPE OF SPONSORING INSTITUTION	NUMBER	PERCENT
University	50	62.50
Four-year college	21	26.25
Community college	3	3.75
Hospital [a]	3	3.75
Military [a]	3	3.75
Total	80	100.00

HIGHEST CREDENTIAL AWARDED	NUMBER	PERCENT
Master	15	18.75
Baccalaureate	49	61.25
Associate	6	7.50
Certificate	10	12.50
Total	80	100.00

[a] Degrees are granted from university or college affiliates. In 1996, the three military programs collapsed into one joint military program.

(Data from A. Simon 1996.)

offer students a Master's degree option, such as the PA program at Northeastern University. Others combine PA education with a related graduate degree program, such as the Physician Assistant/Master of Public Health Program at the George Washington University, and the Physician Assistant Master of Science Program at the University of Iowa.

Historical Roots of PA Education

The creation of the PA and other types of new health practitioners, as well as the expansion of undergraduate medical education, were federal policy approaches that affected health professionals during the 1970s. Policy was aimed toward the broad goals of increasing access to health care, containing costs, and improving the delivery of primary care.

The rationale for the creation of the PA profession was based on the need for a new type of health care provider who would:

1. Compensate for the demise of the general practitioner by augmenting physician capabilities to deliver medical care services and help alleviate the perceived shortage of primary care physicians

2. Help address health care access problems stemming from the geographic and specialty maldistribution of physicians

3. Provide an educational means by which existing health personnel with broad experiences could be channeled into advanced clinical roles

4. Be a positive factor in helping to control health care costs and improve primary care access (Perry 1980; Carter 1984b)

The introduction of the PA had the support of both the medical profession and the federal government, who collaborated in promoting PAs. The medical profession sponsored legal efforts in recognition of PA practice, and the government granted financial support for the development of PA educational programs (NCHSR 1977).

Eugene Stead and Richard Smith are generally credited with being the major developers of the PA concept in the United States. The first educational program was developed at Duke University, soon followed by the Alderson Broaddus Program, the University of Colorado Program, and the Medex Program at the University of Washington. The Duke PA curricula comprised a 20-month, competency-based, generalist program which aimed to prepare clinicians who would perform medical diagnostic and patient management tasks heretofore legally done only by physicians. Duke PAs were intended to be assistants to physicians in all types of practice settings and clinical specialties. The curricula built on the prior clinical experiences of four ex-Navy medical corpsmen recruited for the first class. The Duke curriculum not only drew its educational resources from the multiple academic and clinical departments within the institution, but was linked to medical practices in surrounding community sites as well. This initial program provided 7 months of classroom instruction covering the basic and clinical medical sciences, followed by 13 months of rotating clinical clerkships, culminating in a 2-month primary care, office-based preceptorship. As its first graduates entered practice, the Duke PA program received a great deal of attention in both lay and medical circles and served as a model for the curriculum of many PA programs that followed (Stead 1967a).

Several other PA educational programs developed during this time pioneered innovative approaches to health practitioner education providing a variety of effective models in PA education. The curricula broadly resemble a shorter version of the structure of physician education in the generalist care specialties; maintain a competency-based approach; and include, as part of their primary care emphasis, important elements drawn from the biologic, human behavioral, and preventive care paradigms (Golden 1983).

The Medex model of PA education was pioneered by Richard Smith at the University of

Washington in 1969. Individuals with extensive prior health care experience were admitted to the program often already matched to a physician preceptor, who was often a prospective employer. Medex PA students received 6 to 9 months of intensive didactic medical coursework and are then assigned to serve a 12- to 15-month community-based preceptorship with a physician in practice (Smith RA, 1969; Smith RA, 1971; Smith RA, 1972).

The first medical specialty PA educational program was developed by Henry Silver at the University of Colorado in 1969. The Child Health Associate Program comprised a 3-year course of study set in a medical school that enrolled individuals with a nursing credential and prior pediatric experience. This program was among the first to award the Master's degree for PA education (Silver 1971b).

Another educational model for PAs was developed at Alderson-Broaddus College in 1969, where a PA curriculum was designed within a 4-year liberal arts college. This so-called 2 + 2 approach offers a curriculum that is divided into two phases. The preprofessional phase consists of courses typically taken in the first 2 years of college (i.e., liberal arts, general science courses). This is followed by a professional phase in which the final 2 years of instruction are identical in content to the aforementioned types of PA programs (Meyers 1978; Fasser 1987).

For physicians, most medical education takes place in the university hospital on a very select group of patients—those who have filtered through the system to what is usually a tertiary care center. In contrast, most PA education is primary care and tends to tilt toward ambulatory care settings. Recognizing this, PA educational programs tend to emphasize outpatient more than inpatient skills.

Accreditation

Formal standards for PA educational programs are initially established by the ARC-PA, a Committee on Allied Health Education and Accreditation (CAHEA), formally a division of the American Medical Association (AMA). Standards

for PA programs were first established in 1971 with the publication of *The Essentials and Guidelines of an Approved Educational Program for the Assistant to the Primary Care Physician* (CAHEA 1990). *The Essentials and Guidelines*, now known as the *Standards*, is the reference used as the basis of award of accreditation to PA educational programs. It provides recommendations for the general administrative, organizational, and curricular structure of PA programs. The *Standards* permits PA educational programs and their sponsoring institutions to work within a broad framework to guide the development of PA curriculum. The *Standards* ensures that the core components of PA educational programs (such as levels of institutional support, clinical training affiliations, basic and clinical science course offerings, faculty qualifications, and admission and selection guidelines) are fully met before the award of accreditation. It has also allowed PA educational programs a degree of latitude in which to create curricular configurations based on a structure awarding several types of academic degrees. They have tacitly promoted innovation among educational institutions in developing nontraditional approaches in health professions education. PA educational programs have proven to be successful in creating effective models of health professions curricula, particularly in primary care. Reflecting the multiple changes affecting educational preparation occurring within a rapidly developing field, the *Standards* has been revised and updated in 1978, 1985, 1990, and 1996. The ARC-PA evaluates PA programs and awards accreditation based on compliance with guidelines in the *Standards*. Commission on Accreditation of Allied Health Education Programs (CAAHEP) approval is necessary for PA program eligibility for federal Title VII grant funding, and for graduates to qualify (along with passage of the Physician Assistant National Certifying Examination [PANCE]) to practice in the vast majority of states.

The ARC-PA, one of 17 collaborative committees on accreditation operating under the umbrella of the CAAHEP, is sponsored by the American Academy of Family Physicians, the

American Academy of Pediatrics, the American Academy of Physician Assistants (AAPA), the American College of Physicians, the American College of Surgeons, the AMA, and the APAP. Each of the ARC-PAs sponsoring organizations appoints two members to serve on the committee, with the exceptions of the AAPA and the APAP, which are entitled to appoint three representatives each. The American College of Physicians has elected to send only one representative to the ARC-PA.

CAAHEP, incorporated in June 1994, is a national, voluntary, specialized accreditation agency, independent of any single professional organization or agency, and represents a broad range of health care disciplines. CAAHEP is recognized by the Commission on Recognition of Postsecondary Accreditation through 1997. CAAHEP is also recognized by the US Department of Education (USDE). Its application for continuing recognition by the USDE is reviewed by the USDE's National Advisory Committee on Accreditation and Institution Eligibility.

PA Curriculum

The general philosophy of PA programs includes a broad-based approach to primary care health professions education. This focus has resulted in curricula that give PA students a strong foundation in primary care medicine, yet also prepares them to enter a wide range of other clinical areas.

The format of the typical PA program is an intensive, 2-year medically oriented curriculum that educates the student in primary care (Shelton 1984). Roughly 10 to 12 months are devoted to didactic instruction in the basic and clinical sciences, followed by a similar period of rotating clerkships and preceptorships in all major clinical disciplines. Didactic courses include anatomy, physiology, microbiology, biochemistry, pathology, pharmacology, and the behavioral sciences. Instruction is also provided in the clinical sciences with course work in physical examination, pathophysiology, clinical diagnosis, communication and interpersonal skills,

epidemiology and preventive medicine, clinical procedures and surgical skills, and interpretation of laboratory tests and imaging studies (Oliver 1993b). Courses in the basic medical sciences constitute about 75% of the total didactic portion of PA curricula. Instruction devoted to the behavioral and social sciences averages over 124 contact hours per program. The range of subjects includes topics such as psychosocial dynamics, health promotion/disease prevention, bioethics, medical sociology, death and dying, and cross-cultural medicine.

During their second year, PA students obtain clinical training experiences while serving on rotations, usually 4 to 8 weeks long, conducted over a wide range of inpatient and outpatient care settings. Most PA programs require students to complete rotations in core medical, pediatric, surgical, and primary care clinical disciplines. These typically include experiences in inpatient medicine, primary care/ambulatory medicine, surgery, pediatrics, obstetrics and gynecology, emergency medicine, and psychiatry. Clinical experiences offered also include elective rotations and commonly offer a final preceptorship in a primary care practice setting. In serving on these clinical rotations and preceptorships, PA students are given instruction by practicing physicians, physician residents and house officers, graduate PAs, and a variety of other health care professionals (Oliver 1993b).

Innovations in Primary Care

The curricula of early PA programs were strongly influenced by the expectations expressed by the founders who envisioned PAs serving as primary care and general medical providers. In many instances, the specific curriculum objectives of educational programs were based on addressing the clinical problems most often encountered in primary care practice. This approach differed from the traditional model of medical education, which often relied on departmentally controlled lecture content. PA educators were able to enlist new methods of determining educational program objectives, coordinating courses, lecturers, and instructors. Grant funding in support of these new curricula allowed PA educators to select clinical and basic science department faculty whose teaching complied with program objectives.

Curricular innovations in health professions education that have focused on the clinical preparation of providers for primary care roles originated within now prominent PA programs. Models using decentralized training approaches, such as those seen at the University of Washington Medex Northwest PA Program, the Stanford University Primary Care Associate Program, and the University of Utah Physician Assistant Program, have paved the way for other programs in their efforts to develop effective methods in placing PA graduates in medically underserved areas (Fowkes 1983).

More recently, decentralized satellite training initiatives have been developed at the Medex Northwest PA Program of the University of Washington. Medex Northwest selects students who might not otherwise be able to relocate to urban or academic health centers but who have been deemed to have the potential, based on prior health care experience, to provide primary health care in underserved areas. This model has expanded educational opportunities for PA training in rural sites in Washington and five other states (Alaska, Montana, Idaho, Oregon, and Nevada). At the Medex satellite in Sitka, Alaska, 12 Alaskan Native students were enrolled in 1992 and participated in their clinical educational experiences in rural Alaskan community practices (Ballweg 1994; Hummel 1994a). Other examples of "satellite" educational programs have been developed at the Medical College of Georgia, University of Texas-Galveston, and St. Louis University. A central element in the structure of many of these community-based satellite PA educational programs is a strong tie to regional Area Health Education Centers (AHECs) and the participation of clinical sites that serve medically needy populations.

PA programs remain sensitive to the need to respond to changes in the health care environment, and program curricula undergo regular review and modification. Experience indicates that this flexibility results in newly employed PAs adapting more easily to a wide variety of practice settings. A graduate level educational track that focuses on PA clinical preparation for practice in rural health care, such as the one sponsored by the Alderson-Broaddus College Physician Assistant Program in Philippi, West Virginia, and the rural health curriculum track at the University of Nebraska-Omaha Physician Assistant Program, is a model of innovative curricula that prepares primary health care providers targeted for practices in areas with underserved populations.

In one study of all accredited PA educational programs, it was possible to determine the extent to which they provide students exposure to rural primary care. By merging zip codes of PA program training sites with those of population tracts from federally designated rural areas, investigators were able to determine the location of sites offering clinical training experiences for PA students. While only two PA programs are located in rural counties, 31 of 50 programs (62%) in 1992 offered a total of 288 clinical training sites in 234 nonmetropolitan counties. This represents exposure of PA students to patients in 10% of 2,342 nonmetropolitan counties in the United States, a higher penetration of PA students than medical or nurse practitioner students at that time (Hooker 1994c).

Other examples of innovations of PA programs in health professions education have been the longstanding inclusion of topics such as health education, epidemiology, communication skills, and biomedical ethics. These subjects have only recently been regarded as important in undergraduate medical education. Noting areas essential to the preparation of competent primary care providers, PA programs commonly include instruction on substance abuse prevention and treatment, health care for the homeless, women's health care, geriatric medicine, environmental/occupational medicine, mental health, and a practical orientation to skills in the delivery of clinical preventive services.

PA Program Support

Federal support for PA education first began in 1972 and since then has totaled over $130 million (Table 4-3). Title VII funding in the amount of $5.7 million was available for PA educational program support in FY-94. This figure represents an increase of $1.56 million from FY-93 funding levels, marking the first such boost in the amount of federal funding in more than 10 years. Congressional appropriation of the full level of PA educational program support could promote the desired boost in PA graduate output over the next several years. Increased federal funding will support the expansion of enrollment within existing PA programs, as well as provide start-up funding to support the increasing number of universities, academic health centers, and colleges seeking to establish new PA programs (Finerfrock 1989).

Projected increases in the enrollment capacities of PA educational programs will require that programs take the necessary steps to achieve this goal. These include increasing efforts in the recruitment of new faculty members, strengthening minority recruitment and retention, and adding new clinical training sites and practice affiliations. All of these efforts, linked to expanded enrollments, are dependent on increased financial support from external sources.

Increasing concern has been expressed among leaders in both the nurse practitioner (NP) and PA professions that growth may be too rapid in the annual number of educational program graduates. Level or reduced demand in the marketplace could lead to an oversupply of PAs and, as a consequence, reduce employment opportunities and salaries (Jones 1995). Because the PA (and NP) professions are still relatively new, neither has been forced to pass through severe cyclical fluctuations in market supply and demand as observed in other established professions. An important policy problem is how to determine the number of PA and NP graduates required to meet demand in the future US health system.

Table 4-3 *Federal support for PA education, 1972–1997*

YEAR	TOTAL GRANT AWARDS ($)	NUMBER OF FUNDED PROGRAMS
1972	6,090,109	40
1973	6,208,999	9
1974	8,129,252	43
1975	5,994,002	40
1976	6,247,203	41
1977	8,171,441	39
1978	8,685,074	42
1979	8,453,666	42
1980	8,262,968	43
1981	8,019,000	40
1982	4,752,000	34
1983	4,752,000	34
1984	4,414,850	34
1985	4,442,076	37
1986	4,548,000	37
1987	4,275,000	36
1988	4,549,973	37
1989	4,445,200	37
1990	4,697,680	38
1991	5,000,000	36
1992	5,000,000	34
1993	5,000,000	33
1994	6,500,000	42
1995	6,500,000	34
1996	5,964,000	28
1997	5,725,000	30

Between 1972 and 1976, awards for PA training were provided by contracts under Health Manpower Educational Initiatives, Public Health Service. Since 1977, funding has been authorized under Sections 701, 783, 788, and 750 of Title VII of the Public Health Service Act, Grants for Programs for Physician Assistants, and is administered by the Division of Medicine, Bureau of Health Professions, Health Resources and Services Administration.

(Data from US Department of Health and Human Services, Health Resources and Services Administration, Bureau of Health Professions. *Health Personnel in the United States: Eighth Report of Congress.* Government Printing Office, Rockville, MD, 1992; Cawley 1992a; A. Simon 1996.)

The level of federal support for health professions educational programs of all types will likely be reduced in future Congressional appropriations. The consensus is that there will be too many physicians, nurses, and pharmacists in the future health system. This has led Congressional health policy leaders, whose ideologic adversaries are often anxious to cut discretionary federal spending categories, to shy away from sponsoring health professions education program subsidies. The long-sacred Medicare Graduate Medical Education (physician postgraduate residency) subsidy is in jeopardy. A key question for the PA profession will be continuation of grant award support for PA programs ($5 million in FY-96) under Title VII of the Public Health Service Act. A long-term workforce policy goal for PA professions education could be to attain Medicare-linked support for graduate clinical PA education, similar to the mechanism established for physician graduate medical education (GME).

Table 4-4 *Minority PA students, by percentage of total enrolled, 1983–1996*

ACADEMIC YEAR	NONWHITE PA STUDENTS ENROLLED (%)	AVERAGE NUMBER PER CLASS
1983–1984	13.8	4.0
1984–1985	16.6	4.1
1985–1986	14.7	3.6
1986–1987	21.1	5.3
1987–1988	22.3	5.9
1988–1989	20.3	5.3
1989–1990	19.9	5.2
1990–1991	17.7	5.3
1991–1992	19.0	6.1
1992–1993	17.5	5.7
1993–1994	17.7	6.3
1994–1995	20.9	8.8
1995–1996	22.3	9.3

(Data from A. Simon 1996.)

PA STUDENTS

In 1995, an estimated 5,558 students were enrolled in 71 PA programs. This represents an increase of 450 students over the previous year. The average size of the entering PA class was 43 students. Early demographic patterns observed among PA students show a clear male predominance. However, due to a steady increase in the proportion of women in the PA profession since 1980, they now comprise nearly half (47%) of all practicing PAs. Among presently enrolled PA students, 19% are members of racial and ethnic minorities (COGME 1994; AAPA 1996a; A. Simon 1996) (Table 4-4).

While there is a tendency for students to come from smaller towns and have more education (Brandon 1993), student backgrounds are more diverse than ever before. Most students (72%) admitted to PA educational programs in 1995–1996 held a Baccalaureate (BA, BS) or higher degree on entry. The typical entering student was self-described as white/non-Hispanic, over 27 years of age, with a grade point average of 3.3. Most students possessed substantial previous health care experience (a mean of 53 months as a medical technologist, military corpsman, nurse, etc.). Among the 9.5% of all individuals admitted to PA educational programs with a graduate degree (Master's or Doctoral degree) in 1995, 18 were international medical graduates. The mean age of enrolled students in 1992 was 35.5 years (AAPA 1996a).

Most students plan a career in health care during high school, but the decision to become a PA is usually made later. The majority make the decision independently, after first ruling out medical school and researching the PA profession. Dissatisfaction with a previous health career is a moderate motivator (Currey 1990). Once potential students learn about the profession, it often takes approximately 3 to 4 years before enrollment (Curry 1989). The lag time from learning about the PA profession to enrollment is due to meeting requirements, applying, being accpeted, and finally enrolling. Personal contact with practicing PAs is probably the most effective recruitment tool for the profession. Unfortunately, most high school and college counselors are unaware of the profession (Berry 1989).

Among all enrolled PA students in 1995–1996, 81.2% were white, 7.2% were African American, 5.8% were Hispanic, and 5.8% were either Native American/Alaskan Natives, or Asian/Pacific Islanders (A. Simon 1996). The education of ethnic and racial minorities in PA educational programs since 1970 reflects social progress in providing access to health professions opportunities for these groups. Percentages of minorities enrolled in PA educational programs from 1983 through 1992 averaged 18.3% per enrolled class (Oliver 1993). Expressed differently, the number of minority students has doubled from a mean of four students per program in 1983 to more than nine per program in 1995 (A. Simon 1996).

Only one of the accredited PA educational programs, the Howard University Physician Assistant Program, is set within a historically and predominantly black college and university. It has graduated more than 50% of all African American PAs. Two other programs (Drew University and Harlem Hospital/City University of New York) enroll higher numbers of individuals from racial and ethnic minorities.

Overall attrition among PA students is disproportionate for individuals from racial and ethnic minorities (Lary 1991). The overall attrition rate for PA students was 7.2% in 1992–1993; attrition was 26.1% for African American PA students, 15.4% for Hispanic/Latinos, and 6.7% for other racial and ethnic minorities. The attrition rate for whites/non-Hispanics was 4.6%. Underrepresented racial and ethnic minority persons, in particular African American women, were more likely than nonminority individuals either to be lost to attrition or to be assigned to decelerated tracks in PA programs (Oliver 1993a).

Applicants to PA Programs

In response to forces in the health professions marketplace, PA educational programs have seen a dramatic increase in the number of program applicants (Table 4-5). This has strained the limited resources of many institutions. Because one limiting factor is funding support, and because Title VII grants for PA educational programs have remained essentially level since 1981, resources are stretched to the maximum in many programs. If programs are not funded sufficiently in the future, expansion of PA enrollment may lead to compromise in the quality of educational experiences received by students. For the class that entered in 1995–1996, more than 12,000 applications were received by PA educational programs. The aver-

Table 4-5 *Mean number of applicants, percentage enrolled, enrollment, and matriculants, PA programs, 1989–1996*

ACADEMIC YEAR	APPLICANTS PER PROGRAM (NUMBER)	APPLICANTS ENROLLED (%)	ENROLLMENT	MATRICULANTS
1989–1990	90	29	2,526	
1990–1991	107	28	3,086	
1991–1992	133	24	3,408	
1992–1993	203	17	3,836	
1993–1994	276	13	4,400	
1994–1995	380	11	5,109	
1995–1996	419	10	5,558	2,234

(Data from A. Simon 1996.)

age of 420 applicants per program was up sharply from the 133 applications received in 1991. Forty-three students per program, or roughly 10% of the applicants, were enrolled in 1995 (A. Simon 1996). Between 1988 and 1996, the number of applicants per program increased by 136%.

Since 1984, women have comprised between 58% and 62% of enrolled PA students. When personality measures of PA program applicants were examined at one site, women were more aggressive, autonomous, impulsive, playful, and flexible than male counterparts. They also seem less accepting of social mores and the traditional female role. No sexual bias could be determined by the admissions committee (Crovitz 1975).

Although the number of ethnic minorities enrolled in PA programs has averaged 19% since 1985, these individuals compose only 9.3% of the practicing PA population. These figures, plus the fact that only 3.7% of all practicing PAs are African American, suggest that past federal health professions policy and program strategies supporting the recruitment and retention of ethnic minority and disadvantaged students and faculty within PA educational programs have had only partial success in increasing the number of individuals from these groups. This points out the need for additional efforts and policy directives in this area (Oliver 1993a).

Previous Occupations

Understanding the background of PA students is important not only for recruitment purposes, but also to better understand the underlying influence on PA careers. In the beginning, former military corpsmen and medics were viewed as the most suitable. From a predominance of veterans in the 1970s, this source had shrunk to 5% in 1994. Nurses, comprising RNs, NPs, LPNs, and other types of nurses, made up 19.6% of the 1993 student body. As can be seen in Table 4-6, paramedics account for 10% of the 1994 student body and have ranged from 10% to 15% between 1990 and 1994. An assortment of health care profes-

Table 4-6 *Previous occupations of PA students, 1994*

LISTED OCCUPATION	CASES	PERCENT
Physician (MD/DO)	4	0.1
Athletic trainer	22	0.8
Corpsman (Military)	137	5.0
Paramedic (Civilian)	292	10.6
Emergency room technician	125	4.5
Laboratory technician	186	6.7
Operating room technician	77	2.8
Radiology technician	48	1.7
Nurse practitioner	4	0.1
Registered nurse (RN)	198	7.2
Licensed practical nurse (LPN)	52	1.9
Other type of nurse	166	6.0
Medical assistant	189	6.8
Occupational therapist (OT)	4	0.1
Pharmacist (RPh)	7	0.3
Physical therapist (PT)	25	0.9
Respiratory therapist (RT)	43	1.6
Health care administrator	29	1.0
Other health care professional	658	23.8
Other non-health-care related	162	5.9
No previous employment	339	12.3

(Data from AAPA New Students in PA Programs [1993 and 1994], 1995.)

sionals such as audiologists and health educators made up almost one-fourth of all PA students in 1994 (AAPA 1996a).

Factors Influencing the Decision to Become a PA

In addition to prior occupational background, a number of other factors influence a person's choice to become a PA. Table 4-7, a list compiled by the Research Division at the AAPA, aggregates these factors. Since 1985, dozens of adult children have followed in their PA parents' footsteps, sometimes enrolling at the same time. Having a family member who is a PA accounts for almost 8% of all factors influencing the decision to become a PA. Almost 18% of 1994 students listed PA acquaintances as the most important factor. Other factors included "health-related work"

(19%) and "other health professionals." Each year, the city that hosts the AAPA's national convention designates a day as PA Career Day. On this day, PAs visit inner city classrooms to discuss what PAs are and what they do.

Selection of PA Students

Every PA program uses a unique set of criteria for selecting students. The efficacy of selection measures for predicting successful completion of PA training has been examined. Some of these measures include the Scholastic Aptitude Test (SAT), Minnesota Multiphasic Personality Inventory (MMPI) scores, transcript grade point averages, and records of length of previous health care experience. When these selection criteria are compared, tests of intellectual ability and achievement were the most efficient predictors of success in training programs. Specifically, SAT scores alone predicted excellent or poor student performance in the program. The MMPI tests and previous health care experience had little or no significance in predicting success or failure in the program (Crovitz 1975).

Factors Influencing the Decision to Enroll in PA School

Once a person has made the decision to become a PA, the next step is to enroll in a PA school. The factors that influenced the decision to become a PA (among those accepted in a PA-program) are primarily "health-related work," a "PA acquaintance," or some "other health professional." These three factors account for half of all reasons for choosing a PA career and have important implications for recruitment of additional PAs (Table 4-7).

Once a PA has selected or has been selected by a PA program, the two most influential reasons for almost half of all decisions to enroll in a particular program are "PA program location" and "program reputation." The reputation fac-

Table 4-7 *Factors influencing decision to enroll in PA school, 1994*

INFLUENCING FACTOR	CASES	PERCENT
High school	24	0.4
College	105	1.6
Postbaccalaureate education	41	0.6
Guidance counselor	42	0.7
High school career day	21	0.3
High school library	9	0.1
High school counselor	18	0.3
High school teacher	17	0.3
College career day	85	0.7
College career library	85	1.3
College counselor	121	1.9
College professor	147	2.3
Information poster	42	0.7
Newspaper/magazine	229	3.6
Government publication	35	0.5
National PA programs directory	190	3.0
Other career guide	148	2.3
PA program brochure/catalog	583	9.2
Other media source	64	1.0
PA who treated me or my family	325	5.1
PA acquaintance	1141	17.9
Other health professional	833	13.1
Health-related work	1204	18.9
Illness/accident	217	3.4
Family member	504	7.9
Other personal experience	181	2.8

(Data from AAPA New Students in PA Programs [1993 and 1994], 1995.)

tor is interesting because there is no consensus regarding which programs have the higher reputation. This latter finding may represent a reinforced belief that you have made the correct decision.

Retaining What They Learn

PA curriculum is partially based on the medical school model. The PA program is about 50 weeks shorter than a typical medical school program, but the primary objectives are similar. Both programs provide students with the theoretical knowledge and technical skills needed to perform therapeutic and diagnostic procedures accurately (Estes 1969; Lawrence 1975a; Golden 1983). Like medical schools, PA programs use a format of didactic and clinical training (Wilson 1974; Dobmeyer 1975).

Only a few studies have dealt with the subject of what should be learned. Golden and Cawley found that a majority of PA programs were teaching what had been proposed by medical school educators (Dobmeyer 1975; Golden 1983). Apart from the approach to the patient and certain clinical skills, this included technical skills such as urinalysis, blood analysis, electrocardiogram (ECG) interpretation, hearing and vision screening, Papanicolaou scrapings, applying and removing casts, tuberculosis skin testing, interpreting radiographs, parenteral injections, bacteriology testing, suturing, and pulmonary function testing.

A comprehensive survey of Colorado PAs found that almost all of them learned 39 common procedures. This formed the base for the questionnaire. Eight procedures (including reading chest and long-bone x-ray films, suturing, splinting, interpreting ECGs, pelvic examinations, Papanicolaou tests, and Dipstick urinalysis) were used more than once a month by at least 50% of PAs in their practices. Three procedures (cardiopulmonary resuscitation, lumbar puncture, and suprapubic aspirations) are used less than once a year by more than 90% of PAs (Gray 1995) (Table 4-8).

Although most of the respondents learned the procedures listed in the Colorado survey, they do not report that they necessarily learned them adequately, and most believed the cited procedures needed to be emphasized more in PA education. The authors also note that with the recent enactment of the Clinical Laboratory Improvement Amendments (CLIA), most laboratories have to be certified by the federal government. This has reduced the number of small private laboratories, often in a physician's practice. With fewer laboratory procedures available, PAs and other clinicians will perform fewer laboratory procedures outside of ordering tests in the future (Gray 1995).

Table 4-8 *Skills most frequently learned by PA students*

Procedures
Cardiopulmonary resuscitation
Electrocardiogram (perform, interpret)
Finger stick and heel stick
Fluorescein-Wood's lamp examination
Parenteral injection (intradermal, subcutaneous, intramuscular)
Lumbar puncture
Suprapubic aspiration
Urethral catheterization
Venipuncture

Laboratory techniques
Agglutination test for mononucleosis (read)
Blood smear (perform, read)
Culture (streak out, read)
Gram stain (perform, read)
Sensitivity plate (read)
Stool examination for occult blood
Urinalysis (Dipstick, microscopic)

Patient care
Chest radiograph (read)
Intravenous line (set up, start, monitor)
Long-bone x-ray film (read)
Pap smear (perform)
Pelvic examination
Suturing
Wound care (burns, casts, splints)

Screening tests
Articulation screen
Denver Development Test
Hearing screen
Vision screen

(Data from Gray 1995.)

SOURCE OF SUPPORT FOR PA EDUCATION

Another well-recognized influencing force in PA education is the source of funds that PA stu-

Table 4-9 *Source of support for PA students, 1994*

SOURCE OF FUNDS	CASES	PERCENT
Loans	893	45.7
Savings	382	19.5
Scholarships	253	12.9
Parents	253	10.0
Spouse	161	8.2
Work	66	3.4
Summer job	5	0.3

(Data from AAPA New Students in PA Programs [1993 and 1994], 1995.)

dents need to draw on to complete their education. This generally ranges from $20,000 to more than $40,000; exact figures are not available (Table 4-9).

The mean total annual budget of PA educational programs in 1995 was $556,456 for 50 full-time students. There were wide ranges of total budgets per 50 students, depending on the size of the student body and the region of the country. The average cost per program to educate a PA student was estimated to be $8,822 a year.

The primary source of internal financial support for the majority of programs is the sponsoring institution, providing an average of $374,000 (median = $315,000; SD = $247,000; range = $11,000 to 1,200,000). Federal grant awards to programs during 1995 ranged from $37,000 to $353,000 and averaged $152,000. Over the last decade, when federal funding levels have remained constant at roughly $5 million a year, greater levels of internal support from sponsoring institutions have enabled programs to sustain operations and develop some measure of self-sufficiency. Other sources of support come from state grants (averaging $144,500 a year), research grants, program projects, hospital services, and practice plans (HHS, BrHP 1992; Cawley 1992; A. Simon 1996).

PA educational programs have been responsive to federal grant initiatives that target service in rural areas, medically underserved areas, and delivery of primary care to needy populations (Morris 1977; Finerfrock 1989). Relative to other health professionals, the deployment record of PAs to practices in rural communities and medically underserved areas has been impressive (Goldberg 1984; Hafferty 1986; Shi 1993). More than half of all federally funded PA programs have developed specific curricular content addressing the health and social problems of medically underserved populations. These include people living in inner cities, remote areas, correctional systems, geriatric facilities, or rehabilitation facilities. PA curricula also typically include instruction in topics such as management of persons with HIV/AIDS, counseling regarding the risks of adolescent pregnancy, measures to reduce infant mortality, required schedules of pediatric immunization, health behavior to lower the risk of cancer and heart disease, and skills in the management of health problems which occur disproportionately among medically underserved populations. To ensure that students receive adequate clinical opportunities to complement didactic instruction, most PA educational programs have developed links with Area Health Education Centers, Rural Health Clinics, Community/Migrant Health Centers, and other primary health care agencies within their geographic region.

In 1992, an initiative was developed and jointly sponsored by the Health Resources and Services Administration, the National Rural Health Association, AAPA, and APAP. The purpose of this initiative was to enhance PA clinical practice among underserved populations and in rural communities by providing support for Migrant Health Clinic Fellowships. The broad flexibility that exists within PA educational programs and a demonstrated record of responsiveness to federal incentives to increase the number of primary care providers have resulted in a number of innovative curricular approaches designed to prepare practitioners to meet future societal health care needs. The deployment of PAs to areas of medical need is largely attributable to priorities in federal Title VII grant programs. The emphasis of Title VII funding has been to promote the preparation of PAs for roles working with primary care physicians and for deployment to medically underserved areas. Incentives in Title VII grant awards have encouraged PA programs to educate practitioners with an orientation in primary care. They have also fostered methods of deployment of PA graduates to enter primary care/ambulatory practice, and/or to locate in medically underserved areas. A high proportion of federally funded PA educational programs have developed curricular components that identify clinical training sites and affiliations in rural and medically underserved areas. Qualifications require students to serve a portion of clinical training in such sites.

PA PROGRAM FACULTY

A wide variety of health care professionals and professional educators are utilized within PA educational programs. Approximately 550 individuals work in PA programs nationwide. These include physicians, physician assistants, and Masters and doctoral-level instructors in the basic medical sciences, the behavioral and social sciences, and various other disciplines.

A full-time PA program professional faculty consists of a program director (a person increasingly likely to be a PA who holds a Mas-

Table 4-10 *Credentials of PA program directors, 1993*

CREDENTIAL	NUMBER
Physician (MD or DO)	2
Doctorate (PhD or EdD)	5
Physician Assistant (PA)	10
Physician Assistant with Master's degree (MPA, MEd, MPH)	25
Physician Assistant with doctorate (PhD, EdD)	8
Nursing degree (RN)	1
RN with Master's degree (MSN)	4
NP with doctorate	1
Other Master's degree (MA, MEd, MPA)	2

(Data from Faculty Directory, Association of Physician Assistant Programs, APAP, Alexandria, VA, September, 1993a.)

ter's or Doctorate degree), a medical director, usually a physician serving part-time (0.2 to 0.5 full-time equivalent [FTE]), and an average of 3.3 FTE personnel serving in various PA faculty instructional roles (Table 4-10). The total number of employees per program ranges from 3 to 13, with an average of one employee for every 7.7 students enrolled (A. Simon 1996).

Support staffs average 2.4 FTE noninstructional PA program personnel (Table 4-11). In a mature program, this averages approximately one faculty member to 10 students; however, in the second year, the student is often away on clinical rotations or preceptorship, so contact

Table 4-11 *Faculty structure for a representative PA program with 38 students, 1996*

TITLE	FULL TIME EQUIVALENT	ANNUAL SALARY	ANNUAL BUDGET
Program director	1.0	$67,500	$67,500
Academic coordinator/instructor	1.0	57,400	57,400
Clinic coordinator/instructor	2.8	49,500	138,600
Medical director	0.3	102,500	30,750
Business manager	1.0	30,000	30,000
Secretary/receptionist	1.4	25,000	35,000
Total	7.5		$359,250

Many faculty may be employed part-time by the program.

(Data from A. Simon 1996.)

with the faculty is less intense. Because many programs use part-time faculty, there are usually no more than eight students per faculty member assigned for advisement.

A survey of Medical Directors of PA Programs in 1996 found that they spent a wide range of time working with PA programs. Fifty percent have a time commitment of less than 15%, and one-sixth have a time commitment of more than 50%. As to their respective programs, 100% participate in curriculum planning and committee function, most notably the admissions committee; 100% participate in direct student instruction; rarely do they mentor students or faculty or participate in or guide research (APAP 1996).

Like other relative newcomers in health professions education, PA educational programs have experienced difficulty in identifying, recruiting, and retaining qualified faculty members. The combination of an increasing number of applicants and a growing demand for PA services has resulted in an "academic hourglass" effect. There is a bottleneck in processing PA students because there are not enough programs to train them. This is further complicated by an existing shortage of qualified educators. In addition, consistent rates of faculty attrition in PA programs have averaged 11% per program per year over the last 5 years, and 12% for the 1994–1995 academic year (A. Simon 1996). The chief reasons cited in surveys regarding terminating academic employment include career advancement (31.3%), return to clinical practice (23.3%), geographic relocation (15.3%), and job dissatisfaction (8%) (Oliver 1993b).

If PA educational programs are to meet future workforce requirements, several critical areas must be addressed. To expand enrollment, recruitment, retention, and professional development of qualified faculty (especially faculty from underrepresented minorities) must be expanded. At present, 7.4% of PA program faculty members are from underrepresented racial and ethnic minorities, 4.4% higher than the rate for medical school faculty. In the majority of PA educational programs, the need for faculty role

models and mentors from underrepresented racial and ethnic groups will continue (Vital Signs 1993; Anderson 1993).

PA PROGRAM CURRICULUM

Each PA program seeks to develop within each student a strong foundation in the basic and clinical sciences of medicine appropriate for the delivery of quality health care services. The education process may reflect a traditional medical school curriculum and even share classes with medical students, or it might introduce multidimensional assessment and decision analysis techniques that are unique to a particular PA program. Certain skills taught seem to be common to all programs (Gray 1995).

The basic science curriculum is usually structured to provide an in-depth understanding of structural features characterizing body tissues and organ systems, biochemical mecha-

---

Table 4-12 *Representative PA program curriculum*

Didactic Phase
Anatomy
Biochemistry
Pathophysiology
Health care and professional roles
Patient evaluation
Medical problem solving
Pharmacology
Laboratory sciences
Principles of health and disease prevention

Clinical Phase
Ambulatory care/primary care
General medicine
Pediatrics
Psychiatry and mental health
Surgery
Emergency medicine
Obstetrics and gynecology
Radiology and imaging sciences
Subspecialties and consulting services
Other

nisms regulating body metabolism, and nutrition. Next come the physiologic controls governing body system functions, pathophysiology, and behavioral alterations causing clinical manifestations of illnesses and the management of these illnesses and injuries.

Although there is a great deal of diversity among PA programs, there are a number of similarities. Table 4-12 lists a typical PA program curriculum based on a composite of various familiar programs.

Electives are a modest part of the educational experience and depend on the program. These electives can be in any number of areas including radiology, cardiology, plastic surgery, industrial medicine, geriatrics, and home health (Miller 1994).

THE PA PRECEPTORSHIP

The preceptorship phase of training for PA students is the final step in the professional socialization process. This process usually comes at the end of the training but varies considerably among programs; some programs eliminate it altogether. Because patient management is the essence of medical practice, the future PA must learn the proper attitudes and techniques for handling this career aspect with professionalism and diplomacy. With the science of medicine learned primarily from lectures, books, and laboratory work, the art of relating to patients is acquired through imitative role modeling, intuition, and trial and error. Views about patients will change the most during this time as students gain clinical experience.

Playing the physician role when one is not even a graduate PA can be difficult. Patients are interested in being treated appropriately by seasoned professionals, not in having novices "practice medicine," and both patients and students realize this. Even healthy people may have misgivings about receiving physical examinations from young and inexperienced clinicians. Students may try to counter this by wearing white coats and conspicuously display-

ing a stethoscope or other medical paraphernalia, but patients can usually identify a student. Even if the techniques are faultless, patients usually spot new faces and recognize new names, and staff often inform patients. The most effective method for students to adjust to a rotation or preceptorship is to introduce themselves and explain who they are.

One of the pitfalls of the preceptorship is the conscious and/or subconscious orientation toward certain patients—namely, those most easily dealt with from both a medical and interpersonal standpoint. Although variations are influenced by background and personality, most apprentice clinicians are more comfortable dealing with adults than with children, with patients from middle-class rather than lower-class backgrounds, with the organically ill rather than the emotionally ill, and with the acutely ill rather than the chronically or terminally ill. During the course of medical training, few lasting changes occur in these preferences except that, in some cases, they become stronger. One of the principal roles of the preceptor is to ensure the exposure of the student to all who access clinical practice.

The preceptorship is an expectation shared by the physician mentor and the PA student. The physician provides a lasting role model in the memory of the student. The cardinal experiences of medicine—exploring, examining, and cutting into the human body; dealing with the fears, anger, sense of helplessness, and despair of patients; meeting urgent situations; accepting the limitations of medical science; being confronted with death—will be experiences the physician will guide the PA through to professional self-actualization. How this process is conducted is determined by the precepting physician. This process must take place; there is no substitute.

PA POSTGRADUATE PROGRAMS

Formal educational programs have emerged that offer advanced supervised clinical experiences for

PAs who seek to obtain further training in the specialty disciplines. Physician Assistant Postgraduate Residency programs, most of which are sponsored by and located in teaching hospitals, are typically intensive experiences that provide PA graduates advanced clinical training. In 1996, there were 15 such programs, usually 1-year, paid clinical experiences enrolling highly selected PA graduates (Almanac 1992). The first PA Residency program was developed in surgery at Montefiore Hospital in New York in 1971, just 6 years after the first PA program was initiated (Rosen 1986). Clinical disciplines represented among PA residency programs include surgery, neonatology, pediatrics, emergency medicine, obstetrics/gynecology, and occupational medicine. Most of these programs are clinically based, but a few include a lengthy phase of didactic instruction; most programs award a certificate upon completion. All programs are members of the Association of Postgraduate Physician Assistant Programs (APPAP). The occupational medicine program at the University of Oklahoma awards the Master of Public Health (MPH) degree. Guidelines for uniformity in postgraduate surgical residency programs have been proposed (Timmer 1991).

PAs who have entered clinical practice roles in specialty and subspecialty areas (nearly half of the profession) usually acquire their preparation through on-the-job experiences, learning from employing physicians within their practice or institution. Only a small percentage (6.2%) of PAs have completed PA residency training programs (Table 4-13). The demonstrated capability of PAs to adapt readily to and function effectively in a wide variety of clinical practice specialities is probably attributable to their broad, generalist-oriented educational preparation.

Table 4-13 *PA postgraduate residency programs, 1996*

PROGRAM	LOCATION
Surgery	
Postgraduate Residency in Surgery [a]	Montefiore Medical Center, NY
PA Surgical Residency Porgam	Norwalk Hospital/Yale University, CT
PA Residency Program	St. Vincent's Medical Center, NY
Surgical PA Residency Program	Geisinger Medical Center, PA
PA Cardiothoracic Surgery PA Program	Cedars-Sinai Medical Center, CA
PA Surgical Residency Program	Butterworth Hospital, Western Michigan University, MI
PA Postgraduate Program	King/Drew Medical Center, CA
Residency in Gynecology for PAs [a]	North Central Bronx Hospital, NY
Postgraduate PA Surgical Residency [a]	Sinai Hospital of Baltimore, MD
Pediatrics/Neonatology	
Pediatric PA Postgraduate Program	Norwalk Hospital/Yale University, CT
PA Pediatric Residency Program	USC Medical Center, CA
Emergency Medicine	
Master's Degree Program in Emergency Medicine	Alderson Broaddus College, WV
Occupational Medicine	
Graduate Program in Occupational Health (MPH)	University of Oklahoma, OK
Primary Care	
Master's Degree Program in Primary Care	Alderson Broaddus College, WV

[a] Master's option available.
(Data from AAPA 1996a.)

Since the early 1990s, newer models of PA postgraduate educational programs have emerged. These programs differ from the typical PA residency programs in that they offer an academic-oriented experience. Instead of sharpening clinical inpatient-oriented, often procedural capabilities, the programs focus on skill development for graduate PAs, which spans both clinical and nonclinical areas. Included in curricula are courses in advanced work in clinical areas/clinical training, research methodology, interpretation of the biomedical literature, computer medicine, clinical prevention, health systems management, health policy, clinical decision sciences, and medical ethics. A full-length research paper is usually required. Tracks for clinical, research, PA education, or health administration can be developed. The curriculum emphasizes preparation in those areas that students believe are important in expanding their professional potentials and advancement in the health system. The prototype of this model of PA postgraduate education is the Master of Medical Science (MMS) PA Program sponsored by St. Francis College in Loretto, Pennsylvania. In operation since 1993, this program incorporates inputs from multiple clinical and nonclinical disciplines in its 33-credit curriculum (Table 4-14).

In 1995, Alderson-Broaddus College began to enroll students in two postgraduate Master's degree programs. Students work in clinical settings affiliated with the Alderson-Broaddus College PA Program throughout West Virginia. Two other Master's degree programs are also being developed: Quinnipiac College, Hamden, Connecticut; and The University of Nebraska, Omaha.

To be competitive in the present market, any new PA postgraduate educational program must consider multiple educational, financial, and social factors. Some of the questions include the following: What is the value of a Master's level of education to today's practicing PA? What is the mean cost, the "going rate," for advanced-level health professions education offered by a major academic health center? Finally, a PA postgraduate Master's degree must be weighed against what a more traditional

Table 4-14 *PA postgraduate program curriculum topics*

Research methods/Biostatistics/Epidemiology
Advanced pharmacology
Family medicine/Primary care/Clinical issues
Emergency medicine/Clinical training experiences
Health care systems management
Clinical ethics/Clinical decision making
PA professional issues/PA studies/Health services research
Health care policy/Health policy analysis
Interpretation of biomedical research information
Computer applications in medicine
Medical/Scientific writing/Biomedical communication

degree such as an MPH, MS, or MBA may mean to an employer.

SUPPLY AND DEMAND

From 1989 to 1994, the applications to PA programs increased 300%, and the average PA class size increased 42% (Oliver 1993b). Applicant interest has been steadily increasing because of awareness of the role of the PA in health care delivery systems. Despite the increase in size of accredited programs and new programs coming on line, the PA applicant pool continues to rise. The typical applicant applies to three programs with a range of one to ten program applications per individual and up to ten applicants for every position. The 1996 experience of the George Washington University Physician Assistant Program is typical: 551 applicants, 47 accepted; a mean grade point average of 3.4; and a mean of 2.7 years of experience in some medical role.

This increase in applications has demanded an efficiency in processing the new work. Sophisticated data entry and data analysis techniques have helped some programs seek traits valued in certain programs such as rural home base, graduate degrees, and commitment to primary care. Most programs require 2 years of transferrable college credits, biology, chemistry, and psychology coursework, along with a mini-

Table 4-15 *Representative PA program requirements for admission*

I. Academic achievement
   A. Minimum grade point average 3.0
   B. Minimum of 2 years of transferrable college credits
   C. Select course work (usually two courses of each)
      1. Biology
      2. Chemistry
      3. Psychology
      4. English composition
II. Clinical experience
   A. Patient contact experience in a health field
   B. Two or more years (variable among programs)
III. Letters of recommendation (usually three)
   A. At least one from a PA
   B. Preferably from a physician or someone who works with PAs
IV. Communication
   A. One-page narrative on why you want to be a PA
   B. Demonstrated ability to write and communicate easily and freely
V. Interview
   A. Usually at the site of the PA program
   B. A chance to strengthen the written application
   C. The opportunity for the faculty to observe deportment and communication skills
      Programs will often invite 1.5–3 times more applicants than positions

mum 3.0 grade point average. How clinical experience counts varies widely by program, but many believe it is helpful to have a minimum of 2 years of patient contact experience. Weakness in one area can sometimes be overcome by strengths in another area (Table 4-15).

As the application pool increases and PA programs strive to efficiently select the best applicants, the use of computers and centralized application processing, such as is used by the Association of American Medical Colleges, will become more important. Whether this practice reduces the diversity of students remains to be seen.

The five components listed in Table 4-15 are often weighted and scored by PA programs. How this is done and what value is placed on certain attributes such as geographic location or minority status varies considerably by program, mission, home institution, and changes annually.

The personal interview may be the most important aspect of the admissions evaluation process. This nonacademic assessment allows for spontaneous questions and answers and is believed to measure maturity, motivation, communication skills, creativity, and problem-solving abilities. One applicant may be interviewed for 30 minutes by at least three faculty members individually, or five applicants may be interviewed as a group by three or more faculty members in one room. While this screening process is conducted by almost all programs, the style of interview varies considerably. While programs may have strong opinions about their application process, the reliance and validity of these procedures are untested (Stumpf 1989).

RANKING PA PROGRAMS

One of the questions most frequently asked by applicants, vocation counselors, educational institutions, parents, employers, and the public is which PA programs are the best. There is no formalized or standardized method to rank PA programs in terms of quality of program, pass rate for national certification, or NCCPA scores. Applicants often ask this question when location of the program is not a factor and they want to select a high-quality program. There has been resistance within APAP to use a quantifiable ranking score for a number of reasons. Some programs clearly select only the best qualified applicants based on academic grade point averages, with the expectation that academic success predicts further success. Other programs point out their success in recruiting minorities and placing graduates in federally designated health professional shortage areas.

Programs committed to recruiting minority and rural-committed applicants argue that they may not be able to compete successfully with high academic achievers, and a ranking system would put them near the bottom of a list and influence the overall quality of applicants. Those schools affiliated with academic success argue that PA programs have evolved enough that academic scrutiny will allow competition, and the quality of all programs will benefit by comparative studies.

Other arguments center around elitism, different mission statements, and trying to emulate medical and osteopathic schools that use such ranking systems. One side of the debate that seems to have merit is that both the applicants and the public have a right to know how the PA programs are doing and where they stand in

Table 4-16 *Former PA programs*

PROGRAM	LOCATION	DATES
Alabama Medex	*	1973–1976
Alabama University PA Program	*	1970–1976
Allegheny Community College	Pittsburgh, PA	1978–1985
Catawba Valley	NC	1978–1980
Cerritos Orthopedic PA	Norwalk, CA	*
Chattanooga Orthopedic PA	Chattanooga, TN	*
Cincinnati Technical College	Cincinnati, OH	1974–1977
Cincinnati University Urology PA	Cincinnati, OH	*
Colorado University OB/Gyn	CO	1972–1977
Dartmouth College Medex	Dartmouth,	1971–1975
Highline Orthopedic PA	*	*
Hopkins, Johns, University	Baltimore, MD	1973–1979
Indian Health Service	Gallup, NM	1972–1983
Indiana University	*	1972–1977
Kentucky University Radiology PA Program	KY	*
Kirkwood Orthopedic PA	Cedar Rapids, IA	*
Lake Erie PA Program	Erie, OH	1975–1987
Loma Linda College	Loma Linda, CA	1978–1981
Maricopa College	Maricopa, CA	1974–1982
Marshfield Clinic	Marshfield, WI	1972–1981
Marygrove Ortho	Detroit, MI	*
Medical College of South Carolina	Charleston, SC	1972–1983
Minnesota Urology PA Program	MN	*
Mississippi, the University of	MS	1972–1974
Navy, US at Sheppard AFB	San Antonio, TX	*
Navy, US PA Program	Portsmouth, NH	1975–1987
Navy, US PA Program	San Diego, CA	1979–1983
Navy, US PA Program	San Diego, CA	1990–1996
Normandale Orthopedic PA Program	*	*
North Carolina University SA Prog	NC	1970–1981
North Dakota, University of, Medex	Bismark, ND	1970–1985
Oregon, University of	Portland, OR	1973–1976
Pennsylvania State University, Medex	Hershey, PA	1973–1986
Stephens College	Jefferson City, MO	1975–1978

* Data unknown at time of publication.

(Data from Kevin Marvelle, Research Division, American Academy of Physician Assistants 1996.)

relation to each other. Whichever system is finally adopted, it must be above reproach and operate with the public's best interest in mind.

FORMER PA PROGRAMS

One of the holes in the history of the physician assistant profession is the number of PA programs that have started then ceased. More than 30 programs that are no longer in existence have produced PA graduates. Some of these programs were accredited, while others were developed and functioned under another alliance. Some of the programs began as specialty programs (Orthopedic PA programs) and then disbanded. Others were viable programs (The Johns Hopkins University) and were discontinued for political reasons.

Table 4-16 is a partial listing of those PA programs that at one time had some association with the AAPA. Not all programs produced a primary care PA and some never produced a PA that was recognized by any accrediting agency. Interest remains to complete this part of the history and if information is known that will fill in the blanks in this table, please contact one of the authors.

THE FUTURE OF PA EDUCATION

There is a mounting consensus that the nation is training, and will soon have, too many health care professionals, especially physicians, nurses, and pharmacists. Could PAs soon be joining these crowded ranks? Although the profession still is enjoying a period of strong medical market demand, warning signs on the health workforce horizon indicate that PAs, and perhaps other health providers, could encounter an oversupply relative to future health systems requirements. The US Council on Graduate Medical Education (CoGME), the Physician Payment Review Commission (PPRC), the Institute of Medicine (IOM), and the Pew Health Professions Commission have all predicted that the nation will soon have too many physicians overall, and in particular too many specialist physicians. Currently, more than

675,000 physicians are in the United States, at about 200 physicians per 100,000 population, or 1 for every 500 persons. Medical workforce experts generally agree that, in a health system dominated by managed care delivery systems, the ideal ratio is anywhere between 145 and 185 patient care physicians per 100,000 people. By the year 2010, the Bureau of Health Professions estimates the number of patient care physicians will increase to 219 per 100,000 (Rivo 1996). Thus, by all reasonable estimates, the nation is likely to have too many physicians in practice in the coming years. At the same time, there continues to be a marked expansion of PA education. The number of PA programs and student enrollment have risen sharply, with 78 educational programs holding accreditation from the ARC-PA, an increase of 14 programs since 1995. A total of 5,558 students were enrolled in PA programs in 1995, a 20% increase from the 4,400 enrolled in 1993 (A. Simon 1996). The ARC-PA estimates that as many as 40 additional programs are in various stages of development and at least half will seek to gain accreditation. Similar trends are affecting other nonphysician health care professions. As with PAs, there has been a substantial expansion of NP education in recent years. In 1995, the American Association of Colleges of Nursing reported that more than 11,000 NP students were enrolled in 462 educational programs sponsored by 190 institutions (Bednash 1996).

HEALTH WORKFORCE MARKET REQUIREMENTS

It is fairly easy to determine the supply side of the picture of the future health care workforce. We know with reasonable accuracy how many graduates will be entering the health workforce market in the future; however, it is impossible to determine the workforce demand. Given the tumultuous changes underway in the modern health care system, it is difficult to predict with any certainty what the future requirements will be for specific types of health providers. For PAs, whose scope of work overlaps considerably with physicians, it is particularly difficult to estimate future requirements with any accuracy. While questioned as an inaccurate and probably inflated indicator of real market demand for PA graduates, data based on self-reported estimates by PA program directors of the number of positions available to new PA graduates have been used extensively by the profession and educational institutions to suggest a continuing large-scale market demand for PAs. Even using this overly optimistic measure, marketplace demand for PA graduates appears to be slowing; estimates by directors fell from a mean of 6.8 jobs/PA graduate in 1993 to 5.2 in 1995 (A. Simon 1996). The PA profession seems to be operating under the assumption that the present level of marketplace demand for PAs will continue unabated in the future health system. Many PA programs awaiting ARC-PA accreditation have qualified in part on the basis of a continuing strong market demand for PA graduates. A key question is the degree to which the oversupply of physicians, and the rise in the supply of PAs, will match or overmatch future medical market requirements. Employment of PAs necessitates physician cooperation. The prospect of the underutilization of specialist physicians, coupled with an overproduction of nonphysicians, could lead organized medicine to reassert physician roles in health care delivery based on the argument that because there is a sufficient number of physicians in the system, there is less need for nonphysician providers. Leading workforce policy experts and national advisory bodies predict that underemployment of physician specialists in the next 5 to 7 years is possible and that the "increasing participation of nonphysician professionals in work previously performed only by physicians will make the projected surplus even greater" (Rivo 1996).

Colliding forces in the future health system should suggest that the PA profession proceed cautiously with regard to unlimited continuing expansion of annual graduate output. Some occupations exhibit cyclical fluctuations in supply of personnel relative to market demand (e.g., law, accounting, nursing) and such fluctuations may be inevitable in an ever-changing workforce market in a free society. Yet other occupations have managed to minimize the degree of flux in the supply-demand relationship (e.g., engineering, dentistry, and until recently, medicine). It is well known that the dental profession, recognizing a changing market for services, over the last decade has downsized voluntarily the number of annual dental graduates; dental schools in major universities (for example, Georgetown University) have closed. One PA, now a practicing attorney, warns that the overproliferation of PA educational programs and graduates could follow the pattern observed over the last decade in the legal profession in which the booming number of annual law school graduates has led to lower salaries and tighter entering job market for lawyers (Thompson 1996).

Many ask why the profession cannot do something about this issue. Can the PA profession attempt to effectively manage its success and plan growth so as to avoid glutting the market with PA graduates? Which organization within the profession has the capacity to assume responsibility and leadership: the AAPA, APAP, ARC-PA, or none of these? Unfortunately, none of these organizations has seriously addressed this issue. To some degree, this reluctance is understandable given their differing roles and purposes. The prospect of an oversupply of PAs places the AAPA in a difficult position. As the "guild" of the PA profession, it would be difficult for AAPA to speak out on the issue of a PA glut, as it has a vested interest in expanding the number of practicing PAs and avoiding limiting its membership base. On the other hand, an excess of PAs would undoubtely dilute mean salary levels and reduce employment opportunies, factors that will not be popular among members. AAPA provides staff services and liaison representation to ARC-PA. APAP is not in an ideal position to take action on this issue. It is a loose confederation of PA educational programs and their faculties and does not have direct authority in accrediting decisions. APAP cannot impose binding decisions on member programs or institutions. Like AAPA, APAP sends representatives to ARC-PA.

ARC-PA, as the designated accrediting body of the profession, sets, maintains, and adjusts the PA educational program performance standards required for accreditation. ARC-PA makes recommendations to CAAHEP, which receives its health professions accrediting legitimacy through the US Department of Education. Such legitimacy would be threatened if a CAAHEP-member accrediting agency (such as ARC-PA) were to engage in practices counstrued to be as limiting the right of educational institutions to compete for entry into the PA education market. The PA profession and the ARC-PA apparently believe that the present standards for PA educational programs do not need to be raised or tightened. The old *Essentials,* now the new *Standards,* allows for great diversity in eligibility for sponsoring institutions and program configuration, a policy developed in part as a conscious decision by the founders of the PA profession, and continued perhaps by fear of the loss of this CAAHEP legitimacy. Until recently, CAAHEP was a subdivision of the AMA. ARC-PA has just completed its fourth revision of the *Standards.* While it seemed a perfect opportunity for the profession to tighten accreditation standards, a step that could have moderated new PA program proliferation, only minimal changes were approved. Language on specific eligibility for sponsoring institutions was not changed. ARC-PA states it is in the business of setting a "mark" for PA program accreditation and must award accreditation to any program that meets that mark. The implicit assumption contained in the *Standards* is that a PA educational program can be sponsored by a variety of educational institutions, even community and technical colleges.

Some argue that it is anachronistic to believe that the settings, sponsorship, and institutional resources of educational institutions sponsoring PA programs are all equal in their capability to prepare competent PAs. The clinical performance expectations and roles of PAs in the health workforce are now deemed by most to meet or exceed those of NPs whose education typically is based at the graduate level and now uniformly awards the MSN degree. It can also be argued that the "standard" of the *Standards* must change to keep pace with the PA professional evolution and advancement in medical practice. The current expectations of student performance standards for PAs enrolled in accredited educational institutions, as well as the modern professional clinical performance expectation levels on employing physicians, is at a minimum at or beyond the bachelor's level. In a free and largely capitalist society, educational institutions cannot be barred from seeking to fill what appears to be a market demand for personnel. Accreditation bodies must be as free as possible from outside or inside bias and must faithfully apply and enforce professional standards. As a profession evolves and matures, however, it is also important for such bodies to adjust educational program standards that reflect professional change.

PROJECTING PA SUPPLY

Among the most critical professional issues facing PA education and the profession is managing the newfound public acceptance and success, which has increased marketplace demand. The expanding demand and utilization of PAs in the modern health care workforce has led to a sharp rise in the entry level and mean salary levels and has spawned a boom in the interest of educational institutions to explore sponsorship of new PA educational programs.

The Pew Health Professions Commission Report indicates that there is an increased opportunity in America's future system for nonphysician health professionals such as PAs to assume roles as primary care medical generalists (Pew 1995). PAs are currently in enviable positions in the US health professions marketplace. Market demand now exceeds existing supply. Yet these professions should be cautious with regard to a too rapid expansion of educational programs and the numbers of annual NP and PA graduates, particularly in view of predictions of a physician excess.

PA educational programs have seen a marked increase in applicants, and many programs have taken steps to expand existing enrollment. In some cases, increasing the number of students has stretched existing educational resources to maximal levels. With marketplace demand appearing to be strong, and with calls to significantly expand their utilization in service delivery, PA educational programs face the challenge of responding to the suggestion to increase PA supply, while at the same time maintaining existing standards of educational quality. While an increasing number of academic institutions are now interested in expanding their existing enrollments or in sponsoring new PA educational programs, these efforts could be constrained by the shortage of adequately qualified PAs to serve as educational program faculty.

Areas deemed critical to the capabilities of PA educational programs to successfully accommodate anticipated expansion in student enrollment include the following:

1. The recruitment, retention, and professional development of qualified faculty

2. Efforts to bolster existing programs and to establish new program linkages with clinical teaching institutions and ambulatory-based clinical practice settings

3. Effective strategies to recruit and provide financial support targeted to retain qualified students from underrepresented racial/ethnic groups

Future efforts of PA programs to expand enrollments will require increased levels of federal support to prepare the increased number of PAs required to meet anticipated marketplace demand. Projections of future PA supply through the year 2000, based on estimates of annual PA program graduate output capacities, and certain assumptions under health care reform scenarios, are presented in Table 4-17.

Table 4-17 PA Graduates

YEAR	NEW GRADUATES	CUMULATIVE GRADUATES	PA PROGRAMS
1967	3	3	1
1968	a	a	2
1969	a	a	a
1970	195	237	a
1971	75	312	a
1972	278	590	a
1973	667	1,257	a
1974	1,090	2,347	a
1975	1,357	3,704	a
1976	1,573	5,277	a
1977	1,587	6,864	a
1978	1,345	8,209	a
1979	1,334	9,543	a
1980	1,489	11,032	a
1981	1,519	12,551	a
1982	1,376	13,927	a
1983	1,362	15,289	a
1984	1,236	16,525	a
1985	1,178	17,703	53
1986	1,187	18,890	51
1987	1,081	19,971	49
1988	1,081	21,052	50
1989	1,162	22,214	51
1990	1,195	23,409	51
1991	1,383	24,792	55
1992	1,595	26,387	54
1993	1,737	28,124	56
1994	1,952	30,076	63
1995	2,139	32,215	63
1996	2,500[b]	34,715[b]	68
1997	2,600[b]	37,315[b]	84
1998	2,700[b]	40,015[b]	94[b]
1999	2,850[b]	42,865[b]	98[b]
2000	3,000[b]	45,865[b]	100[b]

[a] The number of PA programs in existence between 1969–1985 is not precisely known.

[b] Estimate based on expanding PA program trend.

(Data from American Academy of Physician Assistants, Research Division, 1996.)

Table 4-18 *First-year enrollments in selected health professions schools, selected academic years 1970–1971 through 1991–1992*

HEALTH OCCUPATION	NUMBER OF STUDENTS				
	1970–1971	1975–1976	1980–1981	1985–1986	1991–1992
Medicine					
Allopathic (MD)	11,348	15,295	17,186	16,963	17,071
Osteopathic (DO)	623	1,038	1,496	1,737	1,974
Podiatric medicine (DPM)	351	641	695	811	725
Dentistry (DDS/DMD)	4,565	5,763	6,030	4,843	4,047
Optometry (OD)	884	1,057	1,258	1,251	1,355
Pharmacy (RPh)	5,694	8,710	7,551	7,084	8,343
Veterinary medicine (DVM)	1,430	1,712	2,239	2,282	2,225
Nursing (RN)	78,524	112,174	110,201	100,791	113,526
Physician assistant (PA)					1,700
Nurse practitioner (NP)					2,500

(Data from American Association of Medical colleges, AAMC Data Book, Statistical Information Related to Medical Education, January, 1992; American Association of Colleges of Osteopathic Medicine, 1992 Annual Statistical Report; American Association of Colleges of Podiatric Medicine, unpublished data; American Dental Association, Council on Dental Education, Annual Report on Dental Education, 1991–1993, also prior annual reports; American Schools and Colleges of Optometry, unpublished data; American Association of Colleges of Pharmacy, profile of Pharmacy Students, 1992, also unpublished data; Association of American Veterinary Medical Colleges, unpublished data; National League for Nursing. Nursing Datasource, 1992: Vol 1; Oliver 1993a; Morgan 1993; Oliver, D. Ninth Annual Report on PA Educational Programs, 1992-1993; APAP, 1993; numbers represent means of figures provided by the 51 PA educational programs reporting.)

PA EDUCATIONAL COSTS

In comparison to allopathic and osteopathic medical student educational costs, the overall expense of PA training is relatively low. The average total cost for educating an allopathic medical student in 1992 is more than $92,000; the average total cost for educating an osteopathic medical student is estimated at $45,600 (Estes 1993) (Table 4-18). Findings in the Twelfth Annual Association of Physician Assistant Program Report by Simon estimates the total costs of education for PA students averages $21,308 per student per program per year, with a range of $2,230 to $50,664 (A. Simon 1996). This figure includes the costs to the student for tuition, fees, books, and equipment, but not living expenses. Costs to enrolled students vary by sponsorship (academic health center-sponsored versus nonacademic health center-sponsored programs) and by state-mandated assistance. Among the 68 PA educational programs who responded to the most recent survey conducted by the APAP during 1995, costs averaged $21,308 for in-state resident PA students, and $26,132 for non-state resident students (A. Simon 1996). In 1996, the total tuition for a PA education ranged from $3,800 in the University of Texas systems to $38,000 at the George Washington University in Washington, DC. The expense for a 2-year degree from the University of

Washington Medex Program in Seattle is estimated to be $28,000. This figure includes moving expenses, transportation, housing, meals, and miscellaneous expenses (R. Ballweg, personal communication, 1996).

ASSOCIATION OF PHYSICIAN ASSISTANT PROGRAMS

The Association of Physician Assistant Programs (APAP) is the national organization representing PA educational programs and was formed in 1972 to facilitate communication and cooperation among PA programs at universities and colleges throughout the United States. APAP's responsibilities from the beginning included activities in training, program accreditation, certification, curriculum development and evaluation, and continuing medical education for the individual health care practitioner.

APAP's mission is to assist PA educational programs in the instruction of highly educated PAs in adequate numbers to meet society's needs. The organization also offers an array of services to PA programs, faculty, students, and the public aimed at fulfilling this mission.

APAP services include two national meetings of PA programs each year, publications, newsletters, consultation services, faculty development, leadership education programs, the systematic collection of pertinent PA program data, and the development of tools to assess and improve the quality of PA education for individuals as well as programs.

History

In July 1976, APAP received a grant of $225,000 from the Robert Wood Johnson (RWJ) Foundation for the period July 1976 through June 1979. The grant provided continued core support for the national office (APAP and AAPA) and established a research division within APAP.

Initially, the RWJ grant funds were used to pay partial salaries for 14 shared staff members and full-time salaries for two researchers. Gen-

eral office expenses were also provided. The first national survey of PAs was conducted as part of the grant. Areas surveyed included demography, distribution, utilization, role/function, curriculum, quality of care, cost of training, economic aspects of utilization, and student selection criteria. The following year, AAPA, under contract from the Health Resources Administration, conducted a national practice profile survey of PA graduates. The data collected described in significant detail those tasks performed by PAs in a variety of health care settings. This information, coupled with data from the first national survey of PAs (APAP), supported previous conjectures about PA education and deployment (i.e., PAs were making a positive contribution to health care delivery in this country).

The RWJ Foundation approved a second grant in 1978, this time to APAP's request for 3 years of additional funding for core support and a second national survey of PA graduates and students. The grant award for $225,000 was for the period July 1979 through July 1982.

The June 1979 Annual Report to the Robert Wood Johnson Foundation stated that

> In November 1973 APAP/AAPA national office had one employee … the total shared staff in 1974 was four. By 1975 staff numbers had doubled and by the following year they had doubled again. In April 1979 two executive staff members resigned. Such changes in the executive staff and the expressed desire by APAP leadership to centralize its functions into fewer persons working one hundred percent of effort for the Association will necessitate the formulation of a new organizational structure for the office during the coming year.

In 1979, the Association separated itself (financially) from the AAPA after the conclusion of research activities on the 1978 national survey. The Association then developed a financial arrangement with the AAPA to cover shared general office expenses and some partial salary support of staff members who continued to have dual responsibilities (i.e., executive director, comptroller, bookkeeper, receptionist) with both organizations. In addition, the AAPA agreed to provide the Association with 15% of the revenue realized from each year's annual conference.

The Association employed a full-time Director of Research and Administration, a full-time Administrative Assistant (salary supported by an 18-month faculty development contract from DHHS), and a full-time secretary. In 1981, the APAP conducted a third national survey of PA graduates and students under the terms of its grant from the RWJ Foundation. APAP currently possesses data from three national surveys of the PA profession. APAP membership addressed the issue of its fiscal solvency. Determined to maintain its independence as an organization, APAP negotiated with the AAPA to absorb the total cost of operating the national office in exchange for which the Association would no longer receive a percentage of profits from the annual conference.

In 1983, the AAPA and APAP developed a shared staffing agreement by which AAPA would pay APAP $15,000 annually in exchange for approximately 20% of APAP staff time to be devoted to a variety of tasks as determined by the Executive Director. According to the revised shared staffing agreement, APAP staff agreed to assume administrative responsibility for the AAPA Education and Research Foundation and the Student Academy of the AAPA, with the arrangement to be reviewed annually.

In 1986, APAP began work on the "PA of the Year 2000" project, which was completed in May 1988. The final report and recommendations resulting from this activity were presented at the 1988 annual meeting. That same year a new category, APAP Associates, was developed and approved to encourage greater involvement of program faculty of all types, including basic science, clinical, and adjunct in APAP. This is a non-voting category. The shared staffing agreement was discontinued; AAPA and APAP entered into a contractual arrangement for AAPA to provide APAP with specified services at

Table 4-19 *APAP Presidents*

1997–1998	Donald Petersen, PA, PhD
1996–1997	Dennis Blessing, PA, PhD
1995–1996	James Hammond, MA, PA
1994–1995	Ronald D. Garcia, PhD
1993–1994	Richard R. Rahr, EdD, PA
1992–1993	Anthony A. Miller, MEd, PA
1991–1992	Albert Simon, MEd, PA
1990–1991	Ruth Ballweg, PA
1989–1990	Steven Shelton, MBA, PA
1988–1989	Suzanne Greenberg, MS
1987–1988	Jesse Edwards, MS
1986–1987	Jack Liskin, MA, PA
1985–1986	Carl Fasser, PA
1984–1985	Denis Oliver, PhD
1983–1984	Robert Curry, MD, MPH
1982–1983	Stephen Gladhart, EdD
1981–1982	Reginald Carter, PhD, PA
1980–1981	David Lewis, EdD
1979–1980	Thomas Godkins, PA
1978–1979	Archie Golden, MD
1977–1978	Frances Horvath, MD
1976–1977	C. Hilmon Castle, MD
1975–1976	Robert Jewett, MD
1974–1975	Thomas Piemme, MD
1973–1974	Alfred Sadler, Jr., MD

(Data from Association of Physician Assistant Programs, 1996.)

a fixed annual fee. These services are provided by appropriate divisions in AAPA's national office and by a part-time Coordinator of APAP Services employed by the Academy.

Physician Assistants for the Future, an in-depth study of PA education and practice in the year 2000 by the Association of Physician Assistant Programs, was published in 1989. *A Guide for Institutions Interested in Creating New Physician Assistant Educational Programs* was published in collaboration with AAPA. *A National Directory of Physician Assistant Programs* is published each year.

For the first 6 years beginning in 1974, the leadership was dominated by physician educators. In 1979, consistent with changes in PA program management shifts to PAs, leadership roles were assumed by PAs (Table 4-19).

Role of APAP

The mission of APAP is "to assist PA educational programs in the instruction of highly educated PAs in adequate numbers to meet society's needs." Within this mission are five fundamental goals.

1. *Foster faculty development.* Improve the recruitment and retention of faculty. Development of workshops to promote the sharing of retention strategies.

2. *Promote excellence within PA programs.* Maximize the use of program resources, continue to promote technical help and services, and develop a test item bank and self-assessment examination. Advocate for student services and facilitate collaborative approaches to curriculum design through workshops and roundtables.

3. *Facilitate research and scholarly activities.* Seek outlets for scholarly activity and support for existing endeavors. Current activities include paper presentations at meetings and publication of faculty newsletters, and an annual report on PA programs. Facilitate ways to bring together people with similar research interests and pursue collaborative projects.

4. *Advocate for PA education.* Educate the public, policy makers, administrators, and others about PA education. Help members address issues, support the accreditation process, maintain and increase liaisons with other organizations, and develop funding resources for PA education.

5. *Maintain organization support.* Meet the needs of increasing membership. Seek diversified sources of income. Promote the association through publications of faculty and staff directory into an association resource manual.

In addition, APAP offers a Leadership Training Institute, conferences and workshops on educational methods, new faculty orientation, and focused retreats for program directors.

Developing a New PA Program

For institutions interested in developing a PA program, the ARC-PA has recommended a step-wise plan for achieving accreditation.

1. Establish internal support of sponsoring institution and formalize the relationship with the academic and clinical centers
    Conduct a feasibility study for justifying a new PA program

2. Contact the Executive Director of ARC-PA for application material

3. *Review the Essentials, Guidelines for the Preparation of the Self-study Report,* and *Information and Procedures*

4. Acquire the necessary resources for developing a PA program:
    Acquire adequate administrative personnel leadership
    Recruit PA program director
    Recruit medical director
    Obtain adequate funds for the planning year and the first year of operation
    Obtain adequate space for administrative offices
    Obtain adequate classroom space
    Obtain adequate laboratory space

5. Develop a PA program mission statement that integrates into the institution's mission
    Adopt goals for the PA program

6. Develop a didactic curriculum plan
    Adapt curriculum materials to institution's resources
    Develop a course syllabus, course objectives, and course description

7. Solicit support from the basic science department
    Recruit and locate basic science instructors
    Recruit members for the advisory/planning committee

8. Solicit support from the medical community to locate educators

> Recruit for core PA faculty
>
> Recruit for clinical preceptors (both physicians and PAs)
>
> Obtain support for clinical training sites for future PA students

9. Formalize all clinical affiliation agreements with supporting institutions

10. Draft of ARC-PA accreditation application to the dean

> Review and revision

11. Finalize Accreditation Application

12. Submission for institutional review and approval

> Obtain signature of highest administrative officer at institution
>
> Mail application and supporting documents and appropriate number of copies to ARC-PA at agreed upon deadline
>
> Mail fee for the first year of accreditation

13. Plan on-site visit, gain support of administration and clinical affiliate participants in the visit

14. Host on-site visit

15. Pay expenses for two site visitors

16. Notification of Award of Provisional Accreditation Status before matriculation of PA students

The timetable for this process depends on the institution's internal approval of the PA program. Historically, most academic institutions need at least 12 months of meetings and discussion before agreeing to begin a PA program. A feasibility study should be a guide and part of this discussion process. The accreditation body no longer grants a review until the program plans to be operational within the year. Most programs require at least 9 months of planning before the on-site visit by the ARC-PA.

The Program Assistance and Technical Help (PATH), a consultative service developed by AAPA with grant funds from the W.K. Kellog Foundation, provides help for developing PA programs. It is a confidential fee-for-service program designed to assist established and developing PA education programs. Some of the types of PATH consultations available include the following:

- *Initial informational consultation:* Provides basic information and perspectives on PA education to institutions considering the feasibility of developing a PA program.

- *General consultation for developing programs:* Designed to assist developing programs to meet PATH standards for excellence.

- *General consultation for existing programs:* Designed for programs seeking an objective, external evaluation to complement their self-study or for programs that have undergone substantial changes.

- *Focused consultation:* Designed to assist programs with a focal problem, such as admissions, minority recruitment/retention, research, resource procurement and utilization, curriculum, and more.

MEDICAL PROFESSIONAL OATHS

Like medical schools, most PA programs do not use the original Oath of Hippocrates. They have dropped it all together or rewritten it to apply to their own particular standards. One reason is that it is not enforceable and, therefore, is more ceremonial. Other documents and procedures provide official licensure, certification, and credentialing. Some PA programs have developed their own oaths and charges as to how they want to charge their graduates with health care responsibility. Below are two of the more common medical professional oaths that are administered to PAs, The Oath of Geneva, followed by the original Hippocratic Oath.

The Oath of Geneva

The Oath of Geneva is as follows:

At the time of being admitted as a member of the medical profession:

I solemnly pledge myself to consecrate my life to the service of humanity;

I will give to my teachers the respect and gratitude which is their due;

I will practice my profession with conscience and dignity;

The health of my patient will be my first consideration;

I will respect the secrets which are confided in me;

I will maintain by all means in my power, the honor and the noble traditions of the medical profession;

My colleagues will be my brothers and sisters;

I will not permit considerations of religion, nationality, race, party politics, or social standing to intervene between my duty and my patient;

I will maintain the utmost respect for human life, even under threat;

I will not use my medical knowledge contrary to the laws of humanity.

I make these promises solemnly, freely and upon my honor.

The Oath of Hippocrates

The Oath of Hippocrates is as follows:

I swear by Apollo, the physician, and Asclepius, and Health, and All-heal, and all the gods and goddesses, that according to my ability and judgement, I will keep this oath and stipulation; to reckon him who taught me this art equally dear to me as my parents, to share my substance with him and relieve his necessities if required; to regard his offspring as on the same footing with my own brothers, and to teach them this art if they should wish to learn it, without fee or stipulation, and that by precept, lecture and every other mode of instruction, I will impart a knowledge of the art to my own sons and to those of my teachers, and to disciples bound by a stipulation and oath, according to the law of medicine, but to none others.

I will follow that method of treatment which, according to my ability and judgement, I consider for the benefit of my patients, and abstain from whatever is deleterious and mischevious. I will give no deadly medicine to anyone if asked nor suggest any such counsel; furthermore, I will not give to a woman an instrument to produce abortion.

With purity and with holiness I will pass my life and practice my art. I will not cut a person who is suffering with a stone, but will leave this to be done by practitioners of this work. Into whatever houses I enter I will go into them for the benefit of the sick and will abstain from every voluntary act of mischief and corruption; and further from the seduction of females and males, bond or free.

Whatever, in connection with my professional practice, or not in connection with it, I may see or hear in the lives of men which ought not to be spoken abroad, I will not divulge, as reckoning that all such should be kept secret.

While I continue to keep this oath unviolated, may it be granted to me to enjoy life and the practice of the art, respected by all men at all times, but should I trespass and violate this oath, may the reverse be my lot.

5

Primary Care

A substantial amount of research identifies physician assistants (PAs) as well-qualified primary care providers. In the first few years this was not clear because the mission of PAs was not necessarily to be primary care providers, but to support the primary care physician. The fundamental role of the PA was initially developed to examine and gather information on the patient (Jacobs 1974). However, the role of the PA quickly transformed from extending or assisting the primary care physician to one of association with the physician employer. Although not planned, this outcome was an inevitable process of delegation and expansion of duties that occurs in almost any apprenticeship. Initially, the PA would see a patient, present the case to the physician, and together they would see the patient. Usually, the physician would decide on the treatment and delegate some treatment plan. Depending on the situation, it may be an antibiotic for an ear infection, or casting for a fracture. The PA would carry out the order of treatment based on level of experience and skill. The next step was seeing the patient and presenting the case without having the patient seen by both clinicians. After seeing numerous middle ear infections, sprained ankles, bicipital tendinitis, and upper respiratory infections, it was only a matter of time before the relationship between physician and PA allowed the delegation of treatment without the physician seeing or reviewing the case of each patient. This relationship is built on trust that the PA will model his or her care for patients after the physician's style.

Inevitably, patients would begin requesting the PA, or were triaged to the PA, and away

from the physician. As physician confidence was reinforced by the skill of the PA, the PA was delegated more work or, in some cases, assumed more roles. The third step was PA management of chronic diseases such as hypertension and diabetes. These began as refilling drugs, evolved to adjusting the medication, and finally to initiating therapy.

Today, in many instances, the PA may see so many common primary care disorders that he or she may have more experience with these conditions than the associated physicians in the same setting. In addition, a more experienced PA may be employed by a recently trained physician who is more familiar with hospital care than ambulatory care. In these instances, there are clearly trade-offs as to who can do what better than the other. As the profession matures, educational programs evolve as well, placing more and more emphasis on independent evaluation and management of common primary care disorders. In some instances the recently graduated PA seems better prepared for primary care than some physicians.

The placement of PAs seemed like a sound policy to many observers. In the 1970s, most were employed in some type of primary care practice (Lawrence 1975b) or ambulatory setting (Steinwachs 1976) and seemed to be fulfilling the ideals of their creators. Some of the early studies of PAs in communities in which they serve demonstrated improvement in the health status of patients beyond what was present before their arrival. Other benefits of PA employment appeared because studies suggested health costs were cheaper, and the financial viability of the clinic's office improved (Anderson 1977).

In 1978, the Institute of Medicine strongly recommended PAs and nurse practitioners (NPs) be given an important role in the delivery of primary care. The report was wide-sweeping and included a number of important issues such as PA prescriptive practices, third-party reimbursement, fee schedules, and pay differentials based on medical education (IOM 1978; Stalker 1978b). These findings were endorsed by the American College of Physicians and were reiterated in many reports over the next few years (DHEW 1979; Peterson 1980; Burnett 1980; Record 1981).

By the early 1980s, the differences in roles between PAs and physicians in primary care were blurring; both seemed to be providing similar services (Repicky 1982; Nelson 1982; OTA 1986; Hooker 1986). Based on these observations, a number of health workforce projections were made. These studies all advocated increased use of PAs and NPs in primary care, ranging from 20% for children to 50% in adult services (Steinwachs 1986; Cawley 1986c; Weiner 1986; Salmon 1986; Synowiez 1986; Johnson 1988). How much traditional primary care could a PA assume? Record examined a representative population of patients managed by physicians and PAs in primary care in a large HMO and, using a number of assumptions, determined that PAs could manage at least 83% of all primary care encounters (Record 1981a). Hooker's study found that, based on diagnoses rendered, there was a 90% overlap in types of patients managed by physicians and PAs in the departments of internal medicine and family practice (Hooker 1986; Hooker 1991c).

Additional evidence showed that PAs could assume a wide variety of care, which had been the traditional domain of primary care physicians. By the 1990s, there was compelling evidence that not only could PAs expand the delivery of primary care services going unfilled by physicians, but national policies should be promulgated to promote this trend (Meikle 1992a; Schroeder 1992; Clawson 1993). This was never more clear than during President Clinton's attempt to reform health care and improve primary care delivery in the mid-1990s. In this plan, the role of primary care PAs, NPs, and certified nurse midwives (CNMs) was expanded dramatically.

Primary care is the raison d'etre of the PA profession. It was the reason for its development and is still the main focus of PA education. Using self-declared specialty in a survey in 1996, 51% of PAs are in practice in the federally designated primary care specialties of Internal Medicine, General/Family Practice, and Pediatrics. Some argue that many primary care services are provided by PAs who are working in clearly defined specialty areas such as correctional medicine and public health. If the percentages of PAs in clinical practice working in emergency medicine (10%), women's health care (3%), and geriatrics (1%) are included, the majority of all PAs are engaged to some degree in primary care clinical activities. Given the demographics and practice characteristics, it is not surprising that the most common clinical disorders seen by PAs reflect the prevalence of those in the general population.

The most frequently reported principal diagnoses are featured in Table 5-1. This is part of a national study on ambulatory visits that has been on-going since 1984. The first 20 diagnoses are the most frequently rendered in ambulatory care and account for 37.4% of all office visits made during 1994 (Schappert 1996).

In 1994, an estimated 857,007,000 drugs were prescribed or recommended. The most frequently prescribed medications in ambulatory care are listed in Table 5-2.

PAs are commonly used in roles as primary care providers by a wide variety of health care organizations and in a variety of settings such as the following:

- Multispecialty group practices expanding primary care service delivery
- Managed care organizations expanding primary care capacities
- Private rural systems of care delivery and small community hospitals seeking to extend ambulatory care/primary care services

Table 5-1 *Number and percent distribution of office visits by principal diagnoses, 1994*

PRINCIPAL DIAGNOSES	NUMBER OF VISITS (THOUSANDS)	PERCENT DISTRIBUTION		
		AVERAGE	FEMALE	MALE
All visits	681,457	100.0	100.0	100.0
Essential hypertension	25,521	3.7	3.6	4.0
Normal pregnancy	22,965	3.4	5.6	
General medical examination	21,719	3.2	3.4	2.8
Health supervision of infant or child	17,503	2.6	2.0	3.4
Acute upper respiratory infection	17,100	2.6	2.0	2.7
Suppurative otitis media	15,968	2.3	1.9	3.0
Chronic sinusitis	12,819	1.9	1.9	1.8
Diabetes mellitus	12,027	1.8	1.7	1.9
Asthma	10,757	1.6	1.3	2.0
Bronchitis (acute and chronic)	10,417	1.5	1.5	1.6
Acute pharyngitis	10,016	1.5	1.5	1.5
Neurotic disorders	9,891	1.5	1.6	1.3
Affective psychoses	9,659	1.4	1.6	1.2
Other postsurgical states	9,300	1.4	1.3	1.4
Allergic rhinitis	9,289	1.4	1.3	1.5
Cataract	8,260	1.2	1.2	1.2
Specific investigations and examinations	8,000	1.2	1.6	0.5
Diseases of sebaceous glands	7,920	1.2	1.2	1.2
Glaucoma	7,657	1.1	1.1	1.2
Contact dermatitis and eczema	6,573	1.0	0.9	1.1
All other diagnoses	428,098	62.6	61.4	64.7

(Data from Schappert 1996-National Ambulatory Medical Care Survey.)

- Public health clinic settings, community and migrant health centers, rural health clinics
- Clinical settings where they may provide clinical preventive services, wellness, and preventive care (i.e., private clinics)
- Geriatric facilities, occupational/work site health settings
- Correctional health systems
- University/college student health facilities
- Residency programs

PA ROLE DELINEATION

PAs have always been aware of the need to communicate what goes on in clinical practice with the designers of educational programs and the certification examinations. A new profession needs a particularly strong self-evaluation to determine how it has evolved from the original concept.

Role delineation studies are one way in which information about a new profession is gathered and analyzed. In 1976, HEW funded a project entitled *The Development of Standards to Ensure the Competency of Physician Assistants* (AAPA 1979). It combined physician assistant task analysis surveys with the opinions of experts about what responsibilities should be considered part of the role of the PA and what is tangential to the role. The results of the study became the basis for the continuing medical education program of the AAPA, as well as its self-assessment examination.

The 1976 study found that the PA role contained three comprehensive areas of compe-

Table 5-2 *Generic substances most frequently prescribed or recommended at office visits in 1994*

GENERIC SUBSTANCE	NUMBER OF OCCURRENCES (THOUSANDS)	PERCENT OF ALL DRUG MENTIONS	THERAPEUTIC CLASSIFICATION
All generic substances	1,001,421	100.0	
Amoxicillin	34,952	4.1	Penicillins
Acetaminophen	27,877	3.3	Analgesics
Albuterol	14,660	1.7	Bronchodilators
Aspirin	13,786	1.6	Analgesics
Ibuprofen	13,260	1.5	Analgesics
Hydrochlorothiazide	12,676	1.5	Diuretics
Multivitamins	11,823	1.4	Vitamins, minerals
Furosemide	11,823	1.4	Diuretics
Erythromycin	11,347	1.3	Antibiotics
Guaifenesin	11,275	1.3	Antitussives
Estrogens	10,642	1.2	Estrogens, progestins
Digoxin	10,033	1.2	Cardiac gylcosides
Prednisone	9,794	1.1	Adrenal corticosteroids
Beclomethasone	9,536	1.1	Bronchodilators
Diltiazem	9,466	1.1	Antihypertensives
Phenylephrine	9,362	1.1	Antihistamines
Phenylpropanolamine	9,205	1.1	Decongestants
Triamcinolone	8,764	1.0	Topical corticosteroids
Codeine	8,465	1.0	Analgesics
Levothyroxine	8,317	1.0	Thyroid supplements

Frequency of mention combines single-ingredient agents with mentions of the agent as an ingredient in a combination drug. Based on an estimated 857,007,000 drug mentions in 1994.

(Data from Schappert 1996-National Ambulatory Medical Care Survey.)

The second role delineation study was conducted by the AAPA in 1985. This project identified distinct differences in practice characteristics among PAs in the various specialties. However, nine general clusters of activities were common to PA practice across specialty lines:

- Gathering data
- Seeing common problems and diseases
- Conducting laboratory and diagnostic studies
- Performing management activities
- Performing surgical procedures
- Managing emergency situations
- Conducting health promotion/disease prevention activities
- Prescribing medications
- Using interpersonal skills

Protocols were developed to standardize the performance of the PA and to ensure physicians and patients that medical treatment provided by the new health practitioner would be adequate. These protocols were written statements that begin with the patient's presenting complaint and follow, step by step, through the questions that should be asked, the tests that should be run, and the medications that should be prescribed. There cannot be a protocol for every situation, but hundreds were written by PA educators and physicians, and were used extensively in training and in practice.

In practice, it is usually not possible for the PA to follow each protocol exactly. A protocol serves as a "security blanket" until the provider's confidence is sufficient to enable him or her to use the skills and judgment gained through experience. As the employing physician comes to feel comfortable with the work of the PA, they are less concerned with the external supports that inform the assistant of correct procedures. They become more concerned with the development of the PA's judgment and critical thinking, particularly knowing when the patient needs to be referred to the physician.

Through role delineation studies and the development of protocols, the PA profession

tence: the *professional role* of the identify of the PA, including the necessary skills and competence to do the work; the *interpersonal role*, which included the ability to communicate effectively; and the *clinical role*, which encompassed the skills and medical knowledge applied to patient problems.

became codified and set into a structured framework of rules and regulations to convince those early innovators that taking an assistant into the physician's practice would be safe and convenient and would not threaten patient confidence.

PAs have displayed an impressive track record in primary care. This has been accomplished through role delineation studies, the education process, and physicians who were willing to apprentice assistants in their offices and places of practice. PAs have shown themselves to be safe and capable providers of primary care services. Ironically, despite the success of the PA, it remains a challenge for practices to attract enough of these providers to rural and other needy areas (OTA 1990). Barriers to their full practice effectiveness remain in place as well (Sekscenski 1994).

PAS AS PRIMARY CARE PROVIDERS: MAKING THE CASE

Should PAs be regarded as primary care providers in future health care delivery scenarios? Central to any discussion of health system policy is the question of workforce supply, distribution, and utilization. The looming oversupply of specialist physicians, the growth of managed care, and issues affecting various types of health care personnel take on greater importance in a changing, market-driven environment. All of this has spurred a critical reexamination of the roles, accountability, cost-effectiveness, and social responsibility of our nation's health professionals (Fryer 1991; Colwill 1992).

PAs are clinicians qualified by formal educational preparation and national credentialing to provide the majority of required medical care tasks in primary care practice when there is a supervised practice relationship with physicians. They were introduced to extend the practice of primary care physicians (Jones 1994a). Although PAs are generally assumed to be primary care clinicians, over the last 30 years, they have gained greater acceptance by physicians and patients and are now recognized as effective medical professionals who work in a wide

variety of physician practice settings (Clawson 1994; PF Larson 1994).

A number of interacting influences in the health workforce explain why the practices of PAs differ so much. One reason is that the demand for PA services is related to external factors such as state licensing and regulation policy, which affect both the scope of practice and prescribing authority. Primary care PAs working in states where legislation enables wider latitude with regard to physician supervisory requirements may be used more effectively (Sekscenski 1994). Another influence is the market forces that shape the demand for PAs to assume different roles than those originally trained for (Hooker 1992).

Before we explain why PAs should be considered part of the primary care workforce in America, we should first define what we mean by primary care. According to Starfield (1992), primary care has four key attributes: (1) first-contact care, (2) longitudinality, (3) coordination, and (4) comprehensiveness. These elements have been incorporated into definitions of primary care considered important by health workforce policy groups.

The Council on Graduate Medical Education (COGME) defines primary care as: "characterized by first-contact care for patients with undifferentiated health concerns; patient-centered comprehensive care that is not organ- or problem-specific; continuous, longitudinal patient care; and coordination of necessary medical, social, mental, and other services through appropriate consultation and referral" (COGME 1994). While there is contention about who should provide primary care, there is also debate regarding the range and content of the clinical activities and tasks specific to primary care practice. Some believe that primary care is more than just a set of specialty-defined clinical tasks; it involves an integrated system of health services delivery. This is based on the fact that such care comprises a majority of the health services required by various populations (Starfield 1992).

More recently, in the initial phase of an in-depth study of primary care in the United

States, the Institute of Medicine Committee on the Future of Primary Care proposed this definition (Donaldson 1995):

> Primary care is the provision of integrated, accessible health care services by clinicians who are accountable for addressing a large majority of personal health care needs, developing a sustained partnership with patients, and practicing in the context of family and community.

Effectiveness of primary care delivery depends, at least in part, on using the correct mix of health care personnel. Starfield believes that this maximizes the clinical capabilities of several types of health professionals. In primary care practice, it is neither necessary nor particularly efficient for each patient to be seen by a physician (Perry 1982). Since PAs are, by definition, physician-supervised clinicians, the very nature of their clinical role is to work with physicians in collaborative interdisciplinary settings.

A number of physician and nonphysician health care professional groups have laid claim to primary care (such as obstetricians and nurse practitioners, asserting that they should be included as primary care providers). Attempts to answer the question of which types of physicians should be defined as primary care providers has prompted systematic analyses of the competencies of various physician specialists to provide the range of medical and preventive care services required (Rivo 1996). The conclusion was that only the disciplines of General/Family Practice, Internal Medicine, and General Pediatrics fulfilled all of the criteria to be considered primary care disciplines.

Using these same criteria, the competency of PAs to provide primary care was assessed (Cawley 1996). We designed a matrix to identify educational preparation, clinical practice, and professional certification measures of competency in the provision of primary care. Four national data sources to be used as indicators of PA clinical practice performance and competency in primary care were identified: educational preparation, national certification examination content, profession-defined role

delineation, and actual data on utilization. The data overwhelmingly indicate that PAs are educated well enough to function as primary care providers and are successfully performing a large proportion of tasks typically required in primary care (Rivo 1997).

PEDIATRICS

Pediatrics is considered one of the three specialties that defines primary care, but attention to pediatrics in this arena is often overshadowed by adult primary care. The role of PAs in child care has a rich history, much of it derived from the Child Health Associate (CHA) program based at the University of Colorado. This program was developed by Henry K. Silver and Loretta Ford in the 1960s and is detailed in Chapter 3.

Throughout the 1970s, several studies examined the role of the CHA or pediatric PA. Many of these studies, performed under the direction of the late Dr. Henry Silver, documented the wide range of diagnostic, preventive, and therapeutic services to children. Working principally in ambulatory settings, CHAs and pediatric PAs have the knowledge and skill to care for more than 90% of patients seen in a pediatric practice (Silver 1973; Fine 1973; Fine 1977a; Fine 1977b). When compared to pediatric residents and medical students, CHA students demonstrate a similar relevant factual knowledge in the pertinent basic sciences and clinical pediatrics (Machotka 1973; Machotka 1975). Patient acceptance and the quality of care associated with pediatric PAs and CHAs are high (Wallen 1982).

One study of CHA care reported favorable marks by all mothers surveyed. Ninety percent indicated a desire to have their future children cared for by a CHA (Dungy 1975).

HEALTH MAINTENANCE ORGANIZATIONS

Health maintenance organizations (HMOs) have usually been quick to seize innovative, cost-containing measures. Their experience with nonphysician providers sharing and offsetting traditional physician responsibilities dates from the 1950s when optometrists began assuming the role of refraction from ophthalmologists, nurse anesthetists began assisting for anesthesiologists, and psychiatrists began shifting mental health patients to psychologists. It was not surprising that when PAs came along, HMOs would embrace them.

Background of HMOs

Although HMOs have existed in this country in some form since the first capitated plan was set up in Elk City, Oklahoma, in 1929, it has only been since the early 1970s that substantial numbers of Americans have had access to this alternative to traditional fee-for-service health care. The first prepaid group practice was started by Sidney Garfield, a physician hired by the industrialist Henry Kaiser, to provide care to workers in the California desert building aqueducts to reach southern California communities. When World War II broke out, Dr. Garfield was recruited to provide the same type of worker health benefit to shipbuilders. A similar program was incorporated in the Kaiser shipyards of Vancouver, Washington (near Portland) under Dr. Ernest Saward. In 1945, with the cessation of the war and the release of workers to other jobs, the two Kaiser plans opened enrollment to the public.

In 1970, 39 prepaid group practices were operating in the United States (Mayer 1985). At this time, most of the legal and political battles against this managed care option had been fought, yet few Americans had access to this kind of plan. The Health Maintenance Act of 1973 seems to have been the impetus for an explosion of growth of HMOs. As a result, by 1985 there were 323 HMOs and by 1996 there were more than 574. The number of preferred provider organizations is almost double this amount (over 1036) and growing. More than 100 million Americans are in some form of managed care plan (GHAA, personal communication, 1996).

As HMOs have developed, several variations on their basic structure have evolved. The primary organizational type is the *staff model*, which is composed of salaried employees and providers and a group of beneficiaries whose health care is provided by the HMO. An example is *Group Health Cooperative of Puget Sound.* Similar in structure is the *group model*, which is organized by a prepaid population of patients; but the physicians are in a separate structure (usually as share holders), who contract with the parent structure. *Kaiser Permanente* is the prototypical group model HMO. A third model, the *network model*, has characteristics of both of the other types.

PAs in HMOs

The first HMO to hire a formally trained PA was Kaiser Permanente based in Portland, Oregon. In 1970, a Duke graduate PA was employed by the Department of Internal Medicine not only to assist in staffing, but also to gain experience for future staffing needs (Lairson 1974). This organization had experience with nurse midwives, psychologists, and nurse anesthetists and believed that PAs and NPs could be useful adjuncts to the primary care physician staff. Within a decade, 10 departments had incorporated a PA or NP and, 25 years from their first hire, more than 160 PAs and NPs work alongside 550 physicians to serve more than 400,000 members.

In some HMOs, the nonphysician providers are organized as a separate department such as the Department of Physician Assistants at the LaGuardia Medical Group in Queens, New York (Goldberg 1983), or the Department of Physician Extenders at Geisinger Medical Center in Pennsylvania (Regan 1991), or as "Affiliated Staff" at Group Health Cooperative of Puget Sound. In others, they are incorporated within the departments that employ them and are considered representative members of that department (Hooker 1993).

HMOs and other types of managed care systems have strong incentives to contain personnel costs, and their structure and size provide the opportunity to capitalize on the economy of scale and division of labor that the use of PAs and NPs can offer.

Based on a 1994 survey of medium-sized plans (45,000 to 100,000 enrollees) and large plans (> 100,000) by the Group Health Association of America (GHAA), a surprisingly high use of PAs and NPs were used in a representative number of group and staff model HMOs (Dial 1995). In Table 5-3, the median number of physicians ranges from 119 to 123 per 100,000 enrollees. In addition, the PA and NP ratios range from 10.6 to 15 per 100,000 enrollees. The PA/NP staffing ratios of about 30 per 100,000 must be taken into consideration when physician ratios are extrapolated as national requirements (Weiner 1996).

Studies also show that NPs and PAs perform at rates of clinical productivity in a manner where quality of care is maintained at levels that are "indistinguishable" from that of physician care. Their practice orientation tends to show an emphasis on interpersonal skills, patient education, and preventive care (NAS-IOM 1978).

Various studies exist regarding how much care a PA or NP can assume in a primary care setting in an HMO. Most percentages are about 81% to 91% (Record 1981b; Hooker 1993; Hummel 1994b; Frampton 1994). Steinwachs and colleagues demonstrated that in one HMO, PAs and NPs tended to manage acute diseases more than chronic diseases (Steinwachs 1976). A study a decade later, however, showed that patients managed by PAs and physicians in adult primary care settings had a 90% overlap of diagnoses (Hooker 1986).

Why have the federal government and HMOs (the two largest employers of PAs) embraced PAs so readily? One theory is that these two forms of health delivery do not have the economic ownership of patients of fee-for-service plans. Therefore, they have greater incentives to use a team approach.

RURAL HEALTH

Access to health care in rural areas in the United States depends on a sufficient supply and distribution of primary care physicians, PAs, NPs, dentists, and a whole host of allied health professions. Although physician supply and distribution have been the focus of this problem, in the late 1980s, attention began shifting to the PA and NP as alternatives when it became apparent that many of them were successfully filling these physician roles (OTA 1990).

Primary care and rural health were the two driving reasons for developing the PA concept, and PAs continue to be a vital part of the health care infrastructure that supports ambulatory and institutional care in rural areas. In 1977, the US Congress enacted the Rural Health Clinics Act (Public Law 95–210) to encourage the use of nonphysician providers such as PAs and NPs in rural areas. This decision was based on a growing realization that many small communities could no longer support a sufficient number of physicians. PL 95–210 facilitated this goal by entitling various health providers to receive reimbursement from Medicare and Medicaid on a cost basis.

Approximately one-third of PAs practice in communities with populations of 50,000 or less, and 18% are in rural areas with 10,000 or fewer people. Even so, more PAs are needed in these areas. The National Health Service Corps believes that PAs and NPs are critical to an

Table 5-3 *Full-time equivalent provider per 100,000 enrollees in group/staff model HMOs*

PROVIDERS	NUMBER OF ENROLLEES	
	45-100,000 (12 PLANS)	>100,000 (16 PLANS)
Total physicians	118.7	122.6
Primary care physicians	68.8	59.1
Specialty care physicians	49.9	63.5
Physician assistants	10.6	11.2
Nurse practitioners	15.0	14.6
Other advanced practice nurses	6.3	2.3

(Data from Dial 1995.)

effort to staff rural areas and have identified a number of strategies to employ more physicians, PAs, and NPs in primary care and rural areas (National Health Service Corps 1991).

According to federal foundation-sponsored initiatives, the supply of PAs and NPs is directly related to the number of training programs (Styles 1990; Shi 1993; Jones 1993).

Certified Rural Health Clinics (RHCs) are located in a health professional shortage area, a medically underserved area, or a governor-designated shortage area. The RHC program was created in 1977 by PL 95–210 to increase access to health care for these areas and to expand the use of PAs, NPs, and CNMs. RHCs make up one of the largest outpatient primary care programs for rural underserved communities. Federally certified "independent" RHCs are reimbursed on a cost basis for their Medicare and Medicaid patients. Currently, RHCs make up one of the largest outpatient primary care programs for rural underserved communities and is one of the fastest growing Medicare programs. By law they must be staffed by PAs, NPs, or CNMs at least half the time the clinic is open (NARHC 1994).

Physician-owned RHCs make up 32% of the clinics. The rest are owned mostly by hospitals and public and private companies (Fig. 5-1). Sixty-six percent of RHCs employ one or more PAs, and 42% of them employ at least one NP.

Although RHCs are required to employ a PA, NP, or CNM, they may receive a waiver of this requirement for up to 1 year. Almost 19% of clinics have operated without a PA/NP/CNM for some period during 1994. More than 18% of clinics had some problem keeping a PA/NP/CNM. But at the same time, more than 35% reported they had problems in general retaining health professionals. Most PAs and NPs were paid between $41,000 and $60,000 annually in 1994 (NARHC 1994).

More recently, evidence has emerged that PAs who remain in rural areas may differ from urban-based PAs. Two studies indicate that PAs practicing in rural areas place considerably more importance on autonomy in selecting the location of their practice than other PAs, perhaps because they spend more time away from

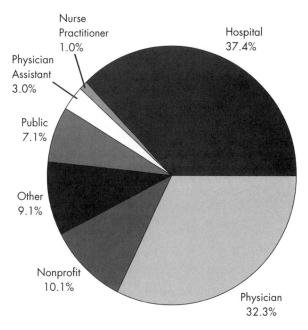

Figure 5-1 Percentage of rural health clinic ownership. (Data from National Association RHCs, 1994.)

their supervising physician. They also have a significantly higher level of satisfaction with role and professional acknowledgment than do urban-based PAs (Singer 1996; Muus 1996).

Another issue of great importance to rural PAs is favorable reimbursement policy. Because state-to-state variability in compensation and Medicaid reimbursement laws affects PA deployment, increased efforts should be directed toward tailoring state policies to compensate PAs adequately (Muus 1996).

As recruitment and retention of physicians in sparsely populated areas become difficult, PAs will be sought in greater numbers to help fill this growing void, especially in primary care. These studies have strong implications for recruitment of PA students for programs trying to fill the needs of medically underserved America.

FEDERAL EMPLOYEES

The federal government is the largest employer of physician assistants (10% of all employed

PAs in 1996). A special category of PAs are those who serve in the US Armed Forces, Veterans Affairs, Bureau of Prisons, Public Health Service, and other federal agencies. The vast majority are in primary care services, and most work in positions previously occupied by a physician. Exact numbers are hard to determine because many agencies and branches of the federal government, including the military, are constantly undergoing change. The estimates in Table 5-4 are based on networking with different employees in different departments and branches of the federal government.

Military

As of 1996, there were approximately 1,300 PAs on active duty in the military worldwide. They are on land or the seas, and many in special hardship situations. In addition, approximately 500 PAs are employed in civilian practice who also serve in the Ready Reserves and National Guard in 50 states and 4 territories. Nor does it include the many nonuniform (civilian) PAs on contract with the different military branches.

Unlike most PA students today, the great majority of military PAs have been medical corpsmen (Perry 1978a). PAs in the military also tend to be male, trained at an older age than civilian counterparts, and mostly in primary care. Job characteristics tend to differ as well; level of responsibility is slightly higher and closeness of supervision is lower for the military PA than for the civilian PA. In 1977, the career opportunities and job security for a PA in the military were considered greater than those of civilians (Table 5-5) (Perry 1978a). Several factors have changed since the study was done: The military has downsized, PAs are commissioned officers, and the role of the PA has expanded universally. Whether these differences continue deserves further study.

Table 5-4 *Federally employed PAs, 1996*

BRANCH	ACTIVE DUTY	BILLETS
Department of Defense		
US Navy	175	275
US Army	430	530
US Air Force	220	320
Department of Transportation		
US Coast Guard	28	30
Federal Aviation Administration	1	2
Department of National Oceanic and Atmospheric Administration	3	3
Department of Justice		
Bureau of Prisons	654	724
Immigration and Naturalization Service	30	40
Department of Health and Human Service		
US Public Health Service	88	100
Indian Health Service		
Food and Drug Administration	2	
Centers for Disease Control and Disease Prevention	4	
National Institutes of Health	6	
National Health Service Corps	16	30
US Coast Guard	2	
Department of Veterans Affairs	1,100	1,200

Billets means available positions. These are highly fluid positions subject to change.

(Data from various sources in the different agencies and branches, 1996.)

Table 5-5 *Differences in job characteristics of PAs employed in the military and civilian health sectors*

	MILITARY PAs	CIVILIAN PAs
Average age of graduates	34.5	29.9
	(n = 99)	(n = 828)
Average number of years of medical experience	11.4	4.4
	(n = 99)	(n = 829)
Level of responsibility	11.1	10.0
	(n = 121)	(n = 818)
Closeness of supervision	22.9	42.1
	(n = 119)	(n = 780)
Career opportunities	2.30	2.65
	(n = 121)	(n = 807)

(Data from Perry 1978a.)

The history of the PA movement began with the corpsman—the returned veteran. The PA as a form of medical officer was introduced in the Army, Navy, and Air Force in 1971 and in the Coast Guard in 1975 (Stuart 1973; Hooker 1991a; Gwinn 1994). Initially, all were noncommissioned officers, usually with senior enlisted rank. Throughout the 1970s, their ranks began to swell. This development was largely in response to the termination of the draft for physicians (Gaudry 1977). Once obligated service was removed for physicians after the draft for military duty for males was abolished, those with little time invested tended to leave, creating a vacuum in medical staffing. The services found it difficult to recruit physicians. With a peace-time military and a need for medical officers, the military turned to PAs as a logical alternative (Hooker 1989).

One of the more interesting footnotes in the evolution of the military PA is the commissioned PAs. While almost all are eligible for commissioned officer status, this was not always so. The first PAs were from the enlisted ranks. PAs were the medics, the corpsmen, or allied health personnel who matriculated through a formal PA training program (Amann 1973). In the early 1970s, their rank status was changed from enlisted to warrant officer to reflect their more technical skills and to avoid conflicts when directing services that involved officers (Hooker 1989). In April 1978, the United States Air Force (USAF)

promoted enlisted PAs to commissioned officer status. This accession was considered consistent with the skill and responsibility of an officer. It also took place because the Air Force warrant officer program had been discontinued since 1958. This left the Army, Navy, and Coast Guard PAs as warrant officers, in contrast to the commissioned officers in the Air Force. This discrepancy in rank, status, and career earnings for military pay was in stark contrast to the uniformity of rank, pay, and hierarchy of physicians, nurses, dentists, pharmacists, and physical therapists in the military. For a 20-year career, the USAF PA was making 25% more than his or her professional peer in the Army (Hooker 1989). This disparity became more apparent after economic research revealed the significant differences commissioning could mean for recruitment and retention. After some intense lobbying by American Academy of Physician Assistants (AAPA) legislative representatives, work by the PA leaders in the different services in the AAPA, and some congressional help, the surgeon generals of the different services eventually commissioned for all military PAs (the Army in 1989, the Navy and the Coast Guard in 1990) (Lott 1989). With the commissioning of the Coast Guard Reserve as the final step achieved in 1991, the AAPA could move on to other professional issues.

There is a strong kinship between the military and PAs. As Admiral Moritsugu once said to a group of Army PAs, "You are the germ plasm of all PAs." The first PA student class at Duke University was made up of four Navy veterans, all hospital corpsmen (Condit 1994). Subsequent classes at Duke and other programs were made up primarily of military veterans, many with Vietnam experience (Hooker 1991b). For the first 10 years, the majority of PA graduates were veterans. With the exception of medics, technicians, and corpsmen coming up through the ranks, the number of civilian-trained PAs entering the military is not very large. At one time, all of the services used their own military schools. To meet demand at different times, some military branches contracted with civilian schools to train military PAs. This took place with the Army at St. Francis College PA Program, and the Coast Guard with Duke University and the George Washington University in Washington DC. In 1996 federal budget cuts forced the Department of Defense to consolidate its military training programs. Mixed classes of PA students from the Army, Navy, Air Force, Coast Guard, and the Federal Bureau of Prisons now train at the Interservice Physician Assistant Training Program at Fort Sam Houston in San Antonio, Texas, the site of the former Army PA Program. The student selection process is the responsibility of each individual service.

The role of the PA in the military has been enhanced in a number of ways, beginning with deployment during international engagements since Vietnam, Panama, the Gulf War, Somalia, Haiti, and Bosnia. PAs have been an integral part of combat-ready troops in the Army, Navy, Marines, and Coast Guard. They also serve in the White House, the Pentagon, and in a number of policy development positions (Harbert 1991; Price 1991). Currently, the highest ranking PA is a lieutenant colonel in the Air Force. In time, a PA will inevitably reach the O-6 pay grade (colonel or captain), or higher.

AIR FORCE

The Air Force has approximately 220 PAs on active duty, serving principally in primary care and family practice clinics. The PAs in the Air Force enjoy strong support from the highest levels of the Air Force medical command. They are part of the Biological Sciences Corps. At one time, the Air Force had its own PA program located at Shephard Air Force Base in Wichita Falls, Texas.

ARMY

The Army, with nearly 430 PAs, has the largest contingent in the military. They are part of the Medical Service Corps. Army PAs work in the field with operational forces, as well as in the primary care setting (O'Hearn 1991). In addition, Army PAs have opportunities to specialize in occupational medicine, orthopedic surgery, emergency medicine (Herrera 1994), and cardioperfusion training. Most Army PAs are trained at Fort Sam Houston in San Antonio, Texas.

NAVY

The 175 active-duty Navy PAs belong to the Medical Services Corps. They are used almost exclusively in primary care. A number of operational billets are available for deep-water vessels, but most are attached to medical centers and shore stations. Navy PAs can be assigned to Marine Corps billets; a few serve on independent duty. The Navy PA school was in San Diego but has now consolidated with the Army program in San Antonio.

Coast Guard

Often overlooked as a military branch, the Coast Guard is part of the Department of Transportation, not the Department of Defense. There are 30 PAs on active duty and 15 in the reserves. All of the ice breakers are staffed by a PA when underway. PAs from the enlisted ranks were trained at the Air Force Physician Assistant Training Program in Wichita Falls, Texas, but are now trained at the combined military program in San Antonio. The US Public Health Service supplies some PAs to the Coast Guard, but the majority are both recruited and trained by the Coast Guard. Because there is no specialty corps in the Coast Guard, PAs are line officers and must compete with these officers for advancement (Hooker 1991a).

National Oceanic and Atmospheric Administration

Only a few PAs wear National Oceanic and Atmospheric Administration (NOAA) uniforms. These PAs are part of the US Public Health Service and are often in the NOAA for only a few years at a time.

US Public Health Service Corps

The US Public Health Service Corps (USPHS) is of one of eight Public Health Service agencies in the US Department of Health and Human Services. PAs serve in the Food and Drug Administration, the Centers for Disease Control and Disease Prevention, the Indian Health Service, the NOAA, the Coast Guard, the National Center for Health Statistics, and other agencies. Some of these are commissioned officers; others are civilian or contract workers. All are recruited, and none are trained at the Uniform Services Medical University.

The National Health Service Corps (NHSC) is one program that has health care professionals in more than 500 neighborhoods suffering from critical shortages of primary health care providers. It is administered by the Health Resources and Services Administration (HRSA) Bureau of Primary Health Care.

A number of recruitment funds support programs that offer financial help for PAs and other medical care professionals in exchange for professional services. These include scholarships, The Federal Loan Repayment Program, The NHCS State Loan Repayment Program, and The Commissioned Officer Student Extern Program (COSTEP).

Bureau of Prisons

The Bureau of Prisons (BOP) is part of the Justice Department and has numerous PAs serving in various federal prisons. The BOP is the fastest growing federal department and is constantly recruiting PAs for correctional medicine. The BOP participates in the Interservice PA Program at Fort Sam Houston in San Antonio, Texas.

Veterans Affairs

One of the principal institutional employers of PAs nationwide is the Veterans Affairs (VA). From the very beginning of the PA profession, the VA has played a vital supporting role in the education and utilization of PAs. For example, the VA Medical Center in Durham, North Carolina, has provided clinical education sites for the first PA students at Duke University and the St. Louis University PA program was initiated by the VA in St. Louis in 1972. The VA first began employing PAs in 1968 (Fox 1983).

Initially, each VA facility largely determined for itself the role of the PAs it employed. In 1972, however, the VA central office issued Circular 10-7-252 entitled, "Utilization Guidelines of Physician Assistants." This document, which represented an effort to standardize the role of the PA within the VA system, defined the areas of the hospital in which the PA could be utilized, as well as specifying the type and level of tasks they could be assigned (Fox 1983). This seems to have opened the door for PAs. Although there are more than 1,100 PAs working in over 130 VA locations, more PAs are needed in the VA system, which includes 172 hospitals, 68 satellite outpatient units, and 127 nursing homes.

Several research projects on PAs in the VA have provided a profile on roles and utilization patterns. These evaluations have enhanced the ability of the VA to establish appropriate PA/NP policies. In 1992, an important study by Alexander and Lipscomb (1992) identified the allocation of time for PAs and NPs (Table 5-6).

Approximately 22% of all PAs are employed by the federal, state, or local government in some capacity (Table 5-7).

Table 5-6 *PA and NP percentage allocation of time to Veterans Affairs Medical Center (VAMC) inpatient, outpatient, and extended care*

UNIT/ACTIVITY	PA (N = 138)	NP (N = 67)
Inpatient		
Medicine	9.8	6.4
Surgery	8.9	0.1
Psychiatry	18.7	2.6
Neurology	0.3	0.5
Rehabilitation Medicine Service (RMS)	2.1	0.0
Spinal Cord Injury (SCI)	3.4	0.0
Intermediate Care	4.0	18.0
Other	2.4	2.1
Subtotal	49.6	29.7
Outpatient		
Medicine	9.8	12.6
Surgery	2.1	0.0
Psychiatry	2.8	0.0
Neurology	0.3	1.5
RMS	0.2	0.0
SCI	0.1	1.5
Other[a]	20.9	30.6
Subtotal	36.2	46.2
Extended Care (nursing home plus other settings)	7.6	14.5
Other (nonclinical) settings[b]	6.6	9.6
Total	100.0	100.0

[a] Includes emergency room, admitting/screening area, compensation and pension examinations, employee health, hospital-based home care, satellite outpatient clinic, hemodialysis, domiciliary, and other outpatient settings.

[b] Includes teaching, administration, and any other units/activities specified by the respondent.

(Data from Alexander 1992.)

Table 5-7 *Distribution of government-employed PAs, 1991*

Not employed full-time by the government	77.9%
Employed full-time by the government	
State governments	5.4
Veterans Administration	4.7
Local governments	2.7
US Air Force	2.6
US Army	2.4
US Navy	1.6
US Coast Guard	0.3
US Public Health Service	0.7
National Guard	0.15
Federal Corrections	0.6
Other federal agencies	1.0
Total	100.0%
Military veteran	
Yes	30.6
No	69.4

(Data from American Academy of Physician Assistants, 1991 General Census Data.)

Other Federal Agencies

PAs are also employed by the State Department, the US Peace Corps, the Central Intelligence Agency, the Federal Bureau of Investigation, and other federal agencies.

CONCLUSIONS

With the exception of the two surgeon assistant programs, all PAs are trained in primary care. This was the underlying reason for the development of PAs and the raison d'être of almost all PA programs today. Because of the pressing need for primary care clinicians and the potential for increasing access while holding down labor costs, the role of the primary care PA is generally believed to be secure for the near term. Health policies determining the future of the health workforce are dictating that PAs and other nonphysician providers need to be part of the labor force mix.

6

Specialization

The physician assistant (PA) profession was created to provide basic medical services to populations that were underserved or that did not receive care at all. Although this is fully recounted in the history of the profession (see Ch. 3), Eugene Stead's original intention in creating the profession may not be well appreciated. He envisioned these new practitioners as assistants to doctors in a very general and literal sense. Stead did not confine the activities of PAs to working only with primary care physicians. Stead and Estes intended that PAs would provide a wide number of services for physicians in all types of medical practice. The original Duke curriculum, for example, not only provided training in the performance and interpretation of electrocardiograms, but also gave instructions on how the machine could be repaired if broken. Thus, the original design of the Duke program was that the PA would perform medical tasks—some involving diagnosis and therapeutic management, and some involving technical and routine procedures—that relieved the busy physician and allowed the doctor more time for continuing professional education, dealing with complex patient illnesses, and seeing more patients (Estes 1968b). The Duke model conceptualized PAs as all-purpose generalist assistants to doctors. This concept became markedly altered as the PA movement gained momentum in the late 1960s.

Another movement in specialization that took place in the late 1960s was a surge of new programs to train nonphysician providers in certain areas of medicine. Some of these programs include the Orthopedic Assistant and the Urologic Physician's Assistant, which were 2 year programs designed to train personnel to work directly for specialists. Another was the 4-month "health assistants" training program. Sponsored by Project Hope in Laredo, Texas, the only requirement was that the student be 18 years old. Eight of the eleven students who entered the first class lacked high school equivalence but were able to earn their General Equivalency Diploma Certificate upon completion of the program (Sadler 1972). Other programs of various duration in length of training were developed in gastroenterology, allergy, dermatology, and radiology. None survived past 1975, with the exception of the surgical assistant, the pathology assistant, and the child health associate program.

Since PAs emulate physicians in many circumstances, it is not surprising that they too would move into specialty practices. Most of the trends observed among physicians are also seen in PA specialization including the trend away from general medicine and the increase in wages for specialization.

As the profession evolved, PAs were diverted into nonprimary care roles so that today the profession is approximately evenly divided (Kole 1991). Why this has occurred is not really clear. Hooker hypothesized that PAs probably respond to the same forces that shape physician specialty choices: the training process, the specialty that fits the lifestyle and geographic preferences of the physician, and market forces (Fig. 6-1) (Hooker 1992). Genova examined the influence of market forces on PA practice settings in Maine and concluded that, at least there, the market was weaker

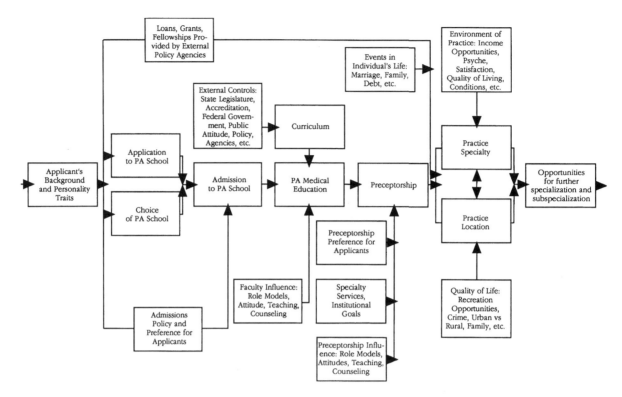

Figure 6-1 The effect of the education process on PA speciality and location. (From Hooker, 1992)

for primary care PAs than for the services of specialty care PAs (Genova 1995).

PAs IN SUBSPECIALTY AREAS

PA utilization in subspecialty practice areas has expanded considerably since 1980. In this chapter we refer to all areas of medical practice outside of primary care (internal medicine, family practice, and pediatrics) as specialty and subspecialties. The trend of increasing demand for and utilization of PAs in specialty and subspecialty roles is likely to continue. Specialty practice areas expected to remain strong for PAs in nonprimary care roles include emergency medicine, cardiovascular surgery, orthopedic surgery, and internal medicine. The trend of utilizing PAs as resident substitutes raises several policy issues in health workforce planning. With relatively small numbers of PA graduates at present, significantly expanding PA utilization in graduate medical education roles diverts them from intended roles in primary care practice in general, and especially in medically underserved settings. Another consideration is that neither PA educational programs nor teaching hospitals provide many financial incentives to participate in the clinical education of PAs in specialty or inpatient care areas. It may be difficult for PA educational programs with curricula focused on primary care to expand numbers and adequately prepare PAs for inpatient care/specialty roles. Table 6-1 is a list of some of the clinical practice specialties and subspecialties in which PAs are utilized.

What are the factors that influence or lead to PAs choosing a particular specialty or practice? Why PAs choose a particular specialty is only partially known. Certainly employment opportunities play a significant role. Studies show

Table 6-1 *Partial listing, clinical subspecialty areas utilizing PAs*

Allergy
Anesthesiology
Cardiothoracic surgery
Clinical research
Critical care units
Dermatology
Emergency medicine
Forensic medicine/pathology
Gastroenterology/endoscopy
Gerontology
Hematology/oncology
Infectious disease/immune deficiency
Interventional radiology
Invasive cardiology
Mental health
Neonatology
Neurosurgery
Obstetrics and gynecology
Occupational health
Oncology/pediatric oncology
Ophthalmology
Organ procurement and transplantation
Orthopedics/sports medicine
Otorhinolaryngology — head and neck surgery
Physical medicine/rehabilitation
Plastic surgery/burn care
Preventive medicine
Rheumatology
Substance abuse/psychiatry
Urology

differences between primary care and nonprimary care PAs. For PAs in nonprimary care roles, the most influential factors determining specialty choice are technical orientation and income/employment. These factors seem to differ from PAs in primary care who identify prevention, academic environment, debt/scholarship, intellectual content, and peer influence as more important factors (Singer 1996).

SURGICAL PAs

In 1967, John W. Kirklin, MD, Chairman of the Department of Surgery at the University of Alabama and an internationally renowned pioneer in cardiac surgery, began the first program to train surgeons' assistants (SAs), or surgical PAs, to assist in the surgical care of patients (Byrnes 1991). Kirklin's decision to train nonphysician individuals to assist in the preoperative, intraoperative, and postoperative care of surgical patients was the culmination of his years of work in medical education and the realization of the value of a trained, professional assistant who was not a physician but who could provide a competent continuity of care (Condit 1992).

Kirklin's program was typical of a number of programs that tried to develop a type of PA who could assist a physician in either primary care or some specialized service. In 1971, the federal government demonstrated interest in the training of PAs when Congress passed the Comprehensive Health Manpower Training Act which placed emphasis on primary care programs (Kress 1971). In 1972, the Bureau of Health Manpower (now known as the Bureau of Health Professionals) assumed responsibility for funding 24 of the existing 31 PA training programs. The intent of this Act was to relieve problems of geographic and specialty maldistribution of health care delivery. This was interpreted as primary care, so the emphasis of specialty care and surgery programs were left without funding. As a consequence, many of the specialty programs either converted to primary care programs or disbanded.

At the same time that policy directives were shaping the PA health workforce, there was much debate over the role of the PA in surgery in the early 1970s. This debate centered around whether or not surgeons should use nonsurgeons as first assistants. In 1973, the American College of Surgeons issued their statement on SAs, in which they supported the concept. This support was published in *Essentials for the Educational Training Programs of Surgeon's Assistants* (American College of Surgeons Bulletin 1973).

Surgical PAs can be trained in one of three ways: formally in a structured SA program, as a graduate PA with on-the-job training, or by entering a postgraduate training program. The first PA postgraduate training program in any specialty was instituted at Montefiore Medical Center/Albert Einstein College of Medicine in 1971 under the direction of Richard G. Rosen, MD. The Montefiore program began as a means of utilizing PAs as surgical house staff. The Yale/Norwalk program was developed by PA faculty members with the Department of Surgery of the Yale University School of Medicine. The first class of 12 students was admitted in 1976 (Beinfield 1991).

The American Association of Surgeon Assistants (AASA) was established by a group of surgical PAs in response to opposition from some primary care PAs in 1972. AASA maintains an active relationship with the American College of Surgeons and the American Academy of Physician Assistants (AAPA). The Association of Physician Assistants in Cardiovascular Surgery maintains a liaison with the American Association for Thoracic Surgery.

As word of the existence of the surgical PA has spread, employment opportunities within the surgical arena have expanded immensely. Today, surgical PAs are widely employed throughout the United States, Europe, and Canada (Table 6-2). They are distributed in rural and urban areas, in community hospitals and major medical centers, in general surgery, and virtually all surgical subspecialties (Condit 1992).

Table 6-2 Distribution of surgical PAs, 1991

SPECIALTY	PERCENT
General surgery	35.4
Orthopedics	26.9
Cardiovascular surgery	19.5
Neurological surgery	4.5
Urologic surgery	4.3
Plastic surgery	2.5
Vascular surgery	1.8
Thoracic surgery	0.8
Traumatic surgery	0.3
Colon/rectal surgery	0.1
Other Surgery	3.1

PRACTICE SETTING	PERCENT
Hospital	55.4
Group office	21.6
Clinic	15.7
Solo office	8.7
HMO	3.0
Inner city	1.9
Rural clinic	0.4
Corrections	0.3
Other setting	4.2

(Data from American Academy of Physician Assistants, 1991 Census Data.)

Surgical PA Profiles

PAs in surgery command the higher end of salaries in the profession. The mean 1995 salary for all surgical PAs was $66,359; the median income was $64,444. For new graduates, the salaries were $51,500 and $52,500 respectively (Table 6-3). The vast majority draw a straight salary, or a salary plus bonus, fewer than 10% have some sort of shared revenue relationship with their employer.

Physician attitudes about surgical PAs have long been positive (Legler 1983). With cost-containment, as well as an increasing acceptance of PAs and SAs, we believe the field of surgery for PAs is likely to grow well into the next century.

OTHER PA SPECIALTIES

A great deal of experimentation has taken place in developing PA programs. While the greatest area of concentration has been in formally preparing PAs for primary care roles, some of this experimentation has been in creating surgical and medical subspecialty roles. This usually occurs because there is a perceived need for a PA in these roles. Other reasons for PAs shifting into specialty roles include an unfilled niche for a provider in this particular specialty or a physician specifically inviting and directing the PA into this specialty.

The following sections present specializations for PAs identified from the literature or in conversations with PAs in these roles. The list is far from complete.

Table 6-3 Surgical PA salaries, 1994

SALARY TYPE	PERCENT OF RESPONDENTS
Straight Salary	53.8
Salary + % Revenue	7.6
Salary + Bonus	37.6
Partnership	1.0

SALARY DISTRIBUTION	OVERALL	NEW GRADUATES
10th Percentile	$44,818	$37,500
25th Percentile	53,523	41,250
50th Percentile	64,444	52,500
75th Percentile	75,893	61,875
90th Percentile	94,500	63,750

(Data from American Association of Surgical Assistants, *Surgical Physician Assistants* 1995.)

Administration

Clinical experience as a PA increases the marketability in health care administration. Nevertheless, little is known about how many PAs are in administrative roles. Many PAs share both clinical duties and administration in offices, and these roles may even fluctuate depending on the demands in either sector. Various attempts have been made to form special interest groups that involve PAs in administration, but these groups do not seem to endure. Many PAs have used their degrees as stepping stones to administrative roles in hospital and clinic administration, sometimes acquiring administrative degrees along the way (Mayer 1988).

Alcohol and Drug Abuse

A small but growing number of PAs provide alcohol and drug abuse management from the clinical side. Often their roles include admission and discharge from detoxification units and the provision of medical management of substance abuse clients in outpatient settings (Srba 1981).

Allergy

A program lasted for 2 years at the University of California, San Diego, which trained PAs in allergy. Developed in 1969, the program trained PAs to prepare, administer, and evaluate allergens for those with suspected allergic conditions. This role has largely been supplanted by nurses skilled in allergy.

Anesthesiology

The concept of an anesthesiologist's assistant (AA) was initiated in 1969 at Case Western Reserve University in Cleveland, Ohio, and at Emory University in Atlanta, Georgia. Having been advised of the programs' purposes and operations, by 1975 the American Society of Anesthesiologists (ASA) was supportive of this emerging occupation. The Emory University curriculum was designed to result in a Master of Science degree. Case Western Reserve offered a Bachelor of Science degree, designed largely as a premedicine curriculum.

In 1976, the ASA petitioned the AMA Council on Medical Education for recognition of the anesthesiologist's assistant as an emerging health profession. The Council's recognition followed in 1978. This authorized the initiation of an ad hoc committee within the ASA to work collaboratively with the American Medical Association's Department of Allied Health Education and Accreditation on the development of a body of educational standards (*Essentials*). Because of differences in opinion about the level of the credential and about the need for graduates in this field, in 1981 the ASA withdrew its collaboration with the AMA in the development of accreditation standards and in the accreditation of educational programs.

By 1982, the Association of Anesthesiologist's Assistants Training Programs (AAATP) was created and incorporated. The next year, the AAATP and the American Academy of Anesthesia Associates (AAAA) petitioned the AMA Council on Medical Education to recognize them as collaborative sponsors for the program designed to educate anesthesiologist's assistants. In 1984, the AMA Council on Medical Education reinstated its recognition of the anesthesiologist's assistant profession. *Essen-*

tials for the education and training of anesthesiologists' assistants were adopted in 1987 by the CME, the AAATP, and the AAAA.

The anesthesiologist's assistant functions under the direction of a licensed and qualified anesthesiologist, principally in academic medical centers. He or she assists the anesthesiologist in collecting preoperative data, such as taking an appropriate health history and performing an appropriate physical examination; in performing various preoperative tasks, such as the insertion of intravenous and arterial lines, central venous pressure monitors, and special catheters; in airway management and drug administration for induction and maintenance of anesthesia; in administering supportive therapy, such as intravenous fluids and vasodilators; in providing recovery room care and in performing other functions or tasks related to care in an intensive care unit or pain clinic; in providing anesthesia monitoring services; and in performing administrative functions and tasks, such as staff education. "Direction" implies the presence of a designated anesthesiologist within the hospital and immediately available to the operating room.

In addition to the duties described in the occupational description, anesthesiologist's assistants provide technical support according to established protocols. This support includes first-level maintenance of anesthesia equipment; skilled operation of special monitors, including echocardiographs, electroencephalographs, special analyzers, evoked-potential apparatuses, autotransfusion devices, mass spectrometers, and intra-aortic balloon pumps; the operation and maintenance of bedside electronic computer-based monitors; supervised laboratory functions associated with anesthesia and operating room care; and cardiopulmonary resuscitation.

Anesthesiologist's assistants are likely to be employed by hospitals with 200 beds and larger and with staffs of 15 or more anesthesiologists, nurse anesthetists, and anesthesiologist's assistants, which use a team approach to anesthesia service, which have facilities for open heart surgery, and which have a graduate medical residency training program for anesthesiologists.

The programs are essentially 2 years, based on a Master's degree model. The programs require a baccalaureate degree with a major in cell biology, chemistry, physics, mathematics, computer science or physiology.

Anesthesiologist's assistants recently sought recognition as PAs, using as justification the premise that the term *physician assistant* includes all assistants to physicians. For many years, anesthesiologists' assistants have been recognized as type B PAs in Georgia. This designation was based on a recommendation by the National Academy of Sciences in 1970 that PAs be classified as types A, B, and C by degree of specialization and level of judgment involved in practice. This outmoded system was abandoned after a year or two.

Cardiology

The cardiology PA includes ambulatory care, hospital admission and discharge evaluation, early myocardial infarction management, treadmill, and other procedures (Mayes 1988).

In at least one institution, the role of the cardiology PA extends to both substituting for and training cardiology fellows in cardiac catheterization (DeMots 1987). Other specialized roles for cardiology PAs are envisioned as cardiology becomes increasingly invasive (O'Rourke 1987).

Cardiovascular and Thoracic Surgery

PAs have been working alongside cardiovascular surgeons since the first Duke class (Cooper 1971; Rothwell 1993). Their roles have evolved along with the fast moving technologic specialty of cardiology and includes the recognition of early postprocedure complications of surgery, ambulatory care, hospital admission evaluation, and early postmyocardial infarction management. Routines include hospital visits, discharge planning, and follow-up appointments (Mayes 1988). They improve operating room efficiency and thus free up the surgeon to consult in other cases (Mauney 1972; Miller 1978b). From 1970 to 1974, a program at the Oregon Health Sciences University in Portland trained approximately 15 PAs in cardiovascular surgery among other specialties.

One of the more important roles for the cardiovascular surgical assistant is harvesting the saphenous veins for coronary artery bypass grafting (Chaffee 1988). Some PAs have further specialized as bypass pump technologists.

Correctional Medicine

PAs have been part of correctional medicine at least since 1973. While often listed as a specialty, in reality, correctional medicine is a primary care discipline that is practiced under extenuating circumstances, challenging behavior, and ethical considerations, along with certain legal constraints (Lombardo 1982; Jarmul 1991; Smith MO 1996). They often work independently and deliver a number of primary care and specialty services depending on the size of the institution (Stalker 1978a; Freeman 1981).

In one study, the employment of a PA in a Baltimore city jail resulted in a decrease in utilization of men's sick call and an increase in duration of encounters. Improvment in prescribing pattern and categories of prisoner complaints was also observed (Freeman 1981).

Each county and state has a prison system with opportunities for PAs. The Department of Justice recruits PAs to staff the Federal Correctional System, better known as the Bureau of Prisons, either as civil service employees or public health service officers. As of 1996 there were 654 PAs working within the Bureau of Prisons (Smith MO 1996) (see Table 5-4). Anecdotal information suggests that this role of medicine offers a great deal of satisfaction for PAs (Brutsche 1986). In one federal correctional institution in Georgia with 1,750 inmates, responsibilities are shared among 10 full-time PAs, two physicians, three administrators, a nurse, and numerous ancillary staff (Smith MO 1996).

There are probably no greater opportunities to examine health care staffing while holding a vast number of variables constant than to practice medicine in this quintessential managed care setting.

Critical Care Medicine

After 3 months of rigorous training, two PAs were assigned to the intensive care unit (ICU) at the Veterans Administration Medical Center in Allen Park, Michigan. Their performance, as well as the operation of the ICU over 2 years, was evaluated and compared to 2 preceding years when it was operated by house officers. There were no changes in occupancy, mortality, or the rate of complications. Instead there seemed to be evidence for more careful evaluation of patients before admission and discharge, manifesting as a slightly fewer admissions and slightly longer duration of hospitalization. The authors concluded that PAs have a role in providing health care in intensive care settings (Dubaybo 1991). Experience in other hospitals is similar (Grabenkort 1991).

Dentistry

In the early 1970s, when the role of the PA was less clear, there was an interest in developing dental associates modeled after PAs (Keith 1974). Unlike many health problems, dental diseases and the procedures commonly used to resolve them require direct practitioner intervention. Many procedures are routine and well suited for delegation. Unfortunately, the dental profession has been generally conservative in employing a dental assistant to assume responsibilities analogous to the contemporary PA, and efforts to promote them has met with strong resistance from organized dentistry (Keith 1974). However, PAs have been used successfully to teach physical diagnosis in a dental school (Devore 1978).

Dermatology

In the late 1960s, a Type C PA program developed briefly at the University of Chicago Pritzker School of Medicine in the Dermatology Department under Stanford I. Lamberg, MD. This 12-month program graduated a certified PA in dermatology. The requirements were a high school diploma plus 3 years of health care experience, such as an RN or medical corpsman (Sadler 1972).

Little is written about what dermatology PAs do, although interest in expanding the role of the primary care PA into dermatology has continued for more than two decades (Krasner 1977; Katterjohn 1982). In one descriptive study, the PA was found to be a useful addition in relieving some of the burden of patient care, but neither patient flow nor income was favorably affected (Laur 1981). The economics of managed care and current emphasis on cost-reduction are making PAs more attractive (Dermatology World 1996).

Eighty-five formally trained PAs identify their clinical practice as dermatology and belong to the Society of Dermatology Physician Assistants, which is part of the AAPA Medical Congress. Their salaries in 1995 ranged from $40,000 to $100,000 (J. Monroe, personal communication, 1996).

Diabetology

The only known diabetes PA program was established by the Diabetes Trust Fund in Birmingham, Alabama in the late 1960s. This 2-year program offered a certified diabetes PA degree (Sadler 1972). Little is known about this program other than that the graduate was a PA in Diabetes.

One book has been written detailing diabetes management in HMOs using primarily PAs (Power 1973). The American Diabetes Association has recognized that a diabetologist is anyone who is involved with the diagnosis and management of diabetes and its complications.

Emergency Medicine

Shortly after the first few PA classes were practicing, PAs were occupying roles in hospitals, and before long they were in the emergency departments (EDs). It seemed a natural fit since many had developed skills in the military, and some had wartime experience that honed their skills further. Others had worked as trauma nurses and technicians. Sometimes they were used to manage the less acute patient. Other times they were seeing undifferentiated patients. There is much consensus that the education process seems to prepare the interested PA for ED services (Gentile 1976; Friedman 1978). In 1993, approximately 8% of PAs reported that they were employed in an ED setting (AAPA 1994).

Only a few studies describe the range of services a PA provides in an ED setting: In a small, rural community hospital, a PA could competently manage 62% of all presenting conditions (Maxfield 1975); in an urban setting, the roles are quite diverse and help bridge complex cultural gaps in medical-surgical services (Goldfrank 1980). No study has identified the range of services that can be provided by an emergency PA or nurse practitioner (NP). Regarding the concentration of both types of practitioners in some EDs, results of a survey of 111 Veterans Affairs Medical Centers showed that a mean of 1.9 full-time equivalent (FTE) PAs are employed in 37 EDs, and a mean of 2.1 FTE NPs are employed in 29 EDs. They work between 43 and 44 hours per week (Young 1993).

Hooker and McCaig analyzed the results of the National Ambulatory Hospital Medical Care Survey that began in 1992. Combining PAs and NPs for statistical purposes, they found that PAs/NPs manage 3.5 million, or 4%, of the approximately 90 million ED visits in the United States. They conclude that there are few differences in the type of patient seen at PA/NP visits compared to all visits when gender, reason for visit, diagnosis, and medications prescribed are compared (Hooker 1996a). Innovative programs have included laceration management by

PAs, which has been shown to improve care and outcome, decrease cost, and seems to be satisfying to patients (Katz 1994).

A few postgraduate programs are available to train the PA in emergency medicine. One at the University of Southern California, in Los Angeles (which closed in 1995) and the other at Montefiore Hospital in New York. The Army implemented a postgraduate program to train Army PAs in emergency medicine in 1992. These programs are located at Brooke Army Medical Center in Texas and Madigan Army Medical Center in the state of Washington (Herrera 1994).

Forensic Medicine

PAs are employed as forensic investigators at the Office of the Medical Examiner, Suffolk County, New York (Golden 1986; Wright 1987), and in New Hampshire (Sylvester 1996). Some are employed full-time and others part-time. That PAs would be attracted to this discipline is interesting since there seems to be little emphasis on forensic pathology as a potential area of practice in the current PA education curriculum (Cardenas 1993) (see Pathology Assistants).

Gastroenterology/Endoscopy

PAs are trained formally and informally in both rigid and flexible sigmoidoscopy, colonoscopy, and gastroscopy. The benefit of a PA in one gastroenterology setting included staff efficiency, improved housestaff education, and ability to perform an increased number of procedures with existing staff over a 3-year period (Lieberman 1992) (Table 6-4). It is probably no coincidence that this study was done at a Veterans Administration center because of the historical role they have played in developing the PA concept, and because the large scale of these medical centers allows them to experiment with alternatives to physician-directed services.

Nonphysician endoscopy is not new. From 1972 to 1976, a Type C PA program in gastroen-

Table 6-4 Impact of a gastroenterology PA on procedure workload

	PROCEDURES/YR			PERCENT CHANGE
	1987 BEFORE PAS	1989 AFTER PAS	1990	1987–1990
Sigmoidoscopy	313	386	442	(+) 41
Panendoscopy	646	810	821	(+) 27
Colonoscopy	373	437	439	(+) 18

(Data from Lieberman 1992.)

terology developed briefly at the University of Washington and the Veterans Administration hospital in Seattle. This 12-month, federally funded program trained about 12 PAs to do rigid sigmoidoscopies, blind biopsies of the esophagus, and manometry; to process tissue; and to assist in other aspects of endoscopy, all of which preceded the development of flexible, fiberoptic instruments. While this program did not survive long, the role of the PA in various endoscopic procedures has persisted. Several screening flexible sigmoidoscopy programs have relied on PAs, NPs, and RNs for more than a decade (Roosevelt 1984; Weissman 1987; Schroy 1988; Cargill 1991). The question of sanctioning independent endoscopy is still being debated in the literature (Palmer 1990; Smith 1992).

Geriatric Medicine

More than 20 studies on the use of PAs in geriatric medicine have been published. The consensus is overwhelming: PAs are very effective in patient management and care in geriatric facilities, contributing to quality care by allowing more patients to be seen and relieving the physician of less pressing problems (Isiadinso 1979; Kraak 1979; Sorem 1983; Romeis 1985). More than one study has demonstrated shorter hospitalization, and overall lower medical costs utilizing PAs in geriatric institutional settings

(Tideiksaar 1982; Tideiksaar 1984). A study by the Rand Corporation demonstrated improvements in care and outcomes when PAs and NPs were introduced into nursing homes. Both nursing home administrators and directors in the demonstration model expressed higher levels of satisfaction with the process of care (Buchanan 1989).

Historically, neither medical schools nor PA program curriculum have emphasized geriatrics (Yturri-Byrd 1984; Tideiksaar 1986a). With the revision on Medicare and Medicaid reimbursement for nursing homes, geriatric health care became center stage, and with it came the renewed interest in and the cost-effectiveness of PAs (Kane 1980; Fox 1980; May 1988). The increase in the geriatric population and the growing medical concerns of this population have increased the need for more PAs in this area (Olson 1983; Gambert 1983; Schafft 1987b; Dychtwald 1988). Since the late 1980s, most PA programs have tended to emphasize gerontology (Ouslander 1989; Kane 1991; Aaronson 1992).

Although less than 2% of all PAs report that geriatrics is their primary clinical responsibility, both students and graduates report a high interest in this area (Bottom 1988; AAPA 1995). Virtually all studies on the aging population of both the United States and the world agree that the health care needs of the elderly will continue to increase. The opportunities for PAs in new and expanded roles in geriatric medicine and administration will increase dramatically in the decades to come (Dieter 1989).

In 1985, the Bureau of Health Professions joined the AAPA to verify the role of the PA in providing geriatric care (Schafft 1987b). The study developed models of geriatric care provided by PAs and suggested appropriate uses of PAs with increasing demands for elderly medical services. Both inpatient and outpatient settings were outlined.

Hospital/Inpatient

PAs are often trained in hospital settings and are utilized extensively in many inpatient arena (see Chapter 7).

Infectious Disease/Immunology/Immunodeficiency

Many PAs are infectious disease specialists, both inpatient and outpatient. Some have assumed this role from the communicable disease nurse in hospital settings; others function as a consultant for both traveler's advice and inpatients. In addition, many PAs are involved with infectious disorders such as acquired immune deficiency syndrome (AIDS). How these roles are formalized and in what capacity they are performed have not been detailed in the literature.

The Physician Assistant AIDS Network (PAAN) is a national HIV/AIDS clinical interest group for PAs who have substantial involvement in HIV/AIDS direct care, education, or research. The network was developed in association with AAPA in 1995 and was designed to facilitate access to current information and the exchange of ideas among PAs who serve people with HIV/AIDS.

Maritime PA

The US Public Health Service Hospital at Staten Island, New York, developed a 12-month PA program for former military medical corpsmen who wanted to continue their medical career. It was operational briefly in the late 1960s as a Type C PA program for the Merchant Marine fleet. The graduates were referred to as Marine Physician's Assistants and were stationed on ships that employed large crews to oversee their health and safety (Sadler 1972). The duration of this program and why it closed are not known.

We know of one PA who served as a Ships Medical Officer on a luxury ocean liner. Responsibilities were divided between passengers and crew.

Mental Health

The mental health field is dominated by non-physician therapists who provide psychiatric services. Most of these workers are psychologists, social workers, and mental health counselors; but increasingly PAs are becoming visible as psychiatric PAs. The PA in the mental health setting is unique since he or she can see clients who need psychological services as well as prescribe psychotropic medication and other medical services. The first documented utilization of a PA functioning in a psychiatric role was in 1977 (Greenlee 1977).

A few studies have evaluated how well PAs perform in the mental health field. One clinical assessment study found that PA interviewers in psychiatric evaluations were comparable to those of physicians for all items, including those thought to require the most clinical and medical judgment (Coryell 1978). Another study found the PA could successfully identify the medical disorders that accompany psychiatric disorders that caused psychiatric symptoms (Mathew 1982). In a third study, PAs detected nearly three times as many physical illnesses as the psychiatrist. The psychiatrists were significantly more likely to miss diagnoses among older patients and women (D'Ercole 1991).

Psychiatry reports critical shortages of trained specialists such as PAs who can work in state hospitals. One institution's addition of PAs to the staff significantly increased the time that psychiatrists had to plan and implement treatment. There was a high degree of acceptance of the PAs in this setting (Matthews 1984). Other cost-effective roles include using PAs to provide primary care and nonpsychiatric inpatient care in psychiatric settings (Morreale 1977).

Neonatology

One formal postgraduate neonatology program exists for PAs at the Physician Assistant Neonatology Residency Program in Los Angeles. Two other residency programs in pediatrics also expose the pediatric PA to neonatology (Norwalk Hospital and the Wolfson Children's Hospital in Jacksonville, Florida).

Evidence suggests that patient care delivered by neonatal PAs and NPs in the intensive care setting is an effective alternative to care delivered by pediatric residents. No significant differences in management, outcome, or charge variables can be demonstrated when comparisons are made between patients cared for by either provider (Carzoli 1994).

Neurology

PAs are practicing neurology both in primary care and in association with neurologists. A 1987 study of members of the American Academy of Neurology revealed that 29% of neurologists used PAs and/or nurse clinicians (NCs) in their practice. Institutionally based neurologists were more likely to use PA/NCs than those in private practice (Gunderson 1988). Many of these physicians are bringing their office PA/NCs into the hospital.

Neurosurgery

Neurosurgery is a labor-intensive surgical subspeciality. It is not surprising that neurosurgical PAs provide some role in this discipline. This surgical specialty tends to be in a higher range of pay. PAs first assist in lieu of another surgeon and sometimes perform certain procedures on their own, such as carpal tunnel releases.

A program in which the PA functions as an intern-equivalent in neurosurgery was described in the late 1970s. This study suggests that patient care and patient acceptance were universally improved. The editor of the journal that published the study cited a number of reasons why he personally was opposed to the use of PAs in this area (Sonntag 1977).

Obstetrics and Gynecology

The shortage of health personnel in obstetrics and gynecology has been cyclic and in the early 1970s was significant (Schneider 1972). The earliest studies of PAs in women's health found that they could care for at least 80% of well patients in family-planning clinics without the need for consultation with a physician (Ostergard 1975). Two programs, Stanford University and the University of Washington, experimented with postgraduate programs to train PAs and NPs as midwives (Briggs 1978; Stark 1984). While these programs did not last long, a third postgraduate program for PAs in gynecology and obstetrics has been present at Montefiore Medical Center in New York since 1986. The 15-month program consists of advanced training in medicine, surgery, gynecology, preoperative and postoperative care, cardiac and trauma life support, and critical care (McGill 1990).

PAs in female reproductive health perform a variety of roles including family planning (Mondy 1986), routine examinations, mammogram interpretation (Hillman 1987), and termination of pregnancies (Freedman 1986; O'Hara 1989; Donovan 1992). The advance practice nurse literature suggests that NPs and CNMs occupy this niche with high levels of employment and that PAs may have trouble entering women's health care provider roles.

Occupational and Industrial Medicine

Occupational and industrial medicine, sometimes referred to as corporate medicine, has utilized PAs as early as 1971 and has been an optional rotation within many PA programs (Lynch 1971; Barnes 1971; Lowe 1971; Howard 1971). The delivery of routine physical examinations for industries and insurance companies by PAs can result in substantial savings compared to the cost when this service is performed by a physician, which makes the PA particularly attractive (Medical World News 1973; Weisenberger 1974; Richmond 1974). Industrial health studies conducted primarily by PAs instead of physicians has been a trend in certain sectors for the last two decades (Harbert 1978; Rom 1979; Elliott 1984).

The role of the industrial/occupational medical PA encompasses the delivery of physical, mental, and emotional health care, as well as preventive medicine. Activities include occupational health and safety, stress reduction, smoking cessation, and wellness. Involvement of PAs in this

area escalated in 1978, as industry responded to cost-containment pressures; PAs perform annual employee physical examinations, exercise stress testing, occupational health education, and treatment of work-related injuries. Work settings initially focused on underserved areas; today they include plant sites, private industrial-medicine clinics, and corporate medical administration. Utilization continues to expand. The American Academy of Physician Assistants in Occupational Medicine, founded in 1981, develops continuing medical education programs and educates industry and the public about PAs in occupational medicine (Ramos 1989). The trend has been for PAs and NPs to become hospital employee health managers, replacing RNs (Hospital Employee Health 1991).

The University of Oklahoma Physician Associate Program has a graduate occupational health program that trains and grants a Master's degree in Public Health and Industrial Medicine.

Orthopedic PAs

There is a great deal of confusion about PAs who work in orthopedic settings, technicians who call themselves orthopedic PAs, and the different organizations of PAs who are specialized in orthopedic medicine. Formally trained PAs who work in an orthopedic setting differ from another group of technicians trained to assist the orthopedic surgeon. Each have "orthopedic" in their title, and many refer to themselves as orthopedic PAs, or OPAs. To add to this confusion, there is the American Society of Orthopedic Physicians (ASOPA), Orthopedic PAs (OPA), and the Physician Assistants in Orthopedic Surgery (PAOS). Approximately 8% of formally trained PAs in 1996 reported they were employed in an orthopedic practice (AAPA 1996a).

The history of orthopedic PAs begins with assistants to the orthopedic surgeon, who have been present since at least 1954 in some capacity, whether to assist applying a cast, or to hold a retractor. It is unclear when the first formal orthopedic technical program started; however, minimum educational standards for orthopedic

PA education were first adopted by the AMA House of Delegates in 1969 upon a recommendation from the American Academy of Orthopedic Surgeons (AAOS). Eight orthopedic PA programs had been accredited by 1973. This proved to be somewhat controversial, and 1 year later AAOS announced its intent to withdraw sponsorship from the accreditation program. After substantial consultation with AAOS, the AMA Council on Medical Education announced a moratorium on the accreditation of any additional orthopedic programs and informed accredited programs that accreditation would be discontinued upon graduation of the classes that would be matriculating in the fall of 1974. It is important to note that accreditation efforts in allied health education are not sponsored by the AMA without the involvement of the medical specialty society or societies and the related allied health organizations most closely associated with the occupation.

During this brief period of AMA-sanctioned orthopedic PAs in the mid 1970s, eight orthopedic PA programs were accredited by the AMA Council on Medical Education (Table 6-5). None of these orthopedic assistant programs are functional today. The one at Kirkwood Community College in Cedar Rapids graduated its last class in 1988. None of the orthopedic PA programs were ever accredited as PA programs by the AMA Committee on Allied Health Education and Accreditation.

The orthopedic assistant programs were confined to training technical orthopedic tasks without the substantial background in the basic medical sciences that the primary care PA programs stress. The educational qualifications of the two groups—orthopedic PAs and NCCPA certified PAs—differ substantially. Orthopedic assistants were trained as technologists in a junior college in an 18-month course that was more closely related to other technical programs, such as respiratory therapy, surgical technology, and medical or dental assisting. From 1,500 to 2,000 graduates are estimated to have matriculated from these eight programs, along with some similar programs in the Air Force.

Graduates of the orthopedic assistant program are *not* eligible to sit for the Physician Assistant National Certifying Examination administered by the NCCPA. An examination for orthopedic PAs is handled by a National Board for Certifying Orthopedic Physician

---

Table 6-5 *Orthopedic PA technical programs*

PROGRAM	LOCATION	GRADUATES
Bismarck Junior College	Bismarck, ND	NA
Cerritos College	Norwalk, CA	3
Chattanooga Technical Institute	Chattanooga, TN	1
City College of San Francisco	San Francisco, CA	2
Highline Community College	Midway, WI	12
Foothills College	Los Altos, CA	NA
Kirkwood Community College	Cedar Rapids, IA	36
Marygrove College	Detroit, MI	62
Normandale Orthopedic Program	*	0

Abbreviation: NA, not available.

* Data unknown at time of publication.

Number of graduates may not be accurate due to lack of verification.

(Data from various sources including conversations with admissions departments of some of the schools.)

Assistants (NBCOPA). This NBCOPA examination is not equivalent to the NCCPA examination, nor are the organizations affiliated in any way (Kappes 1992).

Although both PAs and orthopedic PAs work for orthopedists, Minnesota is the only state with a law regulating orthopedic PAs. In 1978, Michigan included a grandfather title protection for "orthopedic physician's assistants," but orthopedic PAs remain an unlicensed occupation in that state. They were also given a finite period of time to register in Minnesota when regulation of PAs became effective in 1986. In Iowa, home of the Kirkwood Community College program, the 1988 PA Practice Act explicitly states that "orthopedic physician's assistant technologists" are not required to qualify as PAs.

An American Society of Orthopedic Physician Assistants (ASOPAs) represents approximately 400 practicing orthopedic PAs and was formed in 1971. Most states do not regulate the practice of OPAs. The exceptions are New York, where orthopedic PAs must be registered as specialist assistants, and Minnesota, where for 2 years orthopedic PAs were allowed to register as PAs. Services provided by orthopedic PAs are not covered by Medicare (Lindahl 1994).

The PAOS, the most recent special interest group for formally trained PAs, was formed in 1992 at the annual AAPA conference in Nashville. This seems to be the most active organization at present. The PAOS is working with the Southern Orthopedic Association to develop a membership category for PAs (Wallace 1995).

NCCPA-certified PAs in orthopedics provide a host of services that closely juxtapose the orthopedic surgeon. They provide preadmission physical examination, write admitting orders, first assist in surgery, dictate discharge summaries, and conduct fracture clinics (Samsot 1996).

Ophthalmology

There are no formal ophthalmology programs that teach PAs to be ophthalmologists. Two programs developed in the 1960s to train Type C PAs in the management of eye diseases; the Georgetown University Hospital in Washington, DC, and Columbia-Presbyterian Medical Center in New York, each had a 2-year certification program. Both are defunct. The graduate ophthalmology PA could not only refract but could assist in surgery and manage uncomplicated nonsurgical ophthalmologic problems (Sadler 1972).

In 1989, 52 PAs who were members of the AAPA reported that their primary responsibility was in ophthalmology. Most are employed in large practices that specialize in cataract and radial keratotomy procedures (Wilson 1990). The role of PAs in ophthalmology is not viewed positively by optometrists who would like to have expanded roles in eye disease care but are usually prohibited by narrowly defined state laws.

Otolaryngology: Head and Neck Surgery

The Society of Physician Assistants in Otorhinolaryngology—Head and Neck Surgery was founded in Kansas City during the American Academy of Otorhinolaryngology—Head and Neck Surgery's annual meeting in 1991. The Society was developed to enhance the professional growth development of PAs who worked in the field of otolaryngology. These PAs were seeking an organization that would provide an opportunity to meet and interact with PAs who share a common interest and to obtain continuing medical education specific to their field. At least 75 PAs belong to this organization, which has a liaison with the American Academy of Otorhinolaryngology—Head and Neck Surgery.

The roles of PAs in this specialized field include diagnostic tests and procedures such as fine needle aspiration biopsies, tympanostomy tubes, and sinus irrigations. Many assist in surgery, coordinate admissions, dictate discharge summaries, and provide follow-up care. Additional office procedures include cleaning of ear canals and mastoid cavities, electrocautery for the control of epistaxis, insertion of nasal packing, and immediate postoperative care of patients in the inpatient and outpatient setting. They may also perform rhinopharyngolatyngoscopy, videostrobscopy, and vocal/voice recordings.

Approximately 23% of PAs in otolaryngology were employed by a solo otolaryngologist, 57% in a group practice, 4% by hospitals, 7% by the US Government, and 7% by HMOs (Poppen 1996).

Pathology

Pathology assistants are often referred to as PAs. While they are a type of PA, they are not trained in primary care. They are formally trained in pathology and do not have an association with the American Academy of PAs or the Association of Physician Assistant Programs. Formally trained PAs who practice forensic medicine are described in Forensic Medicine.

Pathology Assistant programs developed in the late 1960s; programs at The University of Alabama and Quinnipiac College in Connecticut have been active since 1971. Both are 2-year Master's degree programs and have graduated over 200 individuals. The Quinnipiac College program is affiliated with the VA medical centers in West Haven and with Yale University School of Medicine. A third program is at Duke University. The roles and responsibilities of the Pathology Assistant include histopathology, surgical frozen sections, and general autopsies.

Pediatrics

Pediatrics is considered one of the three specialties that make up primary care. However, many PAs specialize in pediatrics both through formal and on-the-job training. One program specializes in pediatrics and two postgraduate programs are in neonatology.

Since 1971, the University of Colorado Medical Center has been graduating PAs and NPs specialized in pediatrics. These graduates are known as Child Health Associates (CHA), and those who choose to be PAs are eligible to take the NCCPA examination and become certified PAs.

Originally developed as a 3-year program, it has been pared down to a 24-month program.

By completion of their training, CHAs are able to obtain a pertinent medical history, perform a detailed physical examination, diagnose, and formulate an appropriate management plan for more than 80% of the patients seen in an average ambulatory pediatric setting. This includes writing prescriptions for most therapeutic regimens. Other areas emphasized are preventive and psychosocial aspects of comprehensive health care and growth and development from the prenatal period through adolescence.

Pediatric PAs are specialized as well. They are utilized on pediatric bone marrow transplant units (Trigg 1990) and work with the homeless, uninsured, poor, and underserved (Rada-Sidinger 1992). They are members of social service child protection units (Gray 1991) and work with inpatients to address the problems associated with resident overwork and educational needs of hospital services (Giardino 1990).

Plastic/Reconstructive Surgery

Plastic/Reconstructive surgery encompasses the areas of cosmetic surgery, burn management, and hand surgery. PAs in surgery in general, and plastic surgery in particular, can obtain these skills by formal training (i.e., Surgeon Assistant or postgraduate training), or on-the-job training.

The plastic surgeon utilizes the PA in a variety of ways. In the clinic setting, the PA may see patients as postoperative cases. In the hospital, the PA may perform admission histories and physical examinations, order routine laboratory tests, dictate discharge summaries, as well as monitor patients, change dressings, and assist in the operation (Toth 1978; Gittins 1996). Reconstructive microsurgery has relied on trained SAs in this area to reduce operating time (Gould 1984).

Public Health/ Preventive Medicine

The impact of a nonphysician as a health director on full-time public health coverage was first examined in 1980 (Jekel 1980). The experience in Connecticut demonstrates that the public health world does not need to rely solely on physicians. The level of care improved when a nonphysician assumed the role of health director (Atwater 1980).

Radiology

A program to train highly selected, experienced radiologic technologists to become Type C PAs in diagnostic radiology (PA-DRs) was initiated at the University of Kentucky Medical Center in 1970 (Kierman 1977). This 2-year program was underwritten by the federal government and was designed to improve the efficiency of radiologic procedures (DHEW 1977). Approximately 30 individuals graduated before the program closed when the American College of Radiology withdrew its support.

Despite the small number of graduates, six studies have examined the utility of PAs in Diagnostic Radiology. In one study of work activities, including examinations that otherwise would have been performed by a radiologist, and radiographs screened for disease, they performed these activities "accurately and acceptably." Each PA-DR averaged a savings of 34% of the employing radiologist's time (Kierman 1977). Duties were wide ranging and included fluoroscopic procedures, excretory urography, and chest radiographic screening (Thompson 1974). Another study trained primary care PAs to perform competently in screening radiographs, intravenous pyetograms and brain scans. The authors concluded that the PA-DRs performed as well as radiologists (Thompson 1971; Thompson 1972).

At Johns Hopkins Medical Institute, a PA on an interventional radiology staff performs history and physical examinations and Doppler pressures, schedules laboratory work and admissions, answers referring physicians' calls, and obtains preliminary patient information (White 1989). The addition of this person decreased mean length of stay for patients undergoing various procedures and increased the capacity for interventional procedures (White 1988).

Surveys of chiefs of radiology departments were generally favorable when asked if they were willing to delegate traditional radiologist tasks to PAs (Thompson 1971). When private practice radiologists were surveyed, however, at least 60% showed reluctance to delegate these tasks (Parker 1972).

A study on mammograms interpreted by PAs found that the interpretations by PAs were more sensitive and as specific as those made by six HMO radiologists who interpreted the same cases, and as effective as those by radiologists described in the literature. Interpretations by PAs were similar to those made by radiologists. The study concluded that mammogram interpretations by PAs took less time and cost less than did those by performed by radiologists (Hillman 1987).

Anecdotal reports of a few PA-DRs still working for a number of years after the closure of the Kentucky program in the late 1970s have circulated. In 1991, a controversial editorial called for renewed interest in training PAs to work in radiology (Ellis 1991; McCowan 1991). In 1996, the subject was reviewed again after describing a few PAs who provide radiology services in some different settings (Hayes 1996).

Research

Almost as soon as there were more than a handful of PAs, there were researchers to study them. At first medical sociologists, behaviorists, economists, and health services researchers examined the nascent profession (Hooker 1994a). Within a few years, PAs became part of investigative teams, as well as the subjects of research. Since the early 1970s, the PA research agenda has been shaped not only by health researchers interested in the profession, but also by PAs (Jarski 1988). These medical, social, and health services research efforts to involve PAs have been at five levels of activity:

1. Supplying information about ongoing activities as providers

2. Helping to develop new data
3. Participating in data analysis
4. Assisting in research design
5. Co-authoring papers that result from research (Record 1976)

PAs are also clinical investigators who participate in drug trials and biochemical research. They assume roles previously occupied by a physician (Morian 1986). One of us (RSH) has personally participated as a clinical investigator in 14 clinical trials and has been the principal investigator of two of these trials. This experience is not unique since many other PAs around the country conduct clinical trials in many settings, from private firms to university research clinics.

The role of the PA in research is likely to increase as the demand for clinical trials increases and the need for skilled clinicians who can be employed at less cost than a physician also increases. Many PA programs on the Master's level have a research component as part of the curriculum, which is likely to stimulate further research.

Rehabilitation Medicine/Physiatry

PAs function in many rehabilitative roles including employment in hospitals and rehabilitative units. They function essentially as physiatrists.

Rheumatology

Eight members of the AAPA consistently cite their primary medical responsibility as rheumatology. Their role seems to be welcomed as members of the American College of Rheumatology. What rheumatology PAs do is unclear. In one study of rheumatology referrals in an HMO, a PA and two rheumatologists shared approximately equally all of the consultations for that year (Hooker 1985). With the demand for rheumatology service increasing, and the demand for rheumatology service increasing, and the number of training programs for rheumatologists shrinking, it seems that this is an unfilled niche for PAs.

Sports Medicine

Many PAs provide care in sports medicine clinics, are team health providers, and function in a variety of roles that transcends orthopedics and rehabilitation medicine.

Tissue Procurement

Cadaver organ retrieval is an ideal role for PAs because of their training and because it can directly replace a physician. In one 30-month study involving a PA replacing a physician, the total number of kidneys increased threefold, the number of usable kidneys increased dramatically, the number of referral hospitals increased threefold, and the number of kidneys shared with other transplant centers tripled as compared to any period before initiation of the PA approach (Schmittou 1977). PAs are urged to become more active in procurement and transplant programs (Joyner 1984).

Urology

A Type C PA in urology was developed at a time when a number of emerging technologies were requiring a special person trained to manage the tools and instruments of this specialty. In 1970, a program in Cincinnati trained PAs in urology to administer intravenous pyelograms, obtain detailed voided specimens, assist in methods to snare renal stones, perform cystoscopies, and analyze renal calculi. While there is plenty of opportunity for PAs to continue in this vein, a new type of Urology PA has emerged-the medical urology PA. This role tends to be performed in a urology office with one or a group of urologists. This PA often provides the initial consultation, performs a cystoscopy, evaluates the prostate, and manages the impotent patient. An expanded role for PAs in this field is in sexology.

Veterinary Medicine

While we know of no study on PAs formally employed in veterinary medicine, anecdotes abound about rural PAs providing care for both large domestic animals and small animals. This service should be viewed as only an occasional and informal tradition of the rural general practitioner and not taken too seriously as an erosion of the professional animal doctor.

POSTGRADUATE RESIDENCY PROGRAMS

In the first comprehensive book discussing the PA profession Ann Bliss wrote in 1975 (Sadler 1972):

> Immediately upon graduation, the physician's assistant is in considerable danger of being swallowed whole by the whale that is our present entrepreneurial, subspecialty medical practice system. The likely co-option of the newly minted physician's assistant by subspecialty medicine is one of the most serious issues confronting physician's assistants.

Bliss was alluding to the already emerging trend of PAs working with surgeons and other specialists in acute care medicine and surgery in the hospital setting. Instead of threatening the well-being of the profession, however, these trends marked the beginning of expansion of the ways in which PAs were utilized, and also, on a very practical level, indicated that PAs were seeking out and filling the jobs that were becoming frequently available to them.

The first postgraduate program began at Montefiore Medical Center in the Bronx, New York. In 1972 Richard Rosen, MD, a surgeon, was concerned that the large size of the surgical residency training program of that institution was worsening the already apparent overproduction of surgeons. He believed that PAs could be hired to provide the same type of patient care as physician surgical housestaff, thereby limiting the production of future surgeons in what was becoming an overcrowded field. The notion that PAs could substitute for housestaff was quite different from the existing mainstream philosophy of how PAs were to be utilized. Rosen recruited PAs to work on inpatient units, first in surgery and later expanding into other departments. He thought that PAs ought to be used in settings where there were many physicians (i.e., hospitals) and was convinced that PAs should be allowed to provide care that does not have to be given solely by a physician (Rosen 1986).

This unique utilization of PAs pioneered by Rosen led to other postgraduate residency programs for PAs (Table 6-6). The Norwalk Hospital affiliated with the Yale University School of Medicine program began in 1976 and instituted a 1-year training experience that consisted of a 4-month didactic training session of the fundamentals of surgical anatomy and physiology, followed by 8 months of clinical rotations through surgical wards at Norwalk. PA surgical residents perform a full range of inpatient surgical duties, including preoperative care, assisting in surgery, and postoperative care (Heinrich 1980).

The National Association of Postgraduate PA Programs was established in 1988 to assist in the development and organization of postgraduate educational curricula and programs for PAs. This organization assists in the definition of the role of the PA in the specialities and in the development of evaluation methodologies for postgraduate educational curricula and programs. Other activities include information for the public and profession about postgraduate educational curricula and programs.

Despite the remarkably diverse and growing number of PA postgraduate residency programs (Table 6-7), we are unaware of any study that examines where these graduate are dispersed and what they are doing. Whether PAs who are formally trained in surgery, PA who are informally trained in surgery, or postgraduates in surgery perform different duties or see different types of patients is not known. Clearly, research needs to be conducted to answer the charges that PAs in postgraduate residencies are providing anything more than a ready source of labor for institutions.

Table 6-6 *PA postgraduate residency programs*

SPECIALTY	PROGRAM	LENGTH	AWARD
Surgery	Physician Assistant Surgical Residency Program, Montefiore Medical Center/Einstein College of Medicine, NY	15 months	Certificate
Surgery	Physician Assistant Surgical Residency Program, Norwalk Hospital/Yale University School of Medicine, Norwalk, CT	1 year	Certificate
Surgery	Physician Assistant Surgical Residency Program, Sinai Hospital of Baltimore, MD	1 year	Certificate
Surgery	Cedars-Sinai Medical Center, Los Angeles, CA	1 year	Certificate
Surgery	Geisinger Medical Center, Danville, PA	1 year	Certificate
Surgery	Martin Luther King, Jr./Drew Medical Center, Los Angeles, CA	1 year	Certificate
Surgery	Mayo Foundation, Rochester, MN	1 year	Certificate
Surgery	Butterworth Hospital/Western Michigan University	1 year	Certificate
Emergency medicine	Alderson Broaddus College, Phillipi, WV	2 years	Master's degree
Emergency medicine	US Army, Fort Sam Houston, TX	1 year	Certificate
Emergency medicine	Emergency Medicine Physician Assistant Residency, Los Angeles County/University of Southern California Medical Center, Los Angeles, CA	1 year	Certificate
Gynecology/Obstetrics	Montefiore Medical Center, Bronx, NY	15 months	Certificate
Geriatrics	USC School of Medicine, Los Angeles, CA	1 year	Master's Certificate
Neonatology	Physician Assistant Neonatology Residency Program, Los Angeles County/University of Southern California Medical Center, Los Angeles, CA	1 year	Certificate
Rural primary care	Alderson Broaddus College, Phillipi, WV	2 years	Master's degree
Pediatrics	Physician Assistant Postgraduate Residency Program in Pediatrics, Baptist Medical Center, Wolfson Childrens Hospital, Jacksonville, FL	1 year	Certificate
Pediatrics	Physician Assistant Pediatric Residency Program, Norwalk Hospital, Norwalk, CT	1 year	Certificate
Occupational medicine	Program in Occupational Health for Physician Assistants, School of Public Health, University of Oklahoma, Oklahoma City, OK	20 months	Master of Public Health

(Data from 1994 Physician Assistant Program Directory.)

Table 6-7 *Postgraduate residency attendance, 1994 (n = 817)*

SPECIALTY	PERCENT
Anesthesiology	0.7
Emergency medicine	15.2
Geriatrics	1.3
Neonatology	1.5
Gynecology	2.1
Occupational health	3.3
Pediatrics	4.8
Rural primary care	6.1
Surgery	45.9
Other	19.1

(Data from American Academy of Physician Assistants, 1994 Member Census Report, 1995.)

Table 6-8 *PA Specialty Groups*

American Academy of Physician Assistants in Occupational Medicine
American Association of Surgeon Assistants
American Society of Psychiatric Physician Assistants
Association of Neurological Physician Assistants
Association of Physician Assistants in Cardiovascular Surgery
Association of Physician Assistants in Obstetrics and Gynecology
Association of Physician Assistants in Oncology
Physician Assistants in Dermatology
Physician Assistants in Family Practice
Physician Assistants in Orthopedic Surgery
Society of Emergency Medicine Physician Assistants
Society of Physician Assistants in Addiction Medicine
Society of Physician Assistants in Otorhinolaryngology/Head and Neck Surgery
Society of Physician Assistants in Pediatrics
Society of PAs in Physical Medicine and Rehabilitation

(Data from AAPA Membership Directory 1994–1995.)

Specialty Groups in AAPA

PAs practice in a variety of medical and surgical subspecialties. Some have formed independent associations/organizations to share common concerns and interests related to their practice specialty (Table 6-8). A specialty organization may apply for official AAPA recognition if more than 50% of its members are AAPA members.

CONCLUSION

One of the major rationales for the development of the PA profession has been to augment the supply of medically trained providers in those specialties in greatest need of assistance. The diversity of employment settings is an indication of the maturity of the profession. The primary care role of the PA is the root of the profession and remains the basis of PA education, but the PA profession has become much more specialized over the last decade. PAs are widely dispersed throughout the spectrum of medical disciplines and seem to have become well integrated. Many PAs enjoy membership status in physician specialty societies or professional specialties of their own making. These specialty pathways involve PA residencies, Master's degrees in clinical and nonclinical disciplines, and entry into other fields through experience and formal training. Specialization will remain an important component of the PA program, but with the exception of surgery, no one specialty is likely to dominate.

7

Inpatient Settings

Physician assistant (PA) utilization in hospital roles has become commonplace in a wide variety of medical center settings. PAs now work on services within major teaching hospitals, medium and small community and rural hospitals, and other types of inpatient care institutions. Presently about 30% of clinically active PAs, or roughly 8,900 providers, are employed in full-time positions in hospital settings (AAPA 1996a). In a separate earlier survey, nearly 50% of all PAs said they had some hospital responsibility. This ranged from the occasional rounds to seeing patients on a daily basis (AAPA, Council on Professional Practices 1994c).

According to findings from a sample of 1,690 PAs employed in hospital settings who responded to a national survey, 45% of these PAs are "house officers." More than 90% of responding PAs hold formal medical staff privileges and are credentialed under hospital by-laws. A similar percentage of hospital PAs have written job descriptions and are permitted to write diagnostic and therapeutic orders within the institution (AHA 1992). Another national study of teaching hospitals reported 62% use of PAs and/or nurse practitioners (NPs) in at least one of their departments. In 116 programs, PAs were used to perform some tasks previously done by physician residents; NPs were used in 77 programs; both were used in 62 programs. Of the 178 departments using PAs as substitutes for traditional physician services, 42% are surgical, followed by primary care (25%) and medical specialties (21%). In this study, PAs were more likely than NPs to substitute in surgery and emergency departments, while NPs are more likely than PAs to substitute in pediatrics and neonatal care (Riportella-Muller 1995).

PA practice in inpatient settings tends to be focused in specialty and subspecialty areas with 19% working in surgical subspecialties, 19% in medical subspecialties, 15% in emergency medicine, and 10% in general surgery (AAPA 1995). PAs in hospitals also work in non-specialty care areas such as in primary care or ambulatory care departments, in community outreach clinics, in the hospital employee health center, or in the emergency department (Hooker 1996a).

PAs in hospital settings have displayed an extensive range of clinical versatility. Experiences on inpatient services in many institutions demonstrate the safety, skills, and clinical efficacy of PAs (Willis 1993a). Published reports attest to successful experiences in PA utilization in inpatient internal medicine (Frick 1983), surgical and surgical subspecialty (Heinrich 1980; Harris 1987), and pediatric services (Silver 1984). In addition, PAs have been found effective and are employed in critical care units (Grabenkort 1991; Dubaybo 1991); subspecialty services (for example diagnostic radiology) (White 1988), and emergency departments (Goldfrank 1980 Sturman 1990; Hooker 1996a). The addition of PAs to inpatient medical staffs reveal high levels of acceptance by employing physicians and patients, a favorable cost-benefit margin to the institution, and maintenance of high levels of patient care quality (McKelvey 1986).

While PA education typically emphasizes roles in primary care, PAs have adapted readily to clinical inpatient roles and have shown high levels of acceptance and effectiveness in these settings. Residency program cutbacks, the curtailed availability of international medical graduates (IMGs), and reports of the positive experiences in PA use were key factors leading inpatient institutions to employ PAs in staffing efforts to adjust clinical service coverage with less resident availability (Knickman 1992).

Montefiore Medical Center (Bronx, NY) was among the first hospitals to utilize PAs to augment inpatient medical and surgical house staff. More than 25 years ago, PAs were hired for house staff roles at Montefiore on surgical wards to offset reductions in resident numbers. Presently, the institution employs more than 150 PAs not only in surgical areas, but also in internal medicine, the medical subspecialties, emergency medicine, obstetrics and gynecology (OB/GYN), on the employee health service, on transplant services, in burn units, and in a broad range of administrative, education, and research roles (Zarbock 1986; McGill 1990).

Another model of the effectiveness of using PAs on inpatient services was developed and has flourished at Geisinger Medical Center, a 577-bed referral facility located in rural northeastern Pennsylvania. Geisinger began employing PAs more than 20 years ago and now has 110 PAs who serve in clinical roles spanning primary care, as well as in specialty and subspecialty roles. Geisinger utilizes both PAs and NPs to staff family medicine clinics and the emergency department, in general medical internal medicine specialties, in general surgery and surgical subspecialties, in high-technology diagnostic and therapeutic service areas, and in roles in outpatient clinics at satellite settings (Harbert 1994; Walters 1986).

HOUSE OFFICERS

PAs are the primary candidates to substitute for residents because of their skills in physical assessment, medical management, and pharmacology. Many of the PA programs train students in the hospital setting to work alongside residents or house officers. A small but growing body of literature documents the favorable experience teaching hospitals have had using nonphysician providers on the wards, in critical care, and in surgery (Cawley 1988).

The use of PAs and NPs has been especially widespread in surgery to fill positions once filled by residents. In fact, some residency programs have lost accreditation because they lacked sufficient cases to provide adequate clinical experience (Foreman 1992). In other institutions, PAs have assumed responsibility for preoperative and postoperative care, obtaining histories, conducting physical examinations, and performing noninvasive procedures. For example, at Butterworth Hospital in Grand Rapids, Michigan, PAs serve as house officers in cardiothoracic surgery, neurosurgery, urology, and orthopedics (Evenhouse 1992). Nationwide, over 3,000 PAs work as hospital house staff (AAPA 1993b).

Under certain circumstances, PAs may be preferable to residents. Some faculty would rather work with PAs and NPs, who have a lower turnover rate, greater familiarity with departmental procedures, and more clinical experience than first- and second-year residents (Silver 1988). Using PAs may also ensure that residents have richer educational experiences. One time and motion study of residents at three Minnesota teaching hospitals found that residents spent 12% of their time inserting catheters and drawing blood, procedures that can be done by PAs (Lurie 1989). Because these tasks lose their pedagogical value after a certain number of repetitions, delegating them to PAs would free residents to focus on more complex cases (Cawley 1992b).

Clinical, financial, and practical criticisms were raised about the use of PAs as substitute residents. Although PAs may work well as substitutes for first- and second-year residents, some suggest they may require additional training to assume responsibility for more complex cases that call for more advanced medical decision-making or greater technical skill. In a study by Riportella-Muller and colleagues, this was not the case in teaching hospitals. In this national sample, PAs and NPs were filling positions that had been filled by both junior and senior residents (Riportella-Muller 1995). These concerns may lessen in the future with increasing specialization among PAs (Hooker 1992).

Another barrier to using more PAs is the view that they are more expensive to hire than residents and work fewer hours. For example, the 1996 average salary for PAs was $61,000 compared with the average stipend of about $36,000 for second- and third-year residents.

Another financial issue is that, unlike residents who bring Medicare graduate medical education payments to the institution, hospitals do not always receive an explicit payment for the services of the PA. Currently, Medicare pays PAs for hospital services when such services would be covered if furnished by a physician, including assistant-at-surgery services. However, PAs may cost the institution less than salary figures suggest because they may be more efficient than residents and require less faculty supervision. In the long run, the cost utility to the institution may be less when the PA house officer does not need to be retrained each year, is knowledgeable about the system, and operates at a higher level of visibility with the staff. An annual transition to new staff and scheduling arrangements takes time and money. In New York, implementation of resident work hour regulations, coupled with new requirements for continuous supervision of residents and 24-hour availability of intravenous, phlebotomy, and messenger/transport services have cost approximately $225 million. This is about a 2% increase in total hospital expenditures (Thorpe 1990; NY COGME 1991). Economists generally regard the services of a resident as neutral or negative since efficiency is less than that provided by a permanent staff house officer, and the educational commitment to train and pay the resident is expensive. On the other hand, hospitals pay salaries to PAs to be house officers with the expectation that greater continuity and coordination of care will contribute to better outcomes, shorter length of stay, and savings. In a study evaluating the effect of replacing residents with PAs and NPs

in New York City-area hospitals, it was found that, depending on the replacement strategy used, thousands of PA/NPs could be hired costing over $200 million annually to cover patient care services (Green 1995). One limitation of this study assumed that 35% of what a resident physician does is exclusively physician oriented, and that it takes three PAs/NPs to replace one resident because residents work over 80 hours/week and PAs/NPs would work only 40 hours.

Other studies have projected considerable cost savings substituting a percentage of resident slots with PAs and/or NPs. What is unclear is whether a sufficient number of PAs and NPs will be willing or able to step into new jobs that might be created by the loss of 11,000 residents under the reduction envisioned by the Physician Payment Review Commission and the Council on Graduate Medical Education (PPRC 1993b; COGME 1994). Based on one set of substitution estimates, 4,400 physician full-time equivalents (FTEs) and 7,700 PA/NP FTEs would be needed if hospitals maintained current service volumes (Knickman 1992). These estimates were based on a time-motion study at two large New York teaching hospitals where residents spent about 75% of their time providing direct patient care. Using a model in which PAs or NPs would assume responsibility as hour-to-hour managers of patient care, working with physicians to develop and implement a medical plan for each patient, 35% of residents' time could be assumed by PAs and 11% by other hospital personnel, while 20% would have to be assumed by staff physicians. Because residents generally work twice as many hours per week as salaried PAs, these estimates suggest that 0.7 FTE PAs would be required to replace each resident. A conservative estimate of the nonphysician provider workforce from which resident substitutes could be recruited is 80,000. Between 33,500 and 35,000 work in hospitals. About 3,500 PAs graduate annually.

Anecdotal reports suggest that the demand for PAs is already outstripping supply. Hospitals report that vacancy rates for PAs are growing, from about 10% in 1989 to almost 13% in 1991

(Pinckney 1992). Even with its long-standing surgical residency for PAs, Montefiore Medical Center in New York has had a difficult time recruiting PAs to fill its 150 authorized positions (Cawley 1992b). Since at least 1990, there have been more job openings than PAs to fill them (OTA 1990). Whether PAs would be willing to accept jobs created by the loss of residents will depend on the competitiveness of salaries and the attractiveness of these positions relative to other opportunities.

INPATIENT ROLES

Hospital clinical responsibilities assumed by PAs are extensive and vary widely among hospitals. These responsibilities depend on such factors as how many PAs are employed on the service, the extent of resident and attending coverage and supervision, the credentialing policies of the institution, the latitude allowed the hospital and PAs by state medical practice laws, and third-party reimbursement policies. Recently, another factor affecting the use of PAs has been state-mandated limitations on the number of hours worked by physician residents. With these limitations imposed on residency programs, the roles of PAs are expanding.

Frequently, the roles of house staff PAs encompass a fairly standard list of functions (Table 7-1). Duties may go beyond the basic job description depending on the PA's experience and training, pending approval of the hospital credentials committee. House staff PAs on the internal medicine floor have assumed a wide assortment of duties including bone marrow aspiration, thoracentesis, lumbar puncture, coronary angiography, and invasive radiologic procedures, as well as numerous other technical procedures.

House staff PAs may also be involved in clinical research activities, where their duties may include collecting specialized data on patients, monitoring therapeutic effects, participating in the analysis of clinical data, and overseeing professional communication. If the hospital is a teaching institution, the house staff PA may participate in teaching rounds, assist in

the training of third-year medical students and/or second-year PA students, and be involved in other clinical educational activities.

The role of the hospital PA as inpatient house staff has become well established in many hospitals. Institutions often employ 6 to 12 PAs, covering, with physician residents and attending physicians, services of 50 to 150 beds. Sometimes PA house staff duties encompass periods of emergency department (ED) or outpatient-clinic duties, depending on service and institutional needs. Some larger hospitals, may employ 75 or more PAs (Zarbock 1986).

Table 7-1 *Basic job description of a house staff PA*

As a member of the health care team, the PA will provide medical and/or surgical support to the hospital's attending physicians, nurses, and patients and may perform the following functions:

Review patient records to aid in determining health status.

Take patient histories, perform physical examinations, and identify normal and abnormal findings on histories, physicals, and commonly performed laboratory studies.

Perform developmental screening examinations on children.

Record pertinent patient data in the medical record.

Carry out or relay a physician's orders for diagnostic procedures, treatments, and medication in accordance with existing drug laws. The PA may transcribe the orders on the patient chart as a verbal or telephone order from the physician and may then sign it. Orders written by PAs may be reviewed by the physician.

Collect specimens for commonly performed blood counts and laboratory procedures.

Assist in surgery, fulfilling all requirements of a surgical assistant.

Provide preoperative and postoperative surgical and medical care.

Provide patient education, health promotion, and disease prevention instructions.

Screen patients to determine need for medical attention.

Other duties as delegated by the physician and approved by the credentials committee and the by-laws of the institution.

(Data from from Schafft and Cawley 1987a.)

SPECIALTY ROLES

After 1 or 2 years of general house staff experience, PAs may enter more specialized roles in hospital settings. Inpatient PAs are on the staff in many medical and surgical specialties and subspecialties (cardiology, pulmonary medicine, gastroenterology, nephrology, rheumatology, infectious disease, and oncology), in addition to internal medicine and geriatrics. In these disciplines, PAs not only assist physicians in routine patient care duties, but also perform many technical procedures. PAs who work in cardiology, for example, perform or assist in performing exercise stress tests, coronary angiography, and similar invasive and noninvasive diagnostic evaluations.

Hospital-based PAs are also involved in renal transplant teams, burn units, intensive care units, cardiac transplant teams, and neurology and neurologic units, as well as many specialty-oriented technical procedures. A number of PAs work in anesthesiology, and some PAs who specialize in cardiothoracic surgery have obtained additional formal training and certification in cardiac bypass pump technology. In a 1987 study, PAs performing coronary angiograms had a lower rate of complications than did cardiology fellows (Demots 1987). PAs are extensively deployed in neonatology and pediatric intensive care units (DeNicola 1994). For such PAs, three university centers provide extended specialty training programs.

PA roles in cardiothoracic surgery have grown at particularly rapid rates, and it is estimated that there are over 1,000 PAs in this field alone. Nearly all of these PAs are hospital based (typically in academic medical centers or large community medical centers) and perform a wide range of duties. These duties include preoperative evaluation and preparation of the patient, intraoperative assisting (harvesting the saphenous vein, establishing cardiopulmonary bypass, controlling bleeding, and wound closure), postoperative management of the patient in both the intensive care unit and later on the surgical ward, as well as a variety of other clinical, teaching, and administrative functions (Williams 1984). Some of the many other specialties that PAs have entered include neurology, neurosurgery, ENT, ophthalmology, dermatology, urology and urodynamics, renal dialysis, geriatrics, radiology, pathology, allergy and immunology, and infectious diseases.

The distribution of hospital-based PAs differs depending on geographic location. In 1995, the American Academy of Physician Assistants (AAPA) asked members to describe their location of practice. On average, 27% answered that they were located in a hospital setting. In the Northeast more than 40% of PAs work in a hospital setting. In the South and West, less than one in six PAs is hospital based (Fig. 7-1) (K. Kraditor, personal communication, 1996).

The distribution of hospital-based PAs has caught the attention of many health policy analysts, and various explanations for this phenomenon have been advanced. One leading reason for this is the disproportionally high use of international medical graduates as house offices on the East Coast. The increasing difficulty in filling these resident positions has led to replacement by PAs. This trend began in the early 1980s and seems to be increasing.

Another explanation for the difference in geographic distribution is the type of training programs on the East and West Coasts. The Medex model that began in Seattle was strictly outpatient based, both in training and in practice of its early graduates. The Duke model, on the other hand, began in the university hospital setting and continues to expose its students to an inpatient role. Many of the programs that sprang up in the Midwest and on the East Coast have followed the Duke model.

The third hypothesis that explains regional role differences for PAs is that the need for rural providers is far greater in the south central and western part of the United States than in most other regions of the country. The PA seems to be better suited to fill roles in these regions than in inpatient settings. Further research will concentrate on to what extent the PA who identifies a hospital as his or her location of practice actually provides inpatient services.

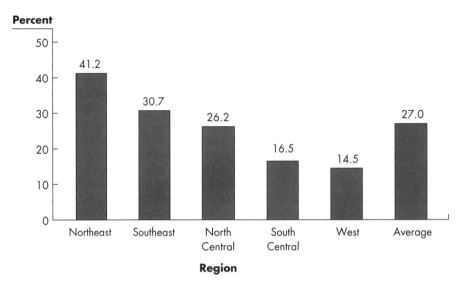

Figure 7-1 Percent of hospital-based PAs by region of the country.

In an effort to describe the roles of PAs in inpatient specialty roles, McKelvey and colleagues (1986) from the University of Iowa conducted a survey of 23 PAs employed by the university's medical center. Using both written questionnaires and personal interviews, McKelvey found that four PAs were in general medicine, one in general surgery, and the rest in various subspecialties: four in cardiothoracic surgery, two in pediatrics cardiology, three in hematology, and one each in radiology, psychiatry, occupational health, gynecologic oncology, urology, burn care, and cardiology. Two other PAs were in urologic oncology. The role activities of these providers and the mean percentage of time spent in each activity covered five areas: technical/procedural (18%), patient care (59.1%), administration (10.7%), research (5.2%), and medical education (6.2%). Patient education was identified as an important component of PA patient-care activities, ranging from 25% of all patient-care time in surgical specialties to 55% of patient-care time in pediatrics. Interestingly, when PAs' estimates of their activities were compared to their physician supervisors' estimates, more than 75% of the physicians significantly underestimated PA activity in patient education.

HOSPITAL CREDENTIALS

Although the PA is a dependent practitioner, he or she must develop and exercise some degree of independent clinical judgment to be effective. The parameters for the application of PA clinical judgments are usually first defined by existing state statutes on PAs and their scope of practice. At present, all states (except Mississippi) have laws regulating PAs. Beyond state regulations, hospitals develop their own institutional guidelines for employed PAs through amendments to the medical staff by-laws.

Hospitals review and approve the qualifications and backgrounds of health professionals before the granting of specific privileges. Since 1980, a wide variety of nonphysician health professionals have been given privileges by hospitals (Darr 1989). Typically, guidelines delineating the duties of a PA are developed by the credentials committee of the medical staff. These guidelines take into consideration the intended clinical duties, the specific needs and requirements of the medical attending staff, the expected training and qualifications of the PA, and provisions regarding supervision and monitoring of the PA's performance. An important part of these guidelines is the PA job description, which is often developed for each type of service on which PAs work (e.g., medicine, surgery, pediatrics). The PA's job description must accommodate both the common tasks and the specific duties on a given service (Morris 1975; Warren 1984).

Some of the basic methods of delineating clinical privileges include:

- A list of procedures
- Categorization according to severity of illness, level of training, or degree of required supervision
- Self-description

Most hospitals use the same form or process for PAs that they use for physicians in granting privileges. The system for granting provisional status for physicians is used for PAs as well. Usually, this requires proctoring until competence is shown. The AAPA's document *Hospital Privileges Summary* includes the major issues that a PA may encounter in seeking hospital privileges and typical hospital responsibilities.

Each state's PA credentialing guidelines specify what type of educational and professional qualifications a PA must have to receive privileges. Typically, a PA candidate is required (1) to be a graduate of an American Medical Association-approved PA training program, (2) to be eligible for or to have passed the national certifying examination administered by the National Commission on Certification of Physician Assistants (NCCPA), and (3) to be properly registered with the state's medical licensing board.

COSTS AND REIMBURSEMENT OF HOSPITAL PAs

Although hospitals employ PAs for many reasons, cost-effectiveness is one of the most important factors in many of these hiring decisions. It is no coincidence that the period of rapid growth of employment of PAs (beginning in the early 1980s) closely parallels the time when hospitals were coming under increasing pressure to contain costs. Even before the intro-

duction of diagnostic-related groups (DRGs) in 1982, many hospitals were faced with the problems of inadequate staffing, rising costs of physician and nursing staffing, and loss of physician-residency training programs. For many hospital administrators, the use of PAs in a restructured staffing pattern was an attractive solution to these problems.

Most PAs who work in hospitals are salaried employees. Their salaries depend on the type of service on which they work, the type of hospital, and the hours worked. Although this amount is slightly higher than salaries paid to interns and residents, it is far below what a fully licensed physician commands. Hospitals have found that by adjusting the mix of attending physicians, residents, and PAs, it is possible to reduce overall salary costs for inpatient staffing, yet preserve adequate levels of medical care. Before 1987, payment for services delivered in inpatient hospital settings by PAs was made either retrospectively on the basis of cost or prospectively on the basis of DRGs. Hospitals paid PAs as salaried employees, and there was no statutory provision under Medicare for or against payment of PA services when they were employed by hospitals.

In late 1986, Congress enacted the Omnibus Budget Reconciliation Act (PL 509), which for the first time permitted Medicare reimbursement to hospitals for services rendered by PAs. The Act modifies Medicare reimbursement policies and authorizes coverage of PAs assisting at surgery at a level of 65% of a physician's reasonable charge and 75% for PAs employed by hospitals. Payment is made to the employing hospital, physician, or physician group.

This legislation has made PAs even more attractive to hospitals and hospital-based physicians. Recognition of the value of PA services by the Medicare program had been a long-sought-after goal for the PA profession. This policy not only allows PAs to firmly justify their roles in institutional settings, but also has promoted the expanded use of PAs by hospitals that were previously reluctant to employ them. Since most third-party payers emulate the Medicare program in terms of reimbursement policies, they tend to reimburse PA services as well.

Another result of this policy change is the public's expanded access to health care and an improvement in quality of care. PAs are well known for being able to spend more time with patients, pay particular attention to patient's psychosocial needs, and place an increased emphasis on patient education and preventive approaches (Cawley 1992a). These attributes and the PA's proven cost-effectiveness should continue to increase the attractiveness of PAs in many institutional health care institutions.

While PAs are trained for roles in primary care, they have readily adapted to inpatient roles showing clinical competency in maintaining quality patient care (Frick 1986; McKelvey 1986).

In response to the interacting forces of predictions of an oversupply of physicians, a service-driven graduate medical education (GME) system, the growth of subspecialization, and the diminishing attraction of internal medicine for recent medical graduates, it is anticipated that teaching hospitals sponsoring residency programs in internal medicine and its subspecialties will reduce the number of available positions within the coming years. Teaching hospitals and academic health centers now face major changes in their medical staffing because of anticipated cutbacks in residency positions. The Council on Graduate Medical Education (COGME) and the Physician Payment Review Commission (PPRC), as well as influential others, have recommended that annual available physician residency slots be limited to 110% of the number of US allopathic and osteopathic medical graduates (COGME 1994; PPRC 1994). This policy approach is part of a larger plan that would restructure the personnel composition of GME and restructure its financing mechanisms, with the objective of reducing the overall number of physician specialists and subspecialists entering America's health care workforce.

If proposed changes affecting GME configuration becomes law, eventually the number of physician residency positions will be reduced from their current levels of 100,000 to roughly 75,000, eliminating about one-fourth of currently existing GME residency positions. The annual number of PG-1 residency positions available to medical school graduates would fall from 24,000 to about 17,000 positions.

Measures reducing the number of residents and shifting positions within subspecialty fields to those in primary care programs will be disruptive to teaching hospitals. Teaching hospitals with downsizing GME programs are likely to compensate for clinical service losses because of fewer residents in one of three ways: (1) by reducing clinical services/eliminating beds, (2) by enlisting community and attending physicians to provide housestaff coverage, or (3) by substituting nonphysician providers to augment clinical service staffing.

With an overall expected loss of about 11,000 residents within GME-sponsoring institutions, the PPRC considered outcomes from the likely consequences of residency downsizing and used data to project that in order to meet the medical staffing requirements within teaching hospitals brought about by GME downsizing, and assuming that most institutions will continue to provide roughly current levels of services, an additional 7,700 nonphysician health practitioners (either PAs or NPs) would be required to meet this workforce demand (PPRC 1994).

The PPRC does not specify how many of each type of nonphysician provider is included in the 7,700 figure. One could assume that this requirement would be equally met by PAs and NPs. To distinguish between PAs and NPs here may be important; based on current evidence from utilization patterns, as well as common perception, PAs seem to be more likely than NPs to be employed by acute care hospitals, particularly in resident-substitute positions. While this is not to ignore the number of NPs presently working in inpatient settings in medical or surgical subspecialties, available data and expert opinion from both professions concur that these trends appear accurate.

If the requirement for an additional 7,700 nonphysician providers is met by an equal number of PAs and NPs, a sizable additional number (3,850) of each type of provider would be needed in the health workforce just to meet GME downsizing needs. This number is greater than the annual number of graduates; in 1996, there were approximately 2,500 PA graduates, and 4,500 NP (including certified nurse midwives [CNM]) graduates. The total number of nonphysician providers in active clinical practice in 1996 in the United States is estimated at 60,000 (28,000 PAs and 32,000 NPs, which includes 4,100 CNMs). Thus, it would appear that if PAs and other types of nonphysicians are expected to plug a large part of the health personnel gap brought about by GME downsizing, a significant increase in the supply of educational program graduates for these professionals will be necessary.

POTENTIAL OF PAs TO FILL RESIDENT ROLES

PAs can fill roles where they essentially substitute for physician residents (Cawley 1991; Ripportella-Muller 1995; Stoddard 1994). PA utilization in the inpatient settings has certain advantages: some faculty prefer to work with PA house staff; PAs may have a lower turnover rate, increased service continuity, be more familiar with departmental routines, and possess greater clinical expertise than junior residents. Using PAs in former resident positions on teaching services in internal medicine programs is not only less costly on an annual basis, but also enriches the residents educational experiences. By redistributing patient care duties among residents and PA house staff, medical staffing reports mention high levels of acceptance by employing physicians and patients, favorable cost-benefit, and maintenance of quality patient care. PA utilization in GME substitution roles results in improvements in clinical efficacy. Additional benefits in using PAs include improvement in continuity of care, richer educational experiences for residents, and overall cost savings for sponsoring institutions (Frick 1983).

Knickman and colleagues from New York University (1992) addressed the clinical potentials for several types of nonphysician providers to fulfill resident roles. While the estimates of PA-specific capacities for resident substitution is not precise, these data offer insight by comparing the proportion of levels of PA capabilities to assume physician-resident inpatient clinical duties in teaching hospitals. The exercise is useful in addressing current workforce issues related to PA roles in the downsizing of GME programs.

In their time-motion study examining the clinical activities of two NPs and eight internal medicine residents in two New York City teaching hospitals, Knickman and colleagues documented the time taken by physicians versus other types of health personnel in performing inpatient medical care tasks traditionally done by physician residents. They compared those times estimated using physicians and nonphysicians under a revised inpatient staffing model. To determine the time per task activity potential for resident substitution, inpatient clinical, educational, personal, and administrative activities were classified by (1) tasks that had to be done by physicians, (2) tasks that were educational only, and (3) tasks that could be done by nonphysician providers or other health personnel. A total of 1,726 specific activities were recorded. Under scenario 1, the traditional model in which the physician serves as the primary medical manager of the patient, about half of a resident's time is spent in activities that must be performed by a physician. Under an alternative model in which a PA or NP would assume an appropriate level of clinical responsibility for day-to-day patient monitoring, only 20% of activities would require a physician (Table 7-2). The study concluded that there is substantial potential for PAs and NPs to assume inpatient medical tasks, that only 20% of each resident's lost time needs to be replaced with other physicians' time, and that to achieve this level of clinical efficiency, inpatient hospital staffing models would need to be restructured in which the contributions of nonphysicians can be used to augment physician services (Knickman 1992).

Table 7-2 *Personnel who could be substituted/needed to perform physician resident activities, two staffing scenarios, by percent time*

	TRADITIONAL MODEL		PA/NP MODEL	
	NUMBER	%	NUMBER	%
Physician only	6,248	46.7	2,693	20.0
None (education activities)	2,778	20.7	2,778	20.8
None (personal time)	1,800	13.3	1,800	13.4
Nurse	588	4.5	449	3.4
Laboratory technician	160	1.2	160	1.2
Unskilled personnel	822	6.1	822	6.0
PA/NP	988	7.4	4,681	35.0
Total	13,384	100.0	13,383	100.0

(Data from Knickman 1992.)

The demand on hospitals is already being felt in the medical personnel marketplace. In recently reported data (AHA 1992) based on an American Hospital Association (AHA) survey of 3,184 US hospitals, the vacancy rate for PAs rose from 10.1% in 1991 to 12.3% in 1992 and was expected to climb even higher in 1993. The 1992 double-digit vacancy rate for PAs was the second highest ranked profession among the 25 health occupations reported in the AHA survey.

FINANCING ISSUES

As policy makers consider reform measures that would change methods of GME financing and structure, PAs may play an increasingly important role in augmenting medical care services in hospital-based settings. PA utilization in hospital-based roles, particularly in institutions sponsoring GME programs, has become commonplace. PAs more than NPs are employed in teaching hospitals, filling positions in which they essentially substitute for physician residents.

For the training of physicians, financial support through Medicare is provided directly to teaching hospitals sponsoring the clinical specialty training of physicians after medical school. The 3- to 8-year process of GME takes place largely in teaching hospital settings and comprises clinical educational experiences in which physicians complete their medical professional preparation and obtain qualification for state medical licensure and specialty board certification. Medicare finances a large proportion of physician residency training (GME) by reimbursing hospital charges through a direct cost "pass through" mechanism and by allowing for an indirect cost educational adjustment for payments to hospitals eligible for reimbursement for educational activities under Medicare Part A DRG payments.

In the 1986 Consolidated Omnibus Budget Reconciliation Act (PL-99-272 Sec 9202), Congress fixed certain limits on the allowable cost per physician resident in an attempt to slow the growth of physician residency programs in certain subspecialties perceived to be overcrowded. The Act established new incentives for the expansion of primary care residency training and contained mild disincentives for the training of future subspecialists at then current levels.

MEDICARE SUPPORT OF HEALTH PROFESSIONS EDUCATION

Teaching institutions now face cutbacks in Medicare subsidies for medical education. These hospitals are compensated for their GME activities under Medicare payments proportional to the number of Medicare-covered patient/days. Medicare direct medical education (DME) and indirect medical education adjustment (IMEA) payments are based on hospital eligibility criteria relative to levels of noncompensated care. These payments do not cover PA-delivered clinical services even when augmenting physician residency services in teaching hospital settings. State-imposed legal limitations on the numbers of hours worked by physician residents are also becoming increasingly common and further accentuate hospitals' problems in adequately staffing inpatient services.

In an effort to assess the financial impact of resident cutbacks stemming from limitation of resident work hours per week in teaching hospitals in New York state a number of options were examined. One option for hospitals included enlisting attending physicians to replace residents, or hiring licensed physicians to serve as house officers, both expensive options. A staffing mix using PAs with physician residents was determined to be far less costly in providing necessary coverage levels for inpatient services ($160 versus $85 million) than the former option. Yet the adoption of such an approach would require about 1,300 additional PAs for New York teaching hospitals alone, when the annual current supply of PAs is 2,000 and where many hospitals already have difficulty in attracting sufficient numbers of PAs (Foreman 1993).

Hospitals employing PAs as general medical house staff and/or in GME substitution roles are believed to be using one of two existing financing methods to obtain reimbursement to cover costs of inpatient PA staffing: (1) by incorporating their costs into per diem charges that are billed and reimbursed under Medicare Part A DRG-based payments, or (2) by billing for the clinical services performed by PAs through eligibility under Medicare Part B, which allows payment when PA services are performed in certain settings. Before Part B eligibility (P.L. 99–509, OBRA, 1986), hospitals employing PAs typically covered their employment costs by building them into the per diem charges hospitals billed under Medicare, DRG-based, Part A allowances. It is believed that many hospitals continue to finance their use of PAs through this mechanism, rather than by billing for PA services under the Medicare Part B option.

SUMMARY

Expansion of the roles of PAs into the hospital setting has been the most significant recent trend in health care's use of these professionals. Initially intended to be primary-care providers, PAs have moved into the institutional setting with ease and in large numbers

to assume roles as medical and surgical inpatient house staff and as assistants to specialists and subspecialists. In most instances, they have adapted to these types of roles without postgraduate training. PAs in hospitals maintain or improve the existing level of quality and access to medical care, are cost-effective in the delivery of inpatient services, and display extensive clinical versatility among the various medical disciplines.

The use of PAs in hospitals emerged from changing forces in the health-personnel supply pool and mandated adjustments in the patterns of GME. Employing PAs has permitted hospitals to maintain cost effectively the required level of patient care, has allowed residency programs to balance the number of specialty-trained physicians, and thereby has contributed to a more balanced supply of specialists in overcrowded fields. The use of PAs has also contributed to increasing the continuity of care on hospital services and to measures that enrich the quality of residency education for physicians in training.

To accommodate PAs as inpatient providers, amended medical staff by-laws now recognize the education and expertise of PAs and provide the institutional sanction necessary to perform inpatient duties under the supervision of physicians. Accrediting groups, such as the Joint Commission on Accreditation of Healthcare Organizations, have acknowledged the roles of PAs as inpatient health providers and have made recommendations about how hospitals can most appropriately recognize, regulate, and utilize them.

Federal legislation has clarified and established policies whereby employing hospitals are now reimbursed for services provided by PAs. The significance of these actions is the recognition by major third-party payers of the value of PAs in rendering quality clinical services in a variety of settings. Such measures solidify the role of the PA as an important member of the health care team.

The demand for PAs in a broad variety of inpatient settings will continue. Employment trends indicate a strong demand for PAs among hospitals and not enough PAs to fill available positions (Rohrs 1988).

The successful incorporation of PAs in the inpatient hospital setting indicates that these providers are well accepted by physicians, administrators, and patients. This acceptance has been earned by PAs who, working with physicians, have adapted to the demands of the hospital environment. There is every reason to believe that PAs will continue to function successfully in the hospital setting.

A cautionary note needs to be interjected here. The role of hospitals is changing as a result of rising health care costs, increasing use of medical technology outside the hospital, managed care, and the implementation of health care reform (either formally or informally), particularly at the state level. Ultimately, there will be fewer hospitals; those remaining will be smaller and much more focused. They will become cost centers rather than revenue centers. Health professionals will be trained to deliver health care services across a continuum of care, and hospitals will no longer be the core business of the American health care system (Shortell 1995).

8

Nonclinical Roles and Opportunities

The issue of physician assistant (PA) career mobility leads to consideration of the attrition of PAs from their original profession. Surveys suggest about 15% of all individuals who have graduated from PA educational programs are no longer in full-time clinical practice as PAs (Cawley 1986b; AAPA 1996b). With 85% of formally trained PAs in some PA-type role, this level of professional retention is higher than that noted for allied health and nursing occupations. Only physician retention is slightly higher (Sibley 1982).

Most of the 15% of PAs who are not considered practicing PAs are individuals who still work within the PA profession or in the health care field but are not directly engaged in clinical services delivery. Some have obtained additional degrees in medically related fields (e.g., public health, health care administration, education, physicians) and have assumed various roles. Others represent PA program faculty. At least 70% of faculty maintain part-time (average of 10 hours/week) clinical practices in addition to their educational duties; 62% of PA program directors remain in clinical practice (A. Simon 1996). Some PAs have combined their years of clinical experience and expertise with graduate degrees in administration and have evolved into roles in health services management; some have assumed public health positions and roles in research and health pol-

icy Table 8-1. About 2% of all persons trained as PAs are either allopathic or osteopathic physicians (Jones 1994b).

It seems clear that the PA credential is becoming increasingly recognized in the health care field as a valuable background, permitting individuals to move into many types of expanded clinical and nonclinical roles. Nor does attrition from the PA profession appear to be a major problem. One can argue that, in any profession, a predictable number of people will migrate to other related roles or explore new and expanding areas of opportunities. Moreover, one could view this as a positive feature that affords individuals in the profession a rather wide degree of career latitude if they decide to seek expanded or alternate roles. As PAs become increasingly accepted in the health care field, it is likely that more opportunities will become open. As Eugene Schneller (1994) writes:

> The fact that some PAs are not satisfied with their level of autonomy and seek career advancement outside of the PA field is not, in my opinion, cause for concern. From its origins the PA occupation has been an "accelerator" occupation, allowing members to work to their potential and to aspire to the tasks performed by their supervisor. This is the essence of the occupation's design. A minority will realize that the PA occupation

is not their final occupation destination. The one-life, one-career imperative is no longer active. Recall that the PA was designed by physicians and that, in the early years, the occupation was "managed" by medicine. PAs have now come to positions of great respect and power as educators and as members of organizations that represent PAs. These advocates for the PA must not become so attached to the desires of some portion of the membership that they jeopardize the most important features of the occupation.

Some nonclinical or alternative roles that PAs have made in their career are described in the following sections.

Table 8-1 *Nonclinical roles of PAs*

Attorney
Academic educator/researcher
Consultant for political candidates
Forensic scientist/legal expert
Hospital administration
Health facility owner/entrepreneur
Health information management
Health insurance management
Health lobbying
Health planner/regulator
Health services administration
Health services research/health policy
Industrial hygienist
Insurance reviewer
Malpractice reviewer
Medical editor/publisher
Medical epidemiologist
Naturopath
PA service/house staff administrator
PA educational faculty/administration
Pharmaceutical representative
Physician
Politician
Professional recruiter
Public health officer
Researcher, clinical and medical social

ATTORNEY

Pursuit of law has become a career move for more than 20 PAs. Many have retained their membership in the American Association of Physician Assistants (AAPA), and the majority have maintained an interest in medicine and risk management. A few have even returned to medicine after finding the role of a general practice lawyer too competitive.

Health care contracting, along with the numerous regulations unique to this field, has been of interest to a number of PAs who have become attorneys (Blaser 1993).

ACADEMIC EDUCATOR

The vast majority of PA programs have PAs in educational roles such as director, academic coordinator, and clinic coordinator (A. Simon 1996). Because these programs are set in academic institutions, the program directors and faculty usually have faculty rank from lecturer to full professor. In many instances, the academic rank carries with it some requirement to periodically publish original research.

BROKER, FINANCIAL

A background in clinical medicine and pharmacology is necessary for certain areas of stock trading and financing. Options are few but exist where PAs have been able to enter this market as stock analysts.

CONSULTANT FOR POLITICAL CANDIDATES

In the early 1990s, most political candidates found that they needed to be particularly informed about health policy and health care reform. As part of a campaign strategy, many candidates and political office holders found they understood some of the issues affecting physician, nurse, hospital, and insurance, but lacked understanding of other health workers such as PAs, NPs, podiatrists, psychologists, and nursing home employees. In some instances, individual PAs were invited to participate in campaigns and help shape health policy positions.

FORENSIC SCIENTIST/
LEGAL EXPERT

The role of the PA in forensic medicine has been documented on a few occasions (Golden 1986; Wright 1987; Cardenas 1993; Sylvester 1996). Sometimes these PAs function as city or county medical examiners or coroners; at other times, they are called on to act as forensic scientists and experts in homicides.

HOSPITAL ADMINISTRATION

Hospital administration is a natural progression for many health workers interested in the management side of health care organization. Many PAs start by assuming some of the administrative roles associated with medical office or department management, often balancing clinical activities with organizational roles. These roles include straight administration, health planning, utilization review, and budgeting. Some may pursue a management degree and move full-time into these roles. Various attempts have been made within the AAPA to create a hospital administration coalition of PAs, but most PAs in these roles find their needs are better met with the myriad number of professional societies devoted to health care organization and management.

HEALTH FACILITY
OWNER/DIRECTOR

PAs have sometimes become owners of health facilities, usually a small medical office. In one scenario, the PA is hired by two physician-owners of a rural clinic. After a time, one of the partners retires and the partnership half is offered to the PA. With more time, the PA may even buy out the second physician or find another physician with whom to partner. In a variation on this theme the PA-owner hires a physician as an employee to act as his or her supervising physician.

Other scenarios include PAs developing or purchasing clinics in small rural towns to run for profit, or purchasing part of the business such as the office equipment or the building. Many times these PAs will become the clinic director/manager (Blaser 1993).

One enterprise was the development of a company made up of Medex-trained PAs who then purchased small hospitals in rural areas and staffed the senior management with PAs.

INSURANCE MANAGEMENT

PAs have been employees and managers in health insurance companies (other than HMOs) for more than a decade. They help to review cases, assign discharge diagnoses (diagnostic-related groups [DRGs]), provide utilization review, analyze reports, summarize the medical literature, and provide advice on policy matters (Webster 1990).

LOBBYING, HEALTH

While health lobbying does not attract too many health professionals, a few PAs do venture into this area on the state level. Most are associated with a health care organization, and are not free-lance lobbyists. Some PAs have become part-time professional lobbyists after trying to modify state laws to enable PAs to practice with fewer barriers and restrictions.

PRACTICE MANAGEMENT
CONSULTANTS

Patient flow and satisfaction of providers are key ingredients to any organization. Numerous

PAs have served as practice management consultants for various organizations. Their roles vary: advising senior managers about how to best use PAs and NPs, working with the PA/NP part of an HMO in negotiations, training support staff in public relations, developing policies and procedures for a new clinic, evaluating staff members, and negotiating salaries for PAs and NPs (Blaser 1993).

RECRUITERS, PA

Recruitment of PAs has become a thriving business for recruitment consultants and placement enterprises. The demand for PAs has increased since 1980, when PAs competed for few jobs. Now every PA graduate has a wide choice of employers in most geographic areas.

The typical search consultant is fairly gregarious and enjoys substantial interaction and communication with people. He or she may be on the telephone 3 to 6 hours a day and will work evenings talking to candidates who prefer being contacted at home. A match with a candidate and employer may require up to 50 calls.

To increase the rate of return for this effort, the consultant networks with clinics, hospitals, providers, and anyone who offers assistance in efforts to locate potential candidates and employers. They will subscribe to dozens of health care publications, and utilize medical literature databases to find authors and other specialists in sought-after fields. They will not only attend seminars and conferences, but often will sponsor or speak at these assemblies.

In the 1970s, as PAs were trying to break into new employment opportunities, many experienced candidates paid fees for assistance in locating new positions. While these situations still exist, they tend to concentrate almost exclusively on entry level positions. Today payment of search fees for recruitment services is almost always borne by the employer. Clients choose from contingency or retained search approaches. Contingency assignments are paid with a one-time fee earned at the successful conclusion of a search (defined as an offer being made by the employer and accepted by the candidate).

In the ideal situation, a medical center desires to hire a PA with certain qualifications, and the search firm identifies a pool of interested candidates. As an example let's suppose the Kansas City Psychiatric Institute wants to hire an experienced psychiatric PA. The firm Medical Associates Unlimited is contracted to conduct the search. The first source they may contact is the AAPA to identify PAs who have identified themselves as psychiatric PAs. Calling these PAs reveals that 20 meet these criteria, but none of them are interested at this time in a change of location. However, contact with these 20 PAs identifies another 10 who may not belong to the AAPA but do practice psychiatry. The American Psychiatric Association identifies another two PAs who are not on the AAPA list. From this list, three PAs are identified who express some interest in a job and location change. The recruiter may facilitate contact with the two parties, or may reveal the names of both and allow them to contact each other. At all times when recruiters call these various psychiatric PAs, they should identify themselves, who they represent, and how they obtained the PA's name. Sometimes this information will be kept confidential, but usually the sources do not mind having their identities revealed.

A small, but growing segment of recruiting firms employ or are owned by PAs. While there is no reason to believe they are any more efficient in recruiting than any other agency, there tends to be a certain appeal by candidates to be called on by a "fellow PA." Perhaps there is a belief that the recruiter will be more versed with your wants and needs (Atwater 1993).

RESEARCH, HEALTH SERVICES/HEALTH POLICY

Only a handful of PAs work in health services research. While it is difficult to break into this field without significant research background and experience, more and more PAs are finding this an area of interest. With more PA programs expanding into graduate level studies, research may become more important for PAs.

Some PAs have established clinical research firms and consulting businesses. These entrepreneurial companies contract with pharmaceutical or research companies to conduct part of a clinical trial or recruit participants. They establish a contract with one or more physicians to be principal investigators, using their practice facilities and recruiting their patients into trials (Blaser 1993).

INDUSTRIAL HYGIENIST

Industrial hygienists are usually employed by industry or large manufacturers to help with the health management of their employees. The petroleum companies were the first to use PAs and, since the late 1970s, many companies have expanded their corporate goal of reducing worker-related injuries and illnesses by employing PAs.

EPIDEMIOLOGIST, MEDICAL

The Centers for Disease Control and Prevention allow PAs to qualify as health officers through their intensive medical epidemiologist course. PAs in this role are prepared to respond to disease outbreaks as members of a medical investigation team.

NATUROPATH

PAs have formally trained as doctors of naturopathy (NDs). Sometimes they combine their roles to allow for prescription writing, and sometimes NDs have gone on to train as PAs.

PHARMACEUTICAL REPRESENTATIVE

Both formally and informally trained PAs have moved into the area of manufacturer representative for pharmaceutical companies. Most major pharmaceutical companies have hired at least one PA for detailing products to prescribers. Sometimes they have remained in the area of sales, but others have found niches within pharmaceutical companies that allow them to specialize as research liaisons to clinical trials.

PHYSICIAN

An estimated 2% of all PAs have matriculated through medical or osteopathic schools (Jones, 1994b). Little is known about where they have located and how they are functioning. Anecdotally, physicians who were formally PAs are generally satisfied with their career as physicians, but those in primary care do not feel they are functioning much differently than they were as PAs.

POLITICIAN

Only a few PAs have ventured into the area of politics, almost always on the local level. They have functioned as city council members, mayors, county commissioners, and state representatives. At least one PA has run for the Congress.

PA JOURNALISM

Journalism within any profession is a reflection of its maturity. How and what a profession says about itself is an evolving process, and the way it promotes itself in journalism and literature is a measurement of its sophistication. Fortunately, this has been a subject of interest to a significant segment of the PA profession, and the increasing numbers of articles authored by PAs has allowed more than one publication to exist at the same time. Cawley (1985b) summed it this way:

> PAs and health care providers communicate with each other through the pages of the professional journals. These journals reflect the thoughts, direction, and vitality of the profession. It follows then, that our profession is judged in part by the quality and content of the PA literature.

The first official journal of the American Academy of Physician Assistants was launched in 1970 by Charles B. Slack, Inc., a publisher in New Jersey. Initially, the volumes were titled *Physician's Associate*. This name reflects the few years that the AAPA was the *American Academy of Physician's Associates*. Later, when the name changed to *American Academy of Physician Assistants*, the name *PA Journal* was adopted.

This first foray into professional journalism contained a number of key members of the profession: Don Detmer, MD; Ann Bliss, MSW; Carl Emil Fasser, PA; Bill Stanhope, PA; David Lawrence, MD, MPH; Steve Turnipseed, MX; John Ott, MD; Bill De'Ak, MD; and others. Later known as the "Green Journal" because of its distinctive cover, the *PA Journal* served "as a forum for the discussion and presentation of important issues related to the advancement of the physician's assistant and other health professional auxiliaries..." (from the masthead of the *PA Journal* – Vol. 4, No 2, 1974).

While the green journal was still in publication, a small independent publisher, United Business Publications, Inc., launched a magazine in 1976 called *Physician Assistant*. Both journals were competing for essentially the same audience and the same advertising revenue. This competition has remained intense ever since. Ultimately neither journal proved particularly viable financially, and the first version of *Physician Assistant* folded a few years later.

Meanwhile, a new prospective publisher, F & F Publications, entered discussion with the AAPA concerning the possibility of a new journal for the profession. An agreement was reached whereby the AAPA granted a 1-year endorsement to *Health Practitioner* (the initial plan was to distribute it to PAs and NPs). As Steve Tiger notes in his history of *Physician Assistant*, the earliest national conferences were designated for "health practitioners," and it was not until a few years later that the annual conference became specifically a PA function (Tiger 1992).

Over the next several years, the name and ownership of the new journal changed a few times. The first issue of *Health Practitioner* was distributed at the May 1977 AAPA conference in Houston. By the end of the year, the tag line "Magazine for Physician Assistants" was added to the title. Next, the defunct title *Physician Assistant* was obtained from its publisher, and that title took the place of the tag line for the March 1978 issue, which was called *Health Practitioner and Physician Assistant Magazine*. Starting with the next issue, the name was simplified to *Health Practitioner/Physician Assistant*. In August 1979, the order was reversed, and the name became *Physician Assistant/Health Practitioner* (reflecting the fact that the audience was primarily PAs). Meanwhile, PW Communications took over publication from F & F Publications. In 1983, *Health Practitioner* was dropped from the title, and the publication became known by its current name *Physician Assistant*. Excerpta Medica purchased *Physician Assistant* from PW Communications and has been listed as the publisher since the October 1989 issue.

During these developments, the AAPA affiliation resumed and ended again. The initial endorsement expired after the March 1978 issue. In January 1983, after the green *PA Journal* had finally folded, *Physician Assistant* again became the official publication of the AAPA; that relationship continued through June 1987, when the Academy was ready to introduce its own new publication, *The Journal of the American Academy of Physician Assistants* (Tiger 1992).

There have been other journals. Peter Frishauf, one of the founders of *Health Practitioner/Physician Assistant*, produced a series of publications that ran for 5 years—*PA 84* through *PA 88*. *PA Drug Update* began in 1980 as a magazine of "continuing medical education for physician assistants." *AAPA Recertification Update* began in 1990 as a special publication to prepare students and graduates for the recertification process under the editorship of Sarah Zarbock, PA. It ended after 4 years of publication. In 1993 *Advance for Physician Assistants*, a new publication "to provide timely and useful information about clinical and practice issues," was launched by Michelle P. Pronsati, Editor. Three publications emerged in the 1990s to market for the recruitment of PAs. *Newsline for Physician Assistants* began publishing in 1991;

PA Today began in 1993; and *PA Career,* an AAPA-generated employment magazine, began in 1992 and merged with *AAPA News* in 1995.

That so many journals are published so frequently speaks for the market attraction of the profession. Some, like *PA Practice* and *AAPA Recertification,* are single pharmaceutical manufacturer's publications that may have some endorsement from the AAPA. Single-sponsored monographs have come and gone. One such example, *PA Drug Update,* has been in the hands of PAs since 1982. Underwritten by Pfizer Pharmaceuticals, it has a number of topics written by specialists in various fields, then wrapped with a cover and distributed to PAs. Other versions similar to *PA Drug Update* are sent to physicians and medical students under different names but with similar contents. This particular publication is a membership benefit for AAPA members.

Advance for PAs is one of the latest publication to seek a niche in the growing PA market. This is the twelfth in a series of 13 "news magazines" by Merion Publications. All are titled *Advance for ...* (e.g., *Advance for Nurse Practitioners, Advance for Physical Therapists, Advance for Occupational Therapists*), and all emphasize day-to-day articles that are clinically relevant for the type of provider they target. *Newsline for Physician Assistants,* similar to *Advance for PAs,* along with *PA Careers,* and *PA Today,* were launched in 1992. Usually they have some short articles on the profession or profile some PA. Recruitment ads and advertisements are the sources of revenue for most journals (Table 8-2).

Clinician Reviews was a break-away publication of *Physician Assistant.* Formed in 1989 by two PAs (David Mittman and Tom Yakeren), *Clinician Reviews* has done what others have failed to do—appeal to a wider audience. This high-quality, bimonthly-glossy journal is marketed to both PAs and NP/CNMs. They claim a subscription distribution of 50,000.

In January 1988, for the first time, the AAPA had a journal with editorial control solely in the hands of the Academy—staff, editorial board, and Leslie Kole, PA, as the editor of the *Journal of the American Academy of Physician Assistants*

Table 8-2 *Current national PA-oriented journals*

AAPA News (for AAPA members)
Journal of the American Academy of Physician Assistants
  (JAAPA)
Physician Assistant (PA Journal)
Clinician Reviews (for PAs and NPs)
Advance for Physician Assistants (PA)
PA Today
Newsline for Physician Assistants

(JAAPA) (Kole 1988). Initially published by Mosby, it has been published by Medical Economics since 1994. As of 1997, *JAAPA* has published over 6,000 pages of clinical articles, policy papers, surveys, scientific studies, editorials, debates, letters, and essays. More than 90% of the contributions have been authored by PAs.

Constituent Chapter Newsletters

Since the development of constituent chapters, there has been an attempt to collect and redistribute information on the decentralized and local PA level. Usually this was by and for PAs in a state affiliation. Like so many fledgling social and professional groups, at first these were just letters typed and mimeographed. Later they would improve along with the technology and be reproduced by photocopying. Now most newsletters are professionally published on word processors and laptop computers. Often the product is reproduced on high-speed printing presses or photocopiers. Little is known about the quality or substance of these early newsletters and publications. Undoubtedly they ranged the full spectrum in scope and readability. A giant boost in these publications came in the mid-1980s when the Leaderle Corporation made unrestricted grants to all 50 chapters to purchase personal computers and other equipment for newsletters. Many of these PCs are currently in use. Today, virtually every special interest group stays in touch by paper; some have ventured into the Internet for better communication.

Books

PAs have authored at least 20 books (Table 8-3), some of which are clinical while others are on the PA profession. Many PAs have been part of special documents and special reports. A few have ventured into fiction and medical history (R. Currey 1992).

ELECTRONIC FORMATS

Through support by Duke University, the Internet is available for PAs in a number of forums: the PA Forum, Student PA Forum, PA Faculty Forum, and PAs in Primary Care Forum. Known as lists, these forums are usually lively exchanges of opinions by PAs and include a wide range of subjects.

As an extension of the Internet, the Academy operates a PA page on the World Wide Web. This is located at the following address: http://www.aapa.org. The Web site provides basic information about the PA profession that PAs can use to educate others and to answer commonly asked questions about PAs and the AAPA. Additional information directed to someone in the Academy can be obtained via the Internet at aapa@aapa.org.

CONCLUSION

Many PAs have found nonclinical positions in health care. Some have used their PA background and experience to branch into related fields, whereas others have acquired further formal education. Employment opportunities and training have led many PAs into more complex and different roles. About 4% of all PAs have moved on to medical/osteopathic school. Employment patterns for PAs are extremely variable, depending on the interests, capabilities, and personalities of the individuals involved. All have used their PA training as a springboard for this change.

Table 8-3 *Books authored by and/or targeted for PAs*

1972	*The Physician's Assistant: Today and Tomorrow*, by Sadler, Sadler, and Bliss. First book on the PA profession.
1975	*The Physician Assistant: a National and Local Analysis*, by Ford.
1977	*The New Health Professionals: Nurse Practitioners and Physician's Assistants*, by Bliss and Cohen.
	The Physician's Assistant: A Baccalaureate Curriculum, by Myers.
1978	*The Physician's Assistant: Innovation in the Medical Division of Labor*, by Schneller.
1981	*Staffing Primary Care in 1990: Physician Replacement and Cost Savings*, by Record, documents that PAs in HMO settings provide 79% of the care of a primary care physician, at 50% of the cost.
	The Art of Teaching Primary Care, by Golden, Hagan, and Carlson.
1982	*Physician Assistants: Their Contribution to Health Care*, by Perry and Breitner.
1984	*First Annual Report on Physician Assistant Educational Programs in the United States*, by Oliver and the Association of Physician Assistant Programs.
	Alternatives in Health Care Delivery, edited by Carter and Perry.
1986	*Physician Assistants: New Models of Utilization*, edited by Zarbock and Harbert.
1987	*The Physician Assistant in a Changing Health Care Environment*, by Schafft and Cawley.
1993	*The Role of the Physician Assistant and Nurse Practitioner in Primary Care*, edited by Clawson and Osterweis.
1994	*Physician Assistant: A Guide to Clinical Practice*, edited by Ballweg, Stolberg, and Sullivan.
1995	*The Physician Assistant Medical Handbook*, by Labus.
1997	*The Physician Assistant in American Medicine*, by Hooker and Cawley.

PA journalism involves both writing and publishing. A number of ventures have been launched with PAs as the target audience. These enterprises have expanded as the profession has grown and will likely continue, an acknowledgment that this profession has come of age and is an important audience to observe.

9

Economic Basis

Are physician assistants (PAs) cost-effective? Are they productive enough to be considered replacements for physicians? If they are cost-effective, do the benefits of employing PAs accrue to the employer, the patient, or society as a whole?

What happens to the output of a physician's practice, inpatient service, or outpatient clinic when a PA is added to the clinical staff? What are the outcomes in terms of access to patient care services, level of quality of care, practice revenues, and productivity? While the practice contributions of PAs are determined by multiple influences, many of which are difficult to measure, a number of PA clinical performance characteristics have been well described in health services research. Many of the findings, some performed years ago, still appear to be valid (Schneider 1977; Greenfield 1978).

Numerous studies have shown that within their spheres of practice competency, PAs provide lower cost health care that is comparable, and in some instances superior, to that provided by physicians (OTA 1986). While PA cost-effectiveness has not been conclusively demonstrated in all clinical practice settings (McCibbin 1978), substantial empirical and health services research evidence confirm the findings that they are cost-effective in most of the settings studied (Romm 1979; Record 1980; Cawley 1986a). Probably more significant, their increasing popularity and utilization in clinical settings would be unlikely if these health providers were not cost-effective.

Evidence indicates that the organizational setting is closely related to the productivity and possible cost benefits of PA utilization. Scheffler documented that PAs employed in institutional settings are more productive than those in private practice in that they see more patients in the same period of time (Scheffler 1979). Record and colleagues noted correlations among productivity, delegation of tasks, and organizational size; they proposed that personnel economies of scale and cost savings incentives were the likely explanations for their observations on PA cost-effectiveness in the health maintenance organization (HMO) setting (Record 1981a).

This chapter examines the central health policy issue of PA cost-effectiveness and the financial impact of utilizing PAs in clinical practice. The major studies that have examined PA productivity and cost-effectiveness and the limitations and generalization of this data are considered. The chapter also assesses the applicability of cost-effectiveness analysis to PA employment and medical care labor. Finally, the beneficiaries of PA employment is reviewed.

BACKGROUND

The performance of PAs in the delivery of medical care services has been extensively studied, beginning in the early 1970s. There was an intense effort to document what was generally regarded as a labor savings device for physicians. Some researchers wanted to document the PA's effectiveness, whereas others thought the stories of PA utilization were overstated. Few professions just beginning have known such scrutiny. Spitzer (1984) notes that

... the introduction of physician assistants has been a responsible policy and ... that many other innovations mediated by medical practitioners have gained widespread acceptance with much less rigorous prior evaluation than was given to ... physician assistants.

The impact of PAs on access to health care services, quality of care, as well as physician and patient acceptance continues to be measured with positive results. The precise degree of productivity and cost-effectiveness of the utilization of PAs, however, remains to be determined; the downstream benefits of PA employment is unclear because the vast majority of PA productivity studies have been viewed as substitutes rather than members of interdisciplinary health care teams (Scheffler 1996).

Almost all the economic research on PAs have examined cost-effectiveness of PA employment. Cost-effectiveness analysis is an economic technique designed to compare the positive and negative consequences of a specific resource allocation. It seeks to measure the comparable benefit of a particular investment versus its cost. In health care, this technique is commonly applied to new medical technologies, diagnostic and laboratory tests, health facilities and delivery systems, and drug treatment and immunization programs.

The application of cost-effectiveness analysis in general to the delivery of medical care services and specifically to the provider of such services is a complex endeavor. It is difficult to measure accurately the content of a medical encounter, given variations in such factors as severity of illness, types of treatment, patient preferences, extent of use of diagnostic tests, level of provider training, and the site and mode of care delivery. Add to these factors the differences in the type of provider delivering a similar service and different styles of task delegation, and it becomes obvious that any efforts to determine cost effectiveness tend to be methodologically difficult and quite expensive.

PAs provide medical care that overlap to a large extent with those services provided by physicians. Understanding what percentage of overlap exists constitutes the heart of the question for physician employers and health planners. Most studies suggest that PAs can substitute for physicians in various ways. What is not clear is which services are included in these percentages and which are left out. The percentages vary considerably depending on practice setting and specialty, the degree of delegation of tasks by an individual physician to a PA, and the amount of supervision the PA requires or needs.

PAs AS SUBSTITUTES OR COMPLEMENTS

Many studies have examined the role of the PA, and many authors have tried to determine whether PAs substitute for or complement physician services. In the classic economic definition, a *substitute* replaces a service with something in kind. For example, a kidney machine replaces a donated kidney, so both are substitutes for the real thing. A bicycle substitutes for an automobile (although not a perfect substitute, it is, nonetheless, a substitute). On the other hand, a *complement* is something that enhances the service being provided. Butter complements a piece of toast. A nurse is generally thought to complement a physician's services.

Paul Feldstein points out that in medical care it is not always easy to know when an input is a complement or a substitute based just on the task to be performed. A PA may be as competent as a physician to perform certain tasks; if the PA works for the physician, however, and the physician determines the performance or directs the task, then the PA is a complement and will increase the physician's productivity. However, if the PA performs the same task and is operating relatively independently of the physician, then the PA is a substitute for the physician in providing that service. The essential element that determines whether an input is a complement or a substitute is who controls the use of that input (Feldstein 1991). Substitutability, as the term is used here, implies that quality of care is not threatened. In examining the literature on this question, Sox (1979) concluded that a PA should be able to "provide the average office patient with primary care that compares very favorably with care given by the physician."

Most studies examining cost-effectiveness of PAs have suffered some flaws based on the preceding constraints. For the most part, they have been small sample sizes, analyzed experiences in only one type of ambulatory setting, compared NPs and nurses instead of physicians, focused on primary care functions, and were incomplete in regard to revenue generation and cost data (Lawrence 1978). Furthermore, the majority of these studies were performed in the 1970s when the role of the PA was still developing. Finally, no study has examined the *cost benefit* of PAs. Do they have downstream effects to society that show that their employment lowers cost overall?

Bearing in mind these limitations and recognizing that the published data are suggestive but not conclusive, it is asserted that the cost-effectiveness of PAs can be reasonably confirmed, and measured to some extent, by the data. Major studies of PA productivity and cost-effectiveness have shown that PAs usually generate practice revenue far beyond the costs of their salaries and overhead (Schneider 1977; Mendenhall 1980). In addition, an important factor not commonly emphasized in major reviews is the nonmonetary contribution made by PAs to medical practice—a factor even more difficult to quantify than cost-effectiveness. Finally, even though one may never be able to precisely measure the cost-effectiveness in every practice setting and specialty, the fact that over 30,000 PAs are currently employed is significant empirical evidence for cost-effectiveness to some degree. Employers— physicians, federal agencies, clinics, hospitals— would not hire them if they were not to some degree cost-effective.

A REVIEW OF THE COST-EFFECTIVENESS LITERATURE

Given satisfactory quality and patient acceptance, the substitutability of PAs for physicians depends on the volume of services delegated and the degree to which the PA's productivity matches that of the physician in performing the delegated services. The delegation and productivity numbers can be combined to produce a physician/PA substitution ratio. For example, if 50% of the physician's services are delegated to a PA, and the PA's productivity is half that of the physician, it will take one PA to substitute for half a physician, and the substitution ratio will be .50 physician/1 PA, or .5.

From the bulk of published studies evaluating PA performance, it is clear that 60% to 100% of the services performed by primary care physicians can be provided by PAs without consultation (Page 1975; Ott 1979; Schleffler 1979; Mendenhall 1980; Record 1980; Johnson 1985; Tirado 1990; Hooker 1993).

The most rigorous of all PA economic studies showed that the substitution ratio of traditional primary care medical office visits is .83, suggesting that it takes one PA to substitute for 0.8 of a physician in primary care ambulatory settings (Record 1980). Other studies confirm that the clinical productivity of PAs in primary care ranges between 75% and 100% (Page 1975; Schleffler 1979; Mendenhall 1980; Hooker 1993).

If we accept the fact that PAs are at least three-fourths as productive as physicians and are capable of managing at least 83% of all primary care encounters, and if we recognize that the mean salary of a PA is half that of a licensed primary care physician, we can begin to appreciate the considerable cost-effectiveness of PAs in clinical practice. These figures tend to become jumbled because of misunderstanding of the terms that economists use: practice arrangements, delegation, supervision, consultation, and cost-effectiveness. Clarification of these terms are presented and the literature reviewed.

Practice Arrangements

Studies have looked at estimates of PA productivity to try to determine the practice arrangements that can best utilize the clinical services of PAs. Past activity analyses used to develop a model of primary care practice organization and productivity consisted of listing the preponderance of tasks that fully describe most typical primary care practices. From this list, a model was developed that estimated that the introduction of a PA can increase medical practice productivity from 49% to 74%. That is, a physician usually producing 147 office visits per week may increase that number to 265 visits per week simply by hiring a PA. Nelson also found that when PA providers were actually studied in medical practices, they increased practice productivity as measured by the number of office visits by 12% during the first year after their introduction, and 37% after their first year in the practice (Nelson 1975).

Reinhardt found that physicians who practiced in groups could manage more patient care visits than those working in solo practices. He noted that medical care services delivery by physicians exhibited clear *economies of scale*, that is, showing patterns that the mean level of clinical productivity for each health care professional working in the practice serves to increase the total productivity output of the practice as more personnel who can substitute for a portion of the physician are added (Reinhardt 1972).

Measures of PA productivity in the health maintenance organization (HMO) setting are consistent with findings observed in studies in rural private practices, urban ambulatory care clinics, and geriatric settings (Frick 1986; Hansen 1992). Scheffler found that PAs spend more of their time in patient care when working closely with three or fewer physicians in general medicine (Scheffler 1977).

Delegation

Delegation is the percentage of primary care medical responsibilities that can be safely handled by a PA under optimal conditions and typically is derived by a panel of experts reasoning from a set of medical criteria. The term *delegability* was adopted by Record to refer to the maximum level of delegation that can be achieved without threat to quality of care (Record 1980).

In one study at Kaiser Permanente, a multidisciplinary panel of health professionals developed a set of medical principles, focusing on the patient's complaint and medical history, for determining the limits of PA substitutability. The team examined an outpatient utilization database for a year of clinical experience to identify the office visits that would have been triaged to PAs had the panel's medical criteria been fully in effect. The team found that the PA-appropriate medical office rate, or delegability, was 83% of the total in adult primary care during the study period (Record 1978). A number of conservative assumptions were used to conduct this study. Significant illnesses such as cancer, renal failure, congestive heart failure, and similar progressive illnesses would be triaged away from PAs; all patients would be given a choice of a physician or a PA at time of appointment; and no patient would be seen more than twice in a row by a PA for the same diagnosis. PAs and physicians were assigned the same number of appointments each day. It was found that 83% of all patients seen in primary care by primary care physicians could be managed without supervision by a PA (Record 1978). No other study has been as rigorous, used as large a pool of physicians and PAs, or had as many encounters to examine.

A review of the literature examining the issue of delegation identified 10 studies that used office visits as an output measure. The findings of these studies are summarized in Table 9-1. In the aggregate, the range of delegation is extremely broad, 6% to 99%, with considerable overlap of the delegation level among the settings.

Because of the economy of scale, large practices seem to be more likely to use PAs/nurse practitioners (NPs), and in these settings physicians tend to delegate a larger percentage of medical services. The positive correlation of size and delegation is further supported by Breslau and colleagues, who studied 70 primary care teams and found delegation of technical tasks to be 24% greater and delegation of patient-care tasks to be 6% greater in large

Table 9-1 *The delegation of office visits to PAs: A summary of the literature*

REFERENCE	STUDY PERIOD	SETTING	PATIENTS	METHOD OF TRIAGE	LEVEL OF DELEGATION (%)
Record 1978	1971–1973	HMO	200,000 health plan enrollees	By receptionist	79
Record 1980	1972	HMO	200,000 health plan enrollees	By receptionist	83
Pondy 1973	1972	HMO Group, solo (2), institution		Not described	81 HMO 36 Group 36 Group 39 Solo 24 Solo
Miles 1976	1971–1974	Solo	27,000 rural Appalachia	N/A	33
Henry 1974	1971–1972	Satellite/ Independent	3.500 in rural FL	All patients seen by PA	80
Riess 1976	1974	Satellite/ Independent	5.300 in rural Pacific Northwest	All patients see by PA	90
Watkins 1978 (unpublished)	1977	Emergency department of an institution	200,000 health plan members	Triaged appropriate patients to PA	45
Ott 1979	1975	Solo and group	Nine practice settings	By receptionist to CHAs	99
Ekwo 1979	1977–1978	Solo, group, and satellite	19 primary care practices in Iowa	By receptionist and independent	87, 87 (satellite)
Weiner 1986	1975	3 HMOs	Over 300,000 health plan members	Varied by health plan	47 15 6

Abbreviation: CHA, Child Health Associate or pediatric PA

(Data from Record 1980.)

medical organizations than in small office-based practices (Breslau 1978).

In a study on the potential for substituting nonphysicians for resident physicians at two New York City hospitals, Knickman conducted a time-motion study analyzing physicians' clinical tasks under two different models: a traditional model in which the physician resident is the primary medical manager, and an alternative model in which a PA or NP performs baseline patient care monitoring. In the traditional model, residents spent almost half their time on tasks that they could not delegate. Under the alternative practice model, only 20% of the resident's time was nondelegatable (Knickman 1992).

The results of the hospital substitution study are applicable to many US teaching hospitals. A recent survey of 144 teaching hospitals found that more than 60% of the medical directors surveyed reported experience with PA or NP substitution in their hospitals. One-third of the hospital departments said they were planning to increase the number of PAs and NPs (Riportella-Mueller 1995).

Consultation

Consultation is the PA's decision to ask for a physician's help in a specific medical office visit. It differs from delegation, which is the physician's decision to assign to the PA some subset of the physician's service. The consultation is some part of the total delegated medical office visits for which the PA is responsible. Many circumstances determine a consultation rate because the consultation can take many forms, with varying time and cost results. Merely signing a prescription, verifying a radiograph finding, or approving a proposed medical management plan may take the PA's supervisory physician only a minute or two, or it may take a prolonged time if a complicated case needs to be reviewed and the physician needs to examine the patient. The summation of the time consulting with the PA decreases the time the physician has for his or her own tasks and decreases the overall productivity of the PA-physician team. A newly graduated PA will seek more consultations from a physician than a PA who has been practicing primary care for 20 years. In a state that forbids PA prescribing or dispensing, the PA may have to consult with the physician on every patient who needs a prescription.

The consultation rate is the number of consultations of any kind over the total number of visits assigned to the PA in a given time period. It may be closely related to the level of delegation in a certain specialty or if the physician wants to use the PA as his or her personal assistant. In other circumstances, willingness to delegate a broad range of services to a PA may be based on the assumption that consultation will be frequent or that the PA needs little supervision. It is important, therefore, to know the consultation rate as well as the delegation level. Because the consultation is usually informal, little is known about the PA consultation rate. Considered higher for inexperienced PAs and lower for experienced PAs, the rate is undoubtedly controlled by many variables such as relationship with the physician, time, availability, and patient mix. When the PA and physician share an office, the rate is undoubtedly higher than when they are separated by distances and office layouts that inhibit formal and informal consultations. Time-motion studies documenting every minute of a physician and PA relationship would need to be conducted over a prolonged time to understand the importance of this labor assessment.

Supervision

Supervision is a state-legislated term (see Ch. 11). It has both legal and economic aspects. Compe-

tent supervision is essential for quality of patient care but can carry with it restriction of delegated tasks, and loss of physician productivity because of the employer administrative tasks associated with this relationship. How much time is devoted to supervision depends largely on the relationship between the PA and the physician. Little study has been devoted to this important function. In 1992, the Veterans Administration surveyed over 100 supervising physicians of PAs and NPs (Alexander 1992). The average time spent supervising a PA or NP in this system ranged from 9.2 to 16.1 hours/week based on a work week of approximately 30 hours of direct patient care (Table 9-2). Although assigned the role of supervising the PA or NP, the supervising physicians were also engaged in patient care, usually in the same setting.

In one large HMO that employed both PAs and NPs, the supervising physician patient load was decreased by 10% per day. This was assigned as administrative time and was inserted into the schedule to compensate the physician for supervising the PA or NP and reviewing a set of medical records used by the PA/NP at the end of the day (Hooker 1991c).

Table 9-2 *Physician survey mean responses to questions on supervision of PAs and NPs*

	PHYSICIAN SUPERVISES	
	PAs (N = 75)[a]	NPs (N = 34)[a]
Hours/week physician spends in direct care	33.0	29.7
Hours/week physician supervises PA/NP	16.1	9.2
Percent time PA/NP takes first call for physician	20.2	26.4
Percent time supervision involves:		
overseeing medical procedures	23.7	27.2
checking orders with PA/NP	25.7	41.5
other activities	50.6	31.3

[a]Number of responding physicians.

(Data from Alexander 1992.)

Clinical Productivity

The noted economist Jane Record (1980) defined productivity this way:

> In theory, productivity is a simple concept: it measures changes in the total output that occur when small changes are made in one factor of production, with all other factors and circumstances held constant. Because these conditions can be met in the real world only rarely, productivity numbers are almost always rough estimates. Certainly that is the case with respect to [PAs].

The findings on PA productivity reflect the changing policy concerns of the American health care system. Initially, emphasis relied on documentation of increased access to services, usually within the organizational framework of solo practice in rural areas. Later investigations focused on issues of costs and delegation in organized health settings. An important contribution of health services research has been the documentation of the multifaceted effects of PAs on clinical productivity, meaning the overall output of a clinic or medical office when a PA is added to the staffing mix. A common measure of productivity, one that can positively affect access to health care, is the number of patient visits performed in a clinical setting. The next question is whether the productivity of PAs compare favorably with physicians.

In virtually every study on productivity, PAs compare favorably to physicians (Crandall 1984; Scheffler 1996). In fact there is evidence in some settings that PAs see more patients per unit time than do physicians (Hooker 1986; Hooker 1993). Generally, PA productivity can be compared to physician productivity in two other ways: (1) on the basis of tasks PAs are qualified to perform and (2) on the full range of tasks performed by a physician. The comparison of the range of these tasks is sometimes known as the *functional delegation* (Record 1981a). For most practices, depending on the degree of task delegation, practice case-mix, the health care delivery system, the context in which the PA performs the clinical service, and

institutional policy on the utilization of PAs results in higher clinical productivity rates.

One study looked at nine medical practices that employed PAs. When these practices were compared to control practices, it was found that the physician-PA team practices increased clinical productivity 40.4% (as measured by the number of office visits), whereas the control practices increased only 1.3% during the same time (Smith 1973). Another study assessed the impact of a PA in a small practice on the distribution of physician time. After employing a PA in primary care, a larger proportion of physician time was spent in seeing older patients, more seriously ill, hospitalized patients, and in communicating with patients (Nelson 1977).

A small scale study of the cost-effectiveness of nonphysician health providers including PAs was conducted in another type of ambulatory care setting. This report describes the performance of four nonphysician providers (PAs and NPs) and five family practice physicians comparing measures of the practice costs of both types of health providers working in a Student Health Clinic, a type of prepaid system, and in a fee-for-service family practice clinic. Total hours worked, numbers of patients seen, revenue generated, and provider salaries were collected for the nine primary care providers over 49 weeks. In the Student Health Clinic, the average cost for salaries to the clinic for each patient visit was $5.49 for nonphysician services, whereas it was $8.53 for each visit to the physician. In the Family Practice Clinic, revenue generated per dollar of salary was $2.68 for nonphysicians and $2.62 for family physicians (Hansen 1980).

Mathematical models have been developed to explore the most efficient contribution of health personnel in different settings. These settings included private group practices, urban medical centers, military settings, and managed health care settings such as health maintenance organizations (Golladay 1973; Zechauser 1974; Golladay 1976; Schneider 1977; Ortiz 1979; Cyr 1985; Hooker 1993) and tertiary centers (Harbert 1994). These models provide the theoretical documentation for the clinical productivity of PAs, with estimates ranging 50% to 95% of physician productivity (where physician productivity equals 100%). These theoretical and carefully documented empirical approaches are similar in their assessment of PA clinical productivity. Hooker studied the hourly, daily, and annual productivity of PAs, NPs, and physicians in the primary care departments of internal medicine, family practice, and pediatrics and found that PAs see more patients than do physicians in the same amount of time (29% more annually). This difference is due in part to PAs being primarily outpatient based, while physicians had hospital responsibilities that took them away from the medical office (Table 9-3). Patient visits to physicians and PAs tended to be similar in 90% of cases (the functional delegation level), but differed in illnesses associated with a hospitalization such as acute cardiac illnesses, cerebral accidents, and cancers (Hooker 1993).

While some practices employ PAs to meet increasing demand, others employ them to relieve physicians of excess workload. Kane noted that after hiring PAs, more patients in the practice are seen by appointment and more patients in the practice have specific plans for follow-up visits (Kane 1978b). Other researchers reached similar findings (Table 9-4).

PA clinical productivity compares favorably to levels of physicians, particularly in organized ambulatory care practice settings that utilize team approaches and structured division of

Table 9-4 *Physician productivity when a PA is added to the clinic*

STUDY BY FIRST AUTHOR	PA/PHYSICIAN RATIO	PERCENT PRODUCTIVITY
Cyr 1985	1:1	80.1
Hooker 1993	1:2	110.0
Greenfield 1978	1:1	92.0

Productivity is defined as the percentage of patients seen in an outpatient setting compared to a physician's patient load.

medical care staffing. While it seems likely that similar levels of PA clinical productivity exist for PAs working in other types of patient care settings, performance measures in newer practice areas such as inpatient hospital settings have not been performed. Additional studies examining levels of PA clinical performance characteristics are needed since the content of clinical care (the specific medical tasks) delivered by PAs differ within various clinical settings. It would be useful to know the number, content, and patient outcomes of clinical services of PAs compared to those of physicians.

One of the many variables that are difficult to control in comparing productivity of PAs in different settings is the population base. Many significant differences exist between groups of PAs depending on the work setting, type of specialty, or years of experience. However, when some of these data are aggregated, it has some interesting findings. Using data collected on the 1995 AAPA membership census, Kraditor with the AAPA Research Division examined the productivity of PAs in terms of number of outpatients seen per day controlling for a number of variables (K. Kraditor, personal communication, 1996.) Tables 9-5 through 9-7 present summary statistics on these measures of outpatient productivity for groups of PAs defined in terms of work setting, years of experience as a PA, and field of practice. All analyses used only data for PAs who reported being in full-time clinical practice and working for a single employer.

Findings from this study include a statistically significant difference observed in the num-

Table 9-3 *PA clinical productivity in an HMO setting*

DEPARTMENT	PATIENTS/HOUR	PATIENTS/DAY
Family practice		
Physician	2.39	17.4
PAs	2.61	19.0
Internal Medicine		
Physician	3.10	22.5
PAs	2.97	21.5
Pediatrics		
Physician	3.14	16.5
PAs	3.07	22.3

(Data from Hooker 1993.)

Table 9-5 *Mean and standard deviation of outpatients per day by work setting for PAs, 1995*

SETTING	RESPONDENTS	MEAN	STANDARD DEVIATION
Clinic	763	21.9	9.6
Group physician practice	517	21.6	7.7
Solo physician practice	190	22.7	9.9
HMO	198	21.3	6.2
Other managed care organization	19	20.1	7.0
University hospital	72	15.0	13.1
Hospital (nonuniversity)	260	23.7	10.7
Inner city clinic	116	19.9	12.2
Military facility	248	24.8	8.3
Corrections facility	51	23.7	12.4
Nursing homes	5	19.4	4.7
Rural clinics	357	20.2	8.9
Self-employed PA	10	35.9	14.5
VA facility	58	16.6	5.5
Industrial facility	44	20.1	9.3
Academic facility	33	22.4	7.9
Public health facility	27	21.0	6.8
Other government facility	14	23.4	20.6
Other clinical setting	109	20.7	10.6
Total	3,091	21.7	9.5

Based on PAs reporting outpatient visits but no inpatient or nursing home visits. Data collected on the 1995 AAPA Member Census.

(Data from American Academy of Physician Assistants, Research Division, 1996b.)

Table 9-6 *Mean and standard deviation of outpatient visits per day by years of experience*

YEARS OF EXPERIENCE	RESPONDENTS	MEAN	STANDARD DEVIATION
Under 1	139	18.6	7.2
1–3	821	20.8	8.8
4–6	505	21.9	10.1
7–9	341	21.2	8.5
10–12	410	21.6	8.6
13–15	371	22.5	10.2
16–18	343	22.8	10.5
>18	296	23.3	10.3
Total	3,226	21.7	9.4

Based on PAs reporting outpatient visits but no inpatient or nursing home visits. Data collected on the 1995 AAPA Member Census.

(Data from American Academy of Physician Assistants, Research Division, 1996b.)

Table 9-7 *Mean and standard deviation of outpatient visits per day by field of practice*

FIELD OF PRACTICE	RESPONDENTS	MEAN	STANDARD DEVIATION
Family/general medicine	1836	22.1	8.2
General internal medicine	255	18.9	8.6
General pediatrics	115	24.4	9.9
Emergency medicine	316	24.6	11.2
General surgery	6	18.3	7.3
Internal medicine specialties	130	16.8	13.6
Pediatric specialties	33	18.7	15.1
Surgical specialties	145	20.0	10.6
Obstetrics/gynecology	88	20.0	10.4
Industrial/occupational medicine	181	21.7	10.3
Other	173	21.4	10.6
Total	3,278	21.7	9.6

Based on PAs reporting outpatient visits but no inpatient or nursing home visits. Data collected on the 1995 AAPA Member Census.

(Data from American Academy of Physician Assistants, Research Division, 1996b.)

ber of outpatients seen per day by work setting with the largest differences reflected by PAs working in military facilities or correction facilities. When years of experience are examined, PAs with more experience see more patients per day than PAs with less experience. Field of experience also seems to make a difference in terms of patients seen per day. The largest differences are found in Emergency medicine, where PAs report seeing 24.6 patients per day on average, with a mean average of 21.7 outpatients per day.

In terms of work week, the vast majority of PAs report working about 40 hours a week. PAs employed in inner city clinics work fewer hours a week, and those in military facilities work more hours per week than all other settings.

The extent of PA productivity cannot be determined without reference to an array of interdependent variables, which, assuming that all of them can be identified, are difficult to evaluate. The classic conceptualization of how productivity should be measured—by observing what happens to total output when small, homogeneous units of one input (in this case, the PA) are added while other inputs and the larger context are held constant—is difficult to measure in a big practice and virtually impossible in a small one (Record 1980).

COSTS OF PAs

Cost implications of the use of PAs can be viewed from two perspectives. The first is that of the entrepreneurial medical practice concerned with whether or not the increase in practice revenue resulting from hiring a PA will exceed the additional costs of adding a provider, and if market conditions warrant, whether it is more desirable to hire a physician or a PA. The second is the societal concern of how to deliver high quality care at minimum cost. The societal view is that all costs, no matter where they come from, is ultimately borne by society. It considers not only employment costs but also training costs. Therefore, all costs must be accounted for.

Employment Costs of PAs

When a PA is employed, a number of costs need to be considered. These include salary, benefits, malpractice insurance, office space, equipment, support staff, supplies, and other direct and indirect expenses. Although data on this subject are sparse, there is little to suggest that the costs other than compensation are different from those associated with employing a physician. Outcome studies evaluating whether a PA uses more laboratory, imaging, and drugs for an episode of care have not been published. Aside from anecdotal reports suggesting that malpractice insurance may be cheaper for the PA

because the litigation rate is less than it is for physicians, there seems to be little to suggest that PAs lose any of their cost-effectiveness by the way they practice medicine.

In contrast to other costs, the income differential for PAs and physicians is clearly quite large. Most PAs are employees and therefore salaried, whereas physicians receive not only a stream of revenue for their own services but also entrepreneurial benefit from employing a revenue-generating provider.

Based on the AAPA data collected in 1996, $55,000 is a reasonable average salary estimate for an experienced primary care PA in 1995 (AAPA 1996b). The figure for a primary care physician in the same year was approximately $129,000 (Simon 1996b). This places the PA at .43 of the salary of physician in primary care.

Compensation/Production Ratio

One of the better ways to examine the net value of a PA is the income generated to the employer in private practice. *Compensation*, which

Table 9-8 *Compensation/production ratio for PAs*

PROVIDER TYPE	NUMBER OF PROVIDERS	MEDICAL PRACTICES	MEAN
Overall for PAs	124	40	.381
Organization type			
Single specialty	19	13	.433
Multispecialty	105	27	.372
Other providers			
Family practice physician	1,117	135	.447
Internal medicine physician	883	134	.447
Pediatric physician	501	107	.409
Nurse practitioner	71	31	.419
Midwife	15	7	.472
Optometrist	57	20	.423
Psychologist	104	32	.477
Podiatrist	31	19	.334

(Data from Medical Group Management Association, 1995.)

includes salary and benefits collectively, is usually examined. The most useful ratio is the amount of compensation the employer foregoes to retain the PA divided by the amount of revenue the PA returns. Basically, the smaller the ratio the more economical the provider is to the practice. The Medical Group Management Association collects this data annually (Table 9-8). In 1994, the compensation/production ratio for PAs was .38. In comparison, the compensation/production ratio was .44 for Family Practice physicians, .40 for pediatricians, .41 for NPs, and .48 for psychologists, suggesting the PA is relatively more economical to employ.

While the number of nonphysician providers used for this study is not large, the relative ratios between providers do give an indication of the efficiency that a PA brings to a practice. For every $1 in revenue generated, the employer pays 38¢ to employ the PA.

Training Costs of PAs

The cost of educating and utilizing PA health care professionals and the annual levels of their compensation are far less than comparable costs for physicians (at least for allopathic physicians). Economic analyses of the utilization of PAs indicate that these, and other nonphysician health care providers, appear to be underutilized in their roles in health care delivery and are limited in their potential to contribute to health delivery (Safriet 1992). Theoretical economic projections of the cost savings that could accrue under optimal conditions of nonphysician utilization are considerable, perhaps as much as $4 to $5 billion for NPs alone (Nichols 1992; Salcido 1993).

The training costs of PAs, like those of virtually all other health professionals, have been borne largely by society through grants to institutions and tuition subsidies to students and trainees. Medicare alone contributes a substantial amount to the postgraduate training of physicians. Typically, the medical practice does not share directly in the cost of training. A PA student, judging the return to medical educa-

tion, perceives "costs" as private costs (tuition, books, and lost income) and is likely to observe a high rate of return on his or her investment in the training because the income as an employed PA is usually substantially higher than that earned from a previous career.

For physicians, the three training-cost components are (1) medical school costs, (2) graduate (resident) training costs, and (3) opportunity costs. The value of services to patients provided during the postgraduate years of training is often debated. There is a high cost of supervision and decreased productivity because of this supervision, as well as staffing costs, inefficiencies in care, and overhead. Most economists tend to consider the value to society during the resident years as a net sum zero. More important, the opportunity cost (foregone years of practice) is large during this training period because productivity is delayed during training.

Because virtually no physician begins practice after graduation, we must consider the cost of medical training as 8 years based on 4 years of medical school and 4 years of residency. The PA chooses a different career path that is only 2 years long. If the medical student had chosen to be a PA, practice income would have begun after 2 years of professional training. If we use the PA salary rather than the potential income of a 4-year postgraduate trained physician, we can estimate the cost differential of physicians and PAs.

Both the PA and medical student start approximately from the same place academically. The average PA student has a baccalaureate degree, and so does the medical student. Most have the same type of background with varying combinations of academic coursework in their undergraduate years. Given the overlapping training periods for physicians and PAs, the opportunity costs for physicians and PAs can be calculated.

In Figure 9-1, the PA and physician student are assumed to begin professional training after completion of 3 to 4 years of undergraduate study. The PA becomes fully productive after 2 years of education and the physician becomes a fully productive provider of care 6 years later

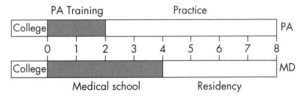

	PA student	MD student
Cost/year	$10,000	25,000
Years of training	2	4
Total	$20,000[a]	100,000[b]

Figure 9-1 Cost comparisons of PA and MD training programs in 1995 dollars. PA student data from Simon 1996; MD student data from Association of American Medical Colleges, 1996. Washington, D.C. (does not include osteopathic colleges).

than the PA. Using the assumption that a provider is valued by his or her salary level, and that the PA salary is $55,000, the PA has delivered $330,000 ($55,000 × 6 years) worth of care before the physician begins practice. This figure is defined as the opportunity cost of additional medical education and training. It is also the value of care that would have been delivered to society had the medical student chosen a PA training course.

Figure 9-1 also illustrates the opportunity cost of additional medical education and training. If direct training costs are assumed to be approximately $20,000 for a PA, and $100,000 for a primary care allopathic physician, the difference between the physician and a PA in total training costs in 1995 may be calculated as $100,000 minus $20,000, plus the protracted training ($100,000 – $20,000 + $330,000). The differential is nearly $410,000 per PA that society gains by having a PA trained instead of a physician. Put another way, the PA produces $410,000 worth of patient care before the physician begins practice.

There is some expected criticism from this set of calculations. The exact training costs for medical and PA students is not known, although the assumptions are considered conservative. Average starting salaries differ and since it takes different times to reach each provider's average earnings potential, the value of each provider may be overstated. In addition, the cost of osteopathic training was not considered. Nevertheless, these calculations, based on Record's original research in 1980, do provide a sense of the differences that society can expect from each type of training program.

If salary costs are used as a proxy for employment costs, the physician-PA differential is $74,000 (the differences between the average primary care salaries of $129,000 for physicians and $55,000 for PAs). This means the salary cost of a PA is .43 of a physician. If it requires 10% of a physician's time to supervise a PA, 10% of $129,000 should be added to the cost of employing a PA. The PA/MD cost ratio as viewed by an employer would then become $67,900/$129,000, or .52. When Record made her original calculations using 1977 data, she found the cost ratio of hiring a PA to be .38 based on a wider disparity between PA and physician salaries (Record 1980). Since that time both physician and PA salaries have steadily climbed, although more recently physician salaries have begun to plateau (Simon 1996b).

Substitution Ratios

The physician/PA substitution ratio is determined primarily by the level of delegation and comparative productivity of physicians and PAs for the delegated services. A substitution ratio of 1.0 implies unity and is achieved when one PA substitutes for one physician. PAs in rural and isolated clinics often function at very high levels, often replacing the physician who was previously occupying that role (DeBarth 1996). These accounts are largely anecdotal, however, and little is known about the types and numbers of patients seen by physicians versus PAs. The best studies occur in large managed care settings where some of the variables can be controlled and physicians and PAs work alongside each other, seeing similar patients.

Using an urban health center as a paradigm, one study constructed production functions that would best exploit the possibilities of substituting PAs for physicians. It was estimated that one PA could replace half of a full-time physician. From data developed in a national survey of physicians, Scheffler estimated that a 10% increase in the medical office visits output of a practice would require, on average, an increase of 3.5% in physician hours or 5.4% in PA hours (Scheffler 1979). These percentages suggest a marginal substitution ratio of .63, as compared to the overall .50 ratio estimated by Zeckhauser and Eliastom (Zeckauser 1974). Another mathematical model tested with data from seven HMOs to demonstrate the potential impact of PAs and NPs on physician requirements found that in adult medicine, the addition of 12.72 PA/NPs would permit physician numbers to drop from 16.44 to 9.74. Thus, the 12.72 PA/NPs could replace 4.59 physicians (Schneider 1977). The respective substitution ratios can be calculated as .53.

Record and colleagues estimated that if enough PAs were hired to perform all of the services for which they were considered competent by physicians in the Department of Internal Medicine at Kaiser Permanente, and if the PA and physician work weeks were equal, the substitution ratio would be .76 (Record 1981a). Steinwachs and colleagues studied ambulatory care in another HMO and found the substitution ratio to be .38 in adult care and .48 in pediatrics (Steinwachs 1976). The ratios might have been higher if the base had been primary care, as it was in the Record study, with outpatient specialty services excluded. Hooker developed data that suggest the ratio was .90, and Page's work in the military was close to unity (1.0) in the military as early as 1975 (Page 1975; Hooker 1993).

Most of the estimates of substitution ratios fall mostly in the range of .75, suggesting it would take, on average, one PA to substitute for three-fourths of a primary care physician. For managers, this suggests that four PAs could replace three physicians.

COST-EFFECTIVENESS OF PAs

How cost-effective is a PA? The answer, while not known exactly, is contained in the difference between the physician/PA substitution ratio (.75) and the PA/physician cost ratio (.43). The meaning of these two numbers is that a PA can substitute for at least 75% of primary care physician services at approximately 43% of the physician's direct cost in salary. If the physician's time is reduced because of supervision, then the ratio is 52%. The social cost figures are even more impressive because the PA/physician ratio including training costs is smaller than the employment cost ratio. Finally, the employment of a PA is fairly economical because the compensation/production ratio at 38% is more efficient than most other types of providers. Table 9-9 presents a summary of the economic exercises in this chapter. These figures, however, must be viewed with caution. They are based on the "best studies" (those studies considered the most rigorous in investigation), or the average of different studies, using fairly conservative figures. Many of the studies use small numbers that may

Table 9-9 *Cost-effectiveness of primary care PAs*

ISSUE EXAMINED	RANGE	AVERAGE OR BEST STUDY
Delegation	.40–1.0	.83
Supervision	.10–.60	.10
Physician/PA substitution ratio	.40–1.0	.75
PA/physician cost ratio (employment)	.40–.50	.43
PA/physican cost ratio (with supervision)		.52
Compensation/production ratio	.25–.52	.38
Societal cost to train a PA (compared to a physician)		.20

Based on a review of the literature up to 1980, using conservative estimates, and extrapolating to 1995 costs.

not be statistically significant, and most of the estimates were derived from studies conducted before 1980.

Reimbursement Issues

Variation in systems of compensation for PA-provided health services through reimbursement by the government or private insurance has also inhibited their practice effectiveness. Federal Medicare policies governing reimbursement for PA services have been long identified as a clear barrier to their full clinical effectiveness (Gara 1989). Differing interpretations of Medicare's "incident to" clause, as defined by the Health Care Finance Administration (HCFA), determines how PAs and other nonphysician services may be paid to employing practices. Historically, under Medicare, services performed by various health care professionals employed in physician practices are eligible for reimbursement under the assumption that such services are "incident to" the services of the physician. Reimbursement is paid at the physician fee level for office or clinic services provided by PAs or other clinicians in the practice whose activities are considered to be integral, although incidental, to the physician-delivered service. The physician must be present when the PA-performed services are delivered, and are billed and paid for as if the physician had performed the service.

The origin of this regulation predates the now well-developed clinical role of the PA in many rural ambulatory practice sites. Following the original intent for PAs to increase primary care access, state medical practice acts affecting these professional were typically written to allow PAs to function where on-site physician supervision was not required at all times. Physicians practicing in rural and medically underserved areas often hire PAs specifically to extend medical care services in such communities.

While PA services are covered if delivered in a federally certified rural health clinic, Medicare will cover PA outpatient services in rural and certain urban clinics at 100% of the physician fee, but only if the supervising physician is present at the time the services are provided. This regulation does not allow for coverage of PA services provided when the patient needs to be seen when the physician is temporarily absent, nor does it allow for flexibility in those states where on-site, continuous supervision is not required. In such instances, rural clinics too small to support a full-time physician may be prevented from utilizing a PA since their services may not be reimbursed.

Private third-party payers compound reimbursement issues for PAs. Although some insurers will cover PA-provided services at physician rates as long as the PA is practicing within the limits of the state law, other third-party payers impose a variety of restrictions on reimbursement in such circumstances. Restrictions include on-site physician supervision (even if not required by state regulation), payment at a lower rate, refusal to pay for certain services (e.g., assisting at surgery, a service commonly covered in other settings by many payers), or refusal to pay for any PA services.

PA clinical services delivered in nonoutpatient settings and practices are reimbursed under Medicare, but at fractional payment rates, depending again on the site of the service delivery. Since 1987, Medicare Part B allows reimbursement for services performed by PAs in a nursing facility (at a rate that may not exceed 85% of the physician fee), in an acute care hospital setting (where it may not exceed 75% of the physician fee), and for PAs assisting at surgery as first assistant (where reimbursement may not exceed 65% of the fee paid to a physician first assistant). PA-rendered services under Medicare and all other third-party payers are billed under, and reimbursed to, the practice or institution employing the PA.

Health policy studies have noted that variation among state Medicaid programs regarding reimbursement for PA services contribute to limitations in PA utilization in the areas most needy of medical care services (Weston 1980; Hoffman 1994). Although improving, policies in some states remain inconsistent. For example, Medicaid reimbursement for PA services, may vary among the states from 100% to 65% of the physician fee. A few states have yet to meet the 1989 federal mandates (Hoffman 1994). Recommended changes in federal and state health services payment policies and regulations, as suggested under proposed heath care reform legislation, aim to increase the clinical practice effectiveness of PAs, particularly in primary care roles, by encouraging health payers to adopt more uniform reimbursement policies for these providers (Mondy 1986).

Prescribing Authority

At present, 39 states, the District of Columbia, and Guam authorize prescribing privileges for PAs. The cluster of 12 southeastern states not authorizing prescribing by PAs represents approximately 37% of the total US rural Health Professional Shortage Areas (HPSAs).

The first state statute to authorize prescribing privileges for PAs was passed in Colorado in 1969. It stipulated that graduates of the University of Colorado Child Health Associate program (pediatric PAs) could prescribe medications without immediate consultation from supervising physicians provided that the latter subsequently approved the script. New York authorized prescribing privilege to PAs in 1972; Maine, New Mexico, and North Carolina followed in 1973. By 1979, 11 states had passed laws allowing PA prescribing privileges. There was a steady trend among states throughout the 1980s to authorize PA prescribing either by statute or regulation in recognition that prescribing medication is part of the PA clinical role and the supervising physician has the authority to delegate such tasks to qualified health professionals (Willis 1990a).

A study in Iowa reported that 95% of physicians and 93% of PAs believed that PAs were qualified to prescribe medications with little or no supervision by the physician (Johnson 1985). Similarly, all 29 Montana physicians who responded to a survey expressed confidence in the ability of the PAs they were supervising to prescribe most therapeutic agents, and 40% had

no reservations at all about their ability to prescribe any agent (Rabin 1980).

Prescribing authority applies generally to the outpatient or nonhospital setting. Medications for patients in the hospital are considered as medical orders and usually fall under the purview of institutional medical staff by-laws. States typically place certain stipulations on PA prescribing activities. These may include (1) requiring physician co-signature for a PA prescription, (2) limitations on the drugs that may be used (i.e., those listed in a specific formulary), (3) excluding selected schedules of drugs (usually schedule II agents (i.e., those defined by the Controlled Substances Act as having the potential for abuse), (4) prescribing using drug treatment protocols, and (5) limiting the quantities of certain drugs that PAs may prescribe.

A 1990 survey administered to PAs working in states having prescribing authority found that 90% of them included prescribing as part of their clinical activities when authorized. Sixty percent of PAs reported that they prescribed urinary/vaginal agents, upper respiratory medications, gastrointestinal agents, antiarthritic/antigout agents, and analgesics. The mean number of prescriptions written per week was 50, and it was estimated that PAs wrote 35.5 million new prescriptions each year; with refill prescriptions, the total approximated 65 million. The most frequently prescribed classes of drugs of PAs were non-narcotic analgesics, antibiotics, antihistamines, antihypertensives, and cough and cold preparations (Willis 1990a).

In 1993, the AAPA estimated that the typical PA in clinical practice in an authorized state wrote an average of 100 outpatient prescriptions per week. Overall, PAs were estimated to provide over 150 million patient visits, and write 165 million (8% of all prescriptions written) prescriptions.

Barriers to Practice Effectiveness

On a public policy level, the term *barriers to practice* refers to factors known to have a significant limiting effect on the practice effectiveness of PAs and other nonphysician health care practitioners. Barriers to practice is commonly used within discussions of the utilization of PAs to denote the multiple health system factors that limit the full capabilities of PAs to provide health services. These factors comprise medical, legal, and economic elements and prevent PAs from discharging the full range of authorized medical tasks for which they are educated and certified to perform (OTA 1990; OIG 1993; Emilio 1994).

PAs are often constrained in their capabilities to augment medical practices because of restrictions imposed by states. Barriers to the full practice effectiveness of PAs may reduce or eliminate the cost benefits that accrue from their utilization and deter them from serving populations in need of medical care services, or from practicing in certain areas. Uneven state medical practice acts, the lack of authorization to prescribe medications, and the absence of Medicare and private third-party reimbursement that exist in many rural ambulatory practice settings (exceptions being Medicare-approved rural health clinics) have been shown to have restrictive effects on PA utilization (Willis 1993b).

While conventionally defined barriers to practice (i.e., state government regulatory policies for supervision requirements and prescribing authority) clearly work to affect levels of PA clinical productivity in a broad sense, on the day-to-day practice level, findings suggest that differences in the delegatory styles of individual employing physicians are also important determinants of PA effectiveness. On a fundamental level, barriers to practice (i.e., practice laws and regulations) represent the parameters drawn for nonphysician providers, usually by physicians. At the margins, since clinical activities between physicians and PAs overlap considerably, scope of practice or "turf" issues arise among these health professionals. Physicians now share a great deal of their medical diagnostic and therapeutic responsibilities with PAs. This willingness to share medical functions is a result of forces affecting the evolution of the division of medical labor in the US health system.

States and their licensing boards have considerable control over the practice activities of PAs and other nonphysician providers through their authority to license and regulate the health occupations. Restrictions to the full practice effectiveness of PAs and similar health care providers may reduce or eliminate the cost benefits that accrue from the utilization of these professionals and may prevent them from serving populations in greatest need of medical care services, or from practicing at all (OIG 1993).

Since states exert considerable control over health practitioner utilization patterns through professional licensing and regulation, Sekscenski and colleagues from the Bureau of Health Professions analyzed variations in the regulation of PAs (as well as NPs and CNMs) and their abilities to practice to full effectiveness in all states and the District of Columbia (Sekscenski 1994). In their approach, key factors related to the licensure and legal status, prescriptive authority, and eligibility for reimbursement for PAs were delineated and quantified according to specific criteria across all 51 jurisdictions. Summary scores estimating the favorability of the practice environment for PAs were derived from points assigned to each of three categories—scope of practice, prescribing authority, and reimbursement eligibility—which were then compared with the numbers of individual practitioners, ratios of generalist physicians, and proportions of underserved persons in each jurisdiction. Only nonfederal PAs and physicians were counted in the analysis (Table 9-10).

PA practice favorability scores ranged from a high (maximum attainable) of 100 points in three states (Washington, Iowa, and Montana) to a low of 0 (lowest attainable) in Mississippi, with a mean score of 73.1. Twenty-one states had practice favorability scores of 90 or greater, and 14 had scores below 50. Lower scores generally correlated with the lack of PA prescriptive authority. A significant relationship ($P < .001$) was observed between practice favorability scores and a state's PA/population ratio. States tended to cluster into three groups, reflecting the association between favorability scores and

Table 9-10 *Provider practice scores for PAs, NPs, and CNMs by state, 1992*

STATE	PAs	NPs	CNMs
Alabama	39	33	32
Alaska	90	93	84
Arizona	99	86	76
Arkansas	54	48	35
California	58	30	80
Colorado	80	59	50
Connecticut	87	58	93
Delaware	55	60	60
District of Columbia	92	53	60
Florida	48	68	98
Georgia	59	32	70
Hawaii	38	27	42
Idaho	89	46	54
Illinois	59	14	31
Indiana	37	34	25
Iowa	99	73	55
Kansas	87	52	68
Kentucky	42	78	68
Louisiana	37	20	37
Maine	94	42	90
Maryland	49	93	69
Massachusetts	83	68	57
Michigan	89	45	70
Minnesota	83	68	100
Mississippi	0	72	59
Missouri	39	63	27
Montana	98	98	98
Nebraska	93	46	50
Nevada	98	73	30
New Hampshire	95	95	70
New Jersey	37	65	54
New Mexico	94	62	78
New York	98	93	67
North Carolina	92	43	90
North Dakota	87	98	55
Ohio	51	14	60
Oklahoma	46	40	54
Oregon	99	100	80
Pennsylvania	86	66	34
Rhode Island	93	50	84
South Carolina	37	41	59
South Dakota	94	65	70
Tennessee	42	27	56
Texas	77	42	54
Utah	93	91	73
Vermont	86	68	57
Virginia	42	38	47
Washington	100	90	70
West Virginia	96	89	47
Wisconsin	95	67	62
Wyoming	97	94	80
Mean	72.5	60.2	62.1
Median	86.0	62.0	60.0
Standard Deviation	25.3	23.8	19.2

(Data from Sekscenski 1994.)

PA/population ratios: states with high favorability scores and high PA/population ratios, states with mid-range scores and mid-range ratios, and states with low scores and, consequently, low ratios. These findings confirm the widely held view that scope of practice regulations, the existence of prescribing authority, and eligibility for reimbursement all affect PA utilization. If these factors are unfavorable, they serve as barriers to PA practice effectiveness.

Prescribing authority has been a particularly troublesome barrier to PA practice effectiveness, and its presence in state law is reflected in the patterns of marketplace demand and utilization of PA providers. State prescribing authority can have a marked influence on the capacity and efficiency of PAs to contribute to health care delivery (Gara 1989). A recent example was seen in Texas where, before the passage of PA prescriptive authority, there were only 26 rural health clinics. By November 1992, only 15 months after the passage of prescriptive authority for PAs in Texas, the number of PAs employed by these clinics had nearly quadrupled to 99. During the same period, the percentage of Texas PAs practicing in rural areas tripled, increasing from 5% to 15% (Willis 1993b).

SUMMARY

For PAs, clear evidence exists that their utilization results in the production of far more revenue than the costs of their employment (Medical Group Management 1995). Yet for various reasons, PAs also tend to be underutilized in many clinical practice settings (Eastaugh 1990).

Knowledge about performance and the potential contribution of PAs is significant and continues to mount. The data suggest strongly that a large portion of primary care services can be safely delegated to PAs at levels that exceed 85%. When PAs provide these services, they perform at high levels of productivity that compares favorably with physicians. When the difference between substitution ratios and cost ratios are compared, even when the ratios are conservatively estimated, the differences are so large as to ensure cost savings for employers.

The societal cost savings of PAs in the form of training suggests that a great deal is gained when PAs are trained because they provide care at substantial savings for 6 years longer than physicians. State barriers in the form of restrictive legislation and reimbursement policies interfere with fuller utilization of PAs. Research is needed to determine whether tax dollars can be saved by employing PAs in Medicare and Medicaid programs. Also, the cost advantages of physician substitution could diminish if the excess supply of physicians significantly reduces the gap between physicians and PA earnings (Scheffler 1996).

Record's work at Kaiser Permanente and data from other studies suggest that physician comfort levels and practice styles in delegating medical tasks to the PAs with whom they work have a significant influence on PA utilization and effectiveness in clinical practices (Record 1981a). In studies of performance and patterns of utilization of nonphysician health providers, Weiner and colleagues noted a marked difference in the observed versus normative rates of delegation of medical tasks by HMO physicians when working with both PAs and NPs (Weiner 1994).

A recent report by the Institute of Medicine (IOM) examined the current characteristics and projected future medical staffing requirements for the health system of the Department of Veterans Affairs (VA). Measures of clinical productivity, professional functions, and anticipated future personnel needs were analyzed for both physicians and several types of nonphysician health providers in the VA health system. The IOM report included information on the clinical activities, staffing relationships, and measures of utilization of four types of nonphysician health providers: PAs, NPs, clinical nurse specialists, and certified registered nurse anesthetists (CRNAs).

Measures of the clinical practice activities and professional characteristics of these health providers were observed in both inpatient and outpatient settings, and a questionnaire was used to obtain their opinions regarding their duties. Results indicate that both physicians and these health practitioners believe that non-physicians are underutilized in the VA system. The factor most critical in determining the effective utilization of nonphysician providers was the medical task delegation style of the supervising physicians. The IOM study recommended that staffing efficiency in the VA system could be increased if physicians were more aware of the clinical roles and practice capabilities of these practitioners and better equipped to delegate tasks appropriately (IOM 1992).

Areas for Further Research

Research activity on the clinical and professional activities of PAs and other nonphysician providers has languished since the extensive health professions investigations conducted in the 1970s. While much about PA utilization and clinical potentials has been learned from both this past body of research, as well as widespread empirical observations, many aspects of PA clinical roles and capabilities remain to be explored. For instance, what is the optimal mix of health care providers to deliver primary care? How can the economic advantages of these providers be best utilized in health systems of the future? No data exist to determine how many PAs and NPs, along with physicians and other health professionals, would be required to staff newly emerging types of managed health systems or to meet anticipated health workforce needs in either primary care or graduate medical education (GME)-related areas. Planning activities regarding the health professions should assess the present capacities of the United States in the health care workforce, consider the short- and long-term population-based need for medical services, and articulate these estimates of need with national goals for providing services required to improve citizen health status (Mullan 1992). The present lack of reliable information on activities in the

health workforce places policy makers at a disadvantage in attempts to either promote the more effective use of PAs or to better coordinate their supply and utilization with those of physicians.

Research on PA practice should focus on (1) determination of physician/PA substitutability ratios and task delegation levels in primary care, managed care, and GME settings and on maximal PA/physician substitution potentials and optimal staffing mix in using PAs in GME positions, (2) description of current practice characteristics and content of care delivered by PAs in primary care including clinical preventive services, measurement of PA levels of clinical productivity and patient care outcomes determined in various settings, comparisons of PA practice performance, and contributions in primary care delivery with those of physicians and other health practitioners, (3) description of the economic aspects of PA practice, including revenue generation, practice costs, and potential for savings, and (4) educational aspects contributing to minority attrition in PA educational programs.

MEDICARE AND MEDICAID POLICIES FOR PAs

Medicare and Medicaid programs began to specify payment for PAs, CNMs, and family and pediatric nurse practitioners in the late 1970s. For the most part, both Medicare and federal Medicaid mandates have been in response to perceived access problems for specific groups of beneficiaries (Table 9-11). In addition, states have always had the discretion to expand coverage of nonphysician provider services beyond the federal Medicaid policies to meet the state's unique needs. Unfortunately, not all states have been as receptive to these nonphysician provider policy expansions as Congress intended (Hoffman 1994).

Since the beginning of the Medicare and Medicaid programs in 1965, services performed by health professionals and allied health personnel employed in physicians' practices have

Table 9-11 *Federal payment policies for PAs*

MEDICARE PART B		FEDERAL MEDICAID MANDATES	
SERVICE	PAYMENT METHOD	SERVICE	PAYMENT METHOD
Rural health clinic services all (P.L.95-210, 1977) services to home-bound patients in areas without home health agency (P.L.95-210, 1977)	Pays clinic reasonable cost, or included in all-services. Pays employer at physician fee level.	Rural health clinic services (P.L. 95-210, 1977)	Pays clinic reasonable cost, or included for all clinic services.
Services in HMO and CMPs that have risk-sharing contracts with HCFA (TEFRA, P.L.97-208)	Capitated payment to HMO or CMP.		
Hospital and nursing facility services if such services would be covered if furnished by physician (OBRA86, P.L. 99-509)	Pays employer. Hospital services not to exceed 75% of physician fee for assisting at surgery; nursing facility services not to exceed 85% of physician fee.		
Services provided in rural HPSAs (OBRA87, P.L.100-203)	Pays employer at 85% of physician fee.		

Abbreviation: CMP, competitive medical plan.

(Data from Physician Payment Review Commission, 1993b.)

been covered, with payment going to the employer. Known as the "incident to" provision, this policy allows payment of the full physician fee for office or clinic services provided by the physician's staff that are integral, although incidental, to the physician's services. The services must be provided under the direct (on-site) supervision of a physician and, therefore, are paid for as if the physician had provided them personally. Because the incident to provision predates the development of most of the non-physician provider (NPP) programs, it does not specifically address payment for NPPs employed in physicians' offices. Most state laws governing the scope of professional practice for PAs, NPs, and CNMs (commonly referred to as practice acts) do not require on-site supervision by physicians. Many NPPs, however, are employed in physicians' offices and clinics. Their services thus may be billed as physicians' services under the incident to provision. In other words, the NPP's employment situation frequently determines the payment method.

When Medicare and Medicaid payment policies began to specifically distinguish NPPs, they were targeted to address beneficiary needs in underserved rural areas. The Rural Health Clinic Services Act of 1977 (RHCSA) made free-standing rural clinics staffed by NPs, PAs, or CNMs eligible for Medicare and Medicaid payments. This was the first federal policy to specify NPP coverage and to separate it from the requirement of employment in a physician's practice. NPP payment is based on a reasonable cost formula, or NPP salaries are bundled into the all-inclusive rates for clinic services. The clinic must be located in a health professional shortage area (HPSA); an NPP must be available at least 50% of the time the clinic is open; and a physician must provide general direction, with a site visit at least once every 2 weeks.

Federal support for services provided by PAs in hospitals and nursing facilities was authorized in the Omnibus Budget Reconciliation Act of 1986 (OBRA86), which allowed Medicare Part B payments to be made to the employing practice group or institution. This provision did not cover PA services in ambulatory or clinic settings. Payment rates were established at 85% of the physician's fee for nursing facility services, 75% for hospital care, and 65% for assistance at surgery. With growing concern about access to care for beneficiaries in nursing facilities, Medicare in OBRA89 expanded coverage in such settings to include NPs. As with the PA provision, payment is made only to the employer and is not to exceed 85% of the physician's fee.

The most recent changes in Medicare NPP payment policy expanded coverage significantly to address perceived access problems in rural areas. First, all PA services provided to beneficiaries in rural HPSAs were covered in OBRA87. As with other payment policies for PAs, the employer is paid; in this case, a payment level of 85% of the physician fee was established. In amendments enacted under OBRA90, NPs and clinical nurse specialists (CNSs) for the first time were permitted to bill Medicare directly, without an employer intermediary, for all services provided in a rural setting.

Because Medicare policy has expanded NPP coverage primarily to meet the needs of beneficiaries in rural areas, NPPs have been restricted in their ability to furnish services to underserved populations in urban areas. For example, PA services delivered in inner-city clinics or offices are not covered unless they are incident to the physician's service and thus require physician supervision.

Both Medicare and Medicaid payment policies for PA services reflect the fact that PAs, by virtue of their practice acts, do not work independently from physicians and are not self-employed. Perhaps because of this and because no federal Medicaid mandate (other than the RHCSA) requires states to cover PA services, more than half of states have not developed specific regulations for PA coverage.

Whether or not a state has specific PA coverage policies, most (but not all) Medicaid programs generally cover all types of PA services, as long as the services are normally covered by their plans when provided by a physician. Furthermore, unlike Medicare statutes, Medicaid regulations do not restrict coverage of PA services or the services of any other NPP to certain regions of the state, such as rural areas or HPSAs. Generally, the amount, duration, and scope of Medicaid program benefits must be the same statewide.

Like Medicare, nearly all state Medicaid programs make payments only to the employer for the services PAs provide. Montana and South Dakota give PAs the option to bill directly for their services, using unique identification numbers when submitting Medicaid claims. They receive a standard percentage of the physician's fee for each service.

Although not allowing PAs to bill directly, many states use either a unique number or a service code modifier to identify PA services on claim forms. More than half the state Medicaid programs have not developed a specific payment policy for PAs. In such states, PA services are covered when provided as incident to physician services. In some states in which the incident to provision is strictly interpreted, Medicaid policy essentially requires on-site physician supervision of services for payment purposes. The exception is when PAs in rural health clinics or federally qualified health centers are not required to be directly supervised according to federal Medicaid mandate. In most states, however, the professional practice act does not require direct supervision. Rather, it allows PAs to work in off-site or remote supervisory arrangement with physicians (see Table 9-11).

Medicaid programs recognize that restricting coverage of PA services to directly supervised settings limits the volume of services and patients the physician-PA team can manage (PPRC 1993a).

JOB SATISFACTION/ATTRITION

A high rate of turnover of professional personnel in a clinic is disruptive to patient care and organizational stability, as well as to the individual clinician. When turnover occurs, productivity and the efficiency of the health care service are negatively affected. The major reason PAs, NPs, and physicians leave an organization is usually management (Pantell 1980).

Research on PAs and job satisfaction is fairly extensive and PAs seem to be reasonably satisfied with their work experience and practice conditions. PAs express an overall level of satisfaction that compares favorably with other professionals such as lawyers, accountants, and engineers (Perry 1978b). They report less stress and have lower turnover rates than nurses and many other health workers (Holmes 1993). PAs also are more satisfied than NPs, who regard themselves as better trained and more effective alternative practitioners. Within the health care hierarchy, PAs tend to have higher status than NPs and see themselves as assistant practitioners. Some analysts suggest that NPs resent the advantageous entry and rapid acceptance of PAs (Wolinsky 1988).

The major determinants of job satisfaction among PAs seem to be the professional and personal support the PA's supervising physician provides, the amount of responsibility for patient care, and opportunities for career advancement (Baker 1989). The strongest correlates of both job performance and job satisfaction are the degree of physician supervisory support and amount of responsibility for patient care (Perry 1976; Engle 1981). Location in smaller communities is also associated with greater satisfaction (Sells 1975), although a more recent study found that satisfaction levels were equally high for PAs practicing in both urban and rural settings (Larson 1994a). Lack of opportunities for career advancement has been frequently cited as a major concern and the main cause of attrition from the PA profession (Clawson 1993). Inadequate financial compensation and control over income are other reported sources of dissatisfaction (Willis 1992). Acceptance by patients and by other health workers has not been found to be a significant problem (Nelson 1974a; Record 1980; Record 1981b).

Among PAs, job satisfaction is highly correlated with the level of clinical responsibility and professional autonomy, the extent of professional and personal support provided by the supervising physician(s), and the opportunities for career advancement. The majority of studies addressing the job/career satisfaction of PAs reveal that they are largely satisfied in their professional roles and quite happy with their career choice, a set of findings a bit surprising in view of the status of PAs as dependent practitioners (Perry 1976, Perry 1978b).

Holmes and Fasser reported findings of occupational stress and professional retention in a survey conducted of 1,360 randomly selected practicing PAs responding to a mailed questionnaire. The typical respondent was male (53%), white (88%), age 37 (mean), and devoted most work time to patient care activities. Job satisfaction was high overall, and it was correlated positively with independence, challenge, and job security. Issues of salary, perceived opportunities for advancement, and the management style of the employer were associated with the highest levels of job dissatisfaction and role stress (Holmes 1993).

In the only study that compares PAs with other occupations that have similar levels of responsibility, Freeborn and Hooker examined PAs in an HMO with NPs, optometrists, mental health workers, and chemical dependency counselors. PAs expressed the most satisfaction with the amount of responsibility, support from co-workers, job security, working hours, supervision, and task variety. They were less satisfied with workload, control over the pace of work, and opportunities for advancement. Chemical dependency counselors expressed the highest levels of satisfaction across various dimensions of work and optometrists the lowest (Table 9-12). NPs also tended to be satisfied with most aspects of practice in this setting. In a number of instances, they were more satisfied than the PAs. Most PAs were also satisfied with pay and fringe benefits (Freeborn 1995; Hooker 1995a).

These findings, along with other studies, suggest that institutions, group practices, and HMOs are favorable settings for PAs (Brady 1980; Perry 1980; Johnson 1988). This is consistent with the PA model of member of a health care team.

Table 9-12 *Comparison of job satisfaction between nonphysician providers*

CHARACTERISTICS	PA	NP	CDC	MH	OD
Responsibility	84.7	89.1	71.0	78.8	51.8
Co-workers	80.0	85.5	90.3	84.6	85.7
Job security	79.9	65.5	60.0	51.9	85.2
Hours	73.3	81.8	64.5	88.5	82.1
Supervision	70.2	69.8	84.4	70.4	59.3
Variety of patients	65.0	74.5	77.4	73.1	35.7
Workload burden	53.3	50.0	55.8	46.1	28.6
Control over pace	40.7	43.6	66.7	44.2	17.9
Advancement	25.0	36.4	38.7	32.7	25.9
Number of respondents	58	54	32	52	29

Abbreviations: PA, physician assistant; NP, nurse practitioner; CDC, chemical dependency counselor; MH, mental health worker; OD, Optometrist.

(Data from Freeborn and Hooker 1995.)

Perry (1984) noted the following:

Little is known about why PAs leave their careers. Clearly some do so to raise families and some may return to resume at least part-time. We estimate that the attrition rate is approximately two percent a year. Background may play a role since men, former military medical corpsmen, and graduates of military PA programs exhibited the lowest attrition in one study.

SUMMARY

Job satisfaction is a significant barrier to cost-effectiveness. If the employee does not feel he or she is being fully utilized, productivity and the confidence of the staff and patients will suffer. It appears PAs are fairly satisfied with their roles as health professionals and the environments in which they are employed.

10

Relationships to Other Health Professions

This chapter describes the different relationships that physician assistants (PAs) have forged as they have sought recognition. The Department of Labor estimates that there are over 1,000 occupations that deal with patients in some aspect of the health workforce. This is a dramatic contrast to the way medicine was originally organized. In the colonial period of America, all medical service was under the purview of the physician. Assistance was provided informally by the patient's family. Formal nursing arose from a need to assist the physician in treatments, and to tend to the sick. Since then there has been a constant genesis of new health care occupations. Virtually all health occupations have taken a common path—an assistant to the physician or nurse. Since the origin of the American PA movement is no different, it is not surprising that the PA profession should try to foster a relationship with medicine and nursing for both support and survival.

PHYSICIANS AND PAS

PAs were born out of a concept developed by physicians—the need for an assistant who could assume physician-type responsibility and extend their usefulness. Because of this concept, a close working relationship with physicians have held PAs in good stead. Therefore, it is not surprising that PAs and their physician employers agree about the degree of supervision and autonomy. Studies find what seems to be greater consensus than conflict in this area, and physicians report that the quality of their lives have improved as a result of hiring a PA (Todd 1992; Johnson 1978).

In the 1970s and 1980s, a number of surveys of attitudes of physicians on PAs examined hypothetical duties and activities of PAs (Legler 1983). These questions were asked both of physicians who employed PAs and those who did not have contact with PAs. Some of the questions centered around taking histories, blood pressure readings, casting, and suturing. All concluded that routine activities were most appropriate and regardless of specialty, type of practice, or community need, most thought it practical to employ a PA (Borland 1972). Sometimes the surveys concluded that a PA could provide appropriate care, but legal and liability questions often arose to suggest that there may be some reluctance to have a PA as an employee (Yanni 1972). Other times the surveys showed a generally favorable attitude towards PAs, but few physicians thought it a solution to the primary care doctor shortage (Haug 1973). A mail survey of Army physicians stationed worldwide found that a majority (74%) would welcome a PA to relieve them of seeing routine or minor problems, and 81% believed that the quality of care would be improved or at least not changed by PA utilization. The majority of Army physicians approved of the assignment of PAs to remote locations with a fairly independent role in the care of active duty personnel, but not of dependents (Stuart 1974). In the rural South, a very high percentage of physicians have a favorable attitude toward PAs even though many had never worked with them (Joiner 1974; Fenn 1987).

The perception of what a PA can do sometimes differs from what they are already providing in patient services. In a study of delegating tasks to hypothetical pediatric PAs, mothers approved the concept of this new health provider by 94%, but when the same question about specific task delegation was presented to the pediatrician, the patient's willingness to accept delegated patient-care services exceeded the pediatrician's willingness to delegate these tasks (Patterson 1969).

In a study of physicians' attitudes toward PAs and nurse practitioners (NPs) as their employment relates to effect on quality of care, risk of malpractice, role threat, and gender bias in a large HMO, internists and pediatricians had favorable attitudes toward both NPs and PAs. Obstetricians/gynecologists had somewhat less favorable attitudes (Fig. 10-1). Several questions were asked to determine whether or not these physicians—who at the time of this study in 1977 were predominantly male—may have had some gender bias, as all the PAs were male and the NPs were predominantly female. Physician responses indicating that PAs more than NPs should be awarded certain privileges and participation would suggest the existence of some gender bias (Johnson 1986).

Physicians were also asked whether it was a good idea to be on a first-name basis with PAs and NPs. These almost all male physicians in general were less likely to think it was a good idea to be on a first name basis with NPs than with PAs. The HMO doctors were also asked about certain privileges such as (1) wearing the same clinical coats except for the identification tag, (2) having access to areas reserved for physicians, (3) participation in decisions about how outpatient care was to be delivered, and (4) sitting on various clinical committees. Physicians were generally accepting of PAs in their attitudes, and no consistent pattern in their acceptance or attitudes toward PAs emerged in this study (Johnson 1986).

However overwhelming the acceptance of PAs by physicians may appear, it is not viewed by all physicians the same way and it would be disingenuous if we did not have some discussion about physician objections to PAs.

For some physicians, professional dominance is jeopardized by PAs and NPs, and they hold that the role of the PA or NP is intended to usurp the role of the physician. One argument is that profit motives and faulty patient satisfaction surveys have contributed to the rise of nonphysician provider demands for expanded scope of practice, often achieved legislatively (Lichter 1995).

Several arguments can be made to counter these views. First is the remarkably opposite view that most policy analysts, economists, and medical sociologists have taken when examining the role of PAs in health care delivery. Their views seem to be endorsed at very high levels, and the utilization of PAs are viewed as an important component in health care reform. At present, America's health care delivery system and personnel are perceived by the public to have a number of problems, prompting the need for major reform measures. Many of these problems relate to the composition of its health workforce and the impact of provider specialty and geographic distribution (White 1992; Pew 1993). In its "Third Report," the Council on Graduate Medical Education (COGME) found the following: The rising physician/population ratio will do little to improve the public's health or increase access to services; moreover, it will hinder cost-containment efforts. There is an imbalance of physician specialty distribution, with too few primary care physicians and too many specialist physicians.

Figure 10-1 Physician attitudes toward PA. (Data from Johnson 1986.)

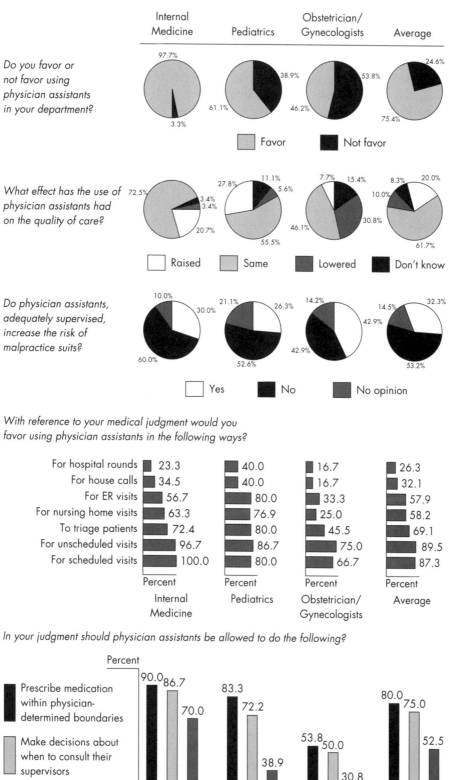

Internal Medicine | Pediatrics | Obstetrician/Gynecologists | Average

Do you favor or not favor using physician assistants in your department?

Internal Medicine: 97.7%, 3.3%
Pediatrics: 38.9%, 61.1%
Obstetrician/Gynecologists: 53.8%, 46.2%
Average: 24.6%, 75.4%

☐ Favor   ■ Not favor

What effect has the use of physician assistants had on the quality of care?

Internal Medicine: 72.5%, 3.4%, 3.4%, 20.7%
Pediatrics: 27.8%, 11.1%, 5.6%, 55.5%
Obstetrician/Gynecologists: 7.7%, 15.4%, 30.8%, 46.1%
Average: 8.3%, 20.0%, 10.0%, 61.7%

☐ Raised   ☐ Same   ■ Lowered   ■ Don't know

Do physician assistants, adequately supervised, increase the risk of malpractice suits?

Internal Medicine: 10.0%, 30.0%, 60.0%
Pediatrics: 21.1%, 26.3%, 52.6%
Obstetrician/Gynecologists: 14.2%, 42.9%, 42.9%
Average: 14.5%, 32.3%, 53.2%

☐ Yes   ■ No   ■ No opinion

With reference to your medical judgment would you favor using physician assistants in the following ways?

	Internal Medicine	Pediatrics	Obstetrician/Gynecologists	Average
For hospital rounds	23.3	40.0	16.7	26.3
For house calls	34.5	40.0	16.7	32.1
For ER visits	56.7	80.0	33.3	57.9
For nursing home visits	63.3	76.9	25.0	58.2
To triage patients	72.4	80.0	45.5	69.1
For unscheduled visits	96.7	86.7	75.0	89.5
For scheduled visits	100.0	80.0	66.7	87.3

Percent — Internal Medicine | Percent — Pediatrics | Percent — Obstetrician/Gynecologists | Percent — Average

In your judgment should physician assistants be allowed to do the following?

Percent

■ Prescribe medication within physician-determined boundaries
☐ Make decisions about when to consult their supervisors
■ Refer patients directly to specialists within the medical offices

Internal Medicine: 90.0, 86.7, 70.0
Pediatrics: 83.3, 72.2, 38.9
Obstetrician/Gynecologists: 53.8, 50.0, 30.8
Average: 80.0, 75.0, 52.5

America's medical educational system is disarticulated between its undergraduate and graduate (GME) components and should be more responsive to regional and national workforce needs. Shortages in the number of primary care physicians contribute to continuing problems in health services access. There continues to be a decline in interest in generalist training among recent medical graduates; only 16% of medical graduates selected residencies in primary care areas and a 57% match rate in internal medicine residency programs in 1993. The preparation of physicians for roles in primary care is often inadequate for future practice responsibilities, particularly in managed care systems. There is a need for better health workforce planning and to restructure financing and reimbursement systems to attain the appropriate specialty mix racial/ethnic composition, and geographic distribution of physicians (COGME 1994).

Strategies aimed at strengthening the ability of the nation's health workforce to deliver primary care and improve effectiveness in reducing costs and increasing access will require many years to attain if physicians are the only professionals assumed to deliver medical care services. If overall policy goals for the workforce put forth by COGME and others are to be achieved, it seems likely that such efforts will require the participation of nonphysicians. Health professions educational planning and clinical delivery systems must increasingly take advantage of the advantages of using PAs. Health care delivery systems in the future have been envisioned where the bulk of primary care services is delivered by PAs and nurse practitioners, as physicians assume an increased amount of staff management, administrative, and clinical consulting duties. Such changes in health care professional roles would likely be economically more efficient for medical practices and be a more rational way to utilize medical training and talent (Meikle 1992a; Meikle 1992b).

Another counter argument is that medicine is being practiced differently and more efficiently now than ever before. We have discarded scalpels that need resharpening and

needles that need sterilization and replaced them with disposable and better quality instruments because of the cost-effectiveness of these innovations. Likewise we have replaced many traditional physician services with alternatives that are more economical than those provided by physicians and in many instances superior to them. History provides us with many examples. Optometrists have taken over the refraction component of ophthalmology care, not because they wanted to, but because physicians were willing to delegate this role to free up their time for other eye services such as surgery. Midwives have been providing birthing services long before there were competent physicians interested enough in assuming this role. A number of studies have shown that contemporary midwifery is not only safe but may be superior, with the cost of a delivery considerably less than an accoucherment assisted by a physician. Other examples abound: nurse anesthetists substitute for anesthesiologists, podiatrists for orthopedic surgeons, and psychologists for psychiatrists.

Lichter also claims that anti-intellectualism has contributed to the rise of PA/NP expanded scope of practice, often achieved legislatively (Lichter 1995). This may be true since PAs make no claim to be elite providers and instead may be more like nurses that are comfortable allying themselves to the needs of consumers. As Paul Starr (1982) points out:

> [Medicine], by its nature, is an inegalitarian institution; it claims to enjoy a dignity not shared by ordinary occupations and a right to set its own rules and standards. These claims go against the democratic grain. They are also exceptionally hard to establish and enforce in a fluid, rapidly expanding society.

The PA role seems more like a blend between the skills of a physician and the patient-oriented role of the nurse. These attributes are attractive to the consumer.

Other arguments contend that the advent of medical boards-guaranteed educational training of practitioners and any movement away from education as the basis of licensure is a step away from medical standards that will have negative long-term consequences (Lichter 1995). What is not accounted for in this view is the superior educational development that has come out of collaboration between PA training programs and physician training programs. As Dr. Estes has stated: "The educational system producing physician assistants is more advanced, efficient, and cost-effective than that producing physicians." (Estes 1993).

Finally, physician attitudes toward an expanded role for the PA in the future is quite favorable (Legler 1983; Lapius 1983).

How receptive physicians are to the effective employment of PAs is questionable since the relationship between physicians and PAs is not always well understood, even by physicians who employ them. Ferraro and Southerland found that physicians are most likely to think that use of PAs should be directed toward caring for the urban poor and least likely to improve care for obstetrics and pediatrics cases (Ferraro 1989). Physicians may seem more willing to employ and delegate tasks to a PA than an NP (Fottler 1979), although this view may be reflective of an older concept of both providers.

Remarkably good relationships now exist between PAs and physicians. These relationships are manifested in the types of positions that PAs occupy, as well as with organized medicine and physician professional societies.

ORGANIZED MEDICINE

A relationship between the American Academy of Physician Assistants (AAPA) and the American Medical Association (AMA) has waxed and waned over the years. In 1994, the AMA granted observer status for the AAPA to sit in on the AMA House of Delegates, a signal that this relationship has recently been strengthened.

In 1995, the AMA House of Delegates adopted a set of guidelines for the working relationship between physicians and PAs. The guide-

lines recognize that PAs practice with physician supervision and that the PA's role in patient care should be determined by the PA and physician together. This recognition came in deference to the practice advocated by NPs. The AMA Board of Trustees wrote that NPs "... use terms like 'collaboration' and 'interdependent' whereas PAs use 'delegation and supervision.' PAs regard themselves as 'agents' of the physicians, legally and practically, and view delegated medical acts and understanding the delegatory style of physicians with whom they work as their particular responsibilities. They define 'collaboration' as synonymous with physician supervision. In contrast, NPs work towards 'independent' practice and decision making under the nurse practice acts." (Gara 1995)

However, this relationship is not entirely mutual, and in 1995 the AMA developed a set of guidelines that establishes the ideal relationship between a physician and a PA (Table 10-1).

Basically these guidelines reflect the AMA belief that in all settings PAs should recognize physician supervision in the delivery of patient care, and that there is no role for PAs either to be in competition with physicians, or to practice medicine independently from physicians.

A similar relationship exists with the American Academy of Family Physicians to work on issues affecting continuing medical education. For now, the relationship between organized medicine and the PA profession seems secure providing it remains as physicians want it.

NURSING

In their first decade of existence, PAs struggled to distinguish themselves from nurses. When assigned to hospital roles, PAs were often placed in nursing departments. In outpatient settings, PAs were often linked with an RN, believing this relationship would strengthen the PA's role (Lairson 1974). Some believe the logical place for PAs is within the nursing profession (Bergman 1971). PAs are sometimes referred to as a *mid-level provider*. This unde-

Table 10-1 *AMA guidelines for physician/PA practice*

1. The physician is responsible for managing the health care of patients in all practice settings.
2. Health care delivered by physicians and physician assistants must be within the scope of each practitioner's authorized practice as defined by state law.
3. The physician is ultimately responsible for coordinating and managing the care of patients and, with the appropriate input of the physician assistant, ensuring the quality of health care provided to patients.
4. The physician is responsible for the supervision of the physician assistant in all settings.
5. The role of the physician assistant(s) in the delivery of care should be defined through mutually agreed upon guidelines that are developed by the physician and the physician assistant and based on the physician's delegatory style.
6. The physician must be available for consultation with the physician assistant at all times either in person or through telecommunication systems or other means.
7. The extent of the involvement by the physician assistant in the assessment and implementation of treatment will depend on the complexity and acuity of the patient's condition and the training and experience and preparation of the physician assistant as adjudged by the physician.
8. Patients should be made clearly aware at all times whether they are being cared for by a physician or a physician assistant.
9. The physician and physician assistant together should review all delegated patient services on a regular basis, as well as the mutually agreed upon guidelines for practice.
10. The physician is responsible for clarifying and familiarizing the physician assistant with his supervising methods and style of delegating patient care.

(Data from AMA House of Delegates, June 1995.)

fined term implies that PAs are somewhere between physicians and nurses. The problem with this term is that nurses feel they are on the same level as physicians as colleagues, not under them; therefore, the term *midlevel* seems inappropriate. Nursing and medicine are occupations that work alongside each other, and although nurses may be employees of physicians, nursing is a profession that assesses the needs of the patient in conjunction with the physician's assessment.

To evaluate nurses' attitudes towards PAs, a survey was conducted in two hospitals. Hospital X employed 19 PAs to work in adult and pediatric ambulatory clinics, the emergency department, neonatal intensive care unit (NICU), and the newborn nursery. Hospital Y employed no PAs (Table 10-2). The results of this study indicate that nurses who have experience working with PAs or have an understanding of the role of the PA in the health care system have more positive attitudes toward them than those who do not have such knowledge or experience (Erkert 1985).

Although some tension exists between PAs and nursing on the academic level, the roots of PAs go deeply into the nurse profession and are likely to remain. Many PAs had their primary introduction to medicine through nursing. The early military corpsmen were often trained in part by nurses and were often under nursing departments in field and stateside hospitals. In 1995, more than 30% of all PA students were from nursing backgrounds.

NURSE PRACTITIONERS

Evolution of patterns in the division of medical labor in US medicine now reveals that important contributions are made by several types of nonphysician health professionals and that utilization of these providers can enhance and expand the services provided to patients. As part of this evolution of health professional roles over the last 30 years, PAs, NPs, and certified nurse midwives (CNMs) have been increasingly incorporated into medical practices and health institutions' staffing.

The NP concept began the same year as PAs, in 1965. Most NP programs are affiliated with nursing schools, and almost all are master's degree programs. Like PAs, NPs are well distributed throughout the medical profession, and in many instances PAs and NPs compete for jobs suggesting parity. NP programs tend to be specialty oriented, but the vast majority are primary care based. They do not consider themselves a physician-dependent profession; they believe their care is an extension of the nursing act. This philosophy has been the source of much debate and comparison between the two professions.

Table 10-2 *Nurses' attitudes towards PAs*

1. *In general, do you believe the PAs with whom you have worked to be professionally competent?*

Hospital [a]	Yes	No
X	91.4%	8.6%
Y	74.2%	25.8%

2. *In general, do you object to performing functions at the request of a PA you believe to be professionally competent?*

Hospital	Yes	No
X	27.9%	72.1%
Y	36.5%	63.5%

3. *In general, are you or would you be comfortable working with a PA?*

Hospital	Yes	No
X	78.4%	21.6%
Y	56.2%	43.8%

4. *Of PAs and NPs, which do you personally prefer?*

Hospital	PA	NP	Both	Neither
X	8.1%	11.1%	58.6%	22.2%
Y	9.6%	35.6%	32.9%	21.9%

5. *How would you describe your overall attitude toward the PA profession?*

Hospital	Positive	Negative	Indifferent
X	52.3%	10.3%	37.4%
Y	35.4%	21.5%	43.1%

6. *I do not clearly understand the need for PAs in the health care system.*

Hospital	True	False
X	37.1%	69.2%
Y	47.9%	52.1%

7. *I do not clearly understand the need for PAs in the hospital.*

Hospital	True	False
X	64.1%	35.9%
Y	74.7%	25.3%

8. *My state Nurse Practice Act:*

	Hospital X	Hospital Y
Allows me to legally take orders from a PA	12.3%	6.0%
Legally requires me to take orders from a PA	2.8%	1.5%
Does not allow me to legally take orders from a PA	34.9%	16.4%
I do not know what the Nurse Practice Act says in regards to PAs	50.0%	76.1%

[a] Hospital X = 19 PAs; Hospital Y = No PAs.

(Data from Erkert 1985.)

Despite divergent training and sometimes acrimonious debate, there is remarkable agreement in how PAs and NPs approach the patient. As a result of this attitude, PAs and NPs are often thought of as similar types of health care providers. In a number of clinical settings, such as managed care health systems and ambulatory clinics, the roles of PAs and NPs are regarded as interchangeable, and jobs are often advertised that can be filled by either one.

Major research reports and policy analyses that have examined both of these health professionals consider them to be equivalent when utilized in ambulatory practice roles (OTA 1986; Morgan 1993). Even on the clinic level, PAs and NPs have similar views about their roles. When PAs and NPs attitudes about jobs and roles are surveyed the results are indistinguishable (Freeborn 1995).

The histories of NPs and PAs have some interesting parallels in their history. In 1965, the first NP demonstration project, funded by the Commonwealth Foundation, was initiated at the University of Colorado Medical Center. Dr. Henry Silver and Loretta Ford, RN, were the developers of this program in pediatrics. The intent was to extend the nurse's role. As a 5-year project it was designed to prepare nurses to provide comprehensive well-child care in noninstitutional settings and to study the program outcomes for their applicability for curriculum changes in collegiate nursing programs (Ford 1979). This course of study was 4 months long followed by 20 months of field experience with a pediatrician. At completion of this program, these nurses were granted a certificate. Graduates of this program were called Pediatric Nurse Practitioners.

Despite their similarity in origins, however, important differences between PAs and NPs do exist (Table 10-3). As health professionals, NPs and PAs possess distinctive professional orientations and educational backgrounds, have different state regulatory systems, and show practice characteristics that appear to be moving in different directions. NPs believe that as nurses, they are empowered to act independently, with the authority to prescribe drugs without physician oversight. They want nurse reimbursement rates to be brought up to physician rates for a "like service" (Safriet 1992). Patients view them differently as well (Conant 1971). These differences have important implications for the future roles of both professions in a reformed health system. About 49,500 NPs have received formal training. In 1994 about 27,500 were in active clinical practice (Moses 1993). NPs represent 1.3% of the total pool of licensed nurses; of all NPs, about 4,500 are CNMs. NPs are distributed mostly in the primary care fields of adult medicine, pediatrics, women's health, student health, and geriatrics. The practice patterns of NPs are largely based in these primary care areas and in the future can be expected to expand their profiles in nursing homes, home care, and community-clinic settings (Morgan 1993). There are almost 500 accredited educational programs for NPs and 17 CNM programs. NP and CNM programs shared federal support under Title VIII Division of Nursing grants, funding 81 programs in 1992 and 83 in 1993, at a total of $14.2 million per year (Moses 1993).

Even in the absence of far-reaching health care reform, it is anticipated that requirements for the utilization of PAs and NPs is expected to increase in the future health system. A commission to the Council on Graduate Medical Education (COGME) reported that the PA supply is far less than current demand, and this demand may increase sharply between 1995 and 2005 (AGPAW 1995). Similar changes are also envisioned for NPs and CNMs, particularly in helping to meet primary care delivery needs under a reformed system providing universal access (Harper 1996). Projections include requirements for higher numbers of both PAs and NPs to fulfill roles as primary care practitioners, in private practices, in expanding managed care systems, and in institutional settings.

Unique to nurse practitioners are resources that relate to the nursing professional base. Social appeal, political potential through numbers, lower level practice, and substitution opportunities all relate to nursing origins. For PAs, the lack of these origins and some of their related phenomena can either benefit or hinder them. Unencumbered by "doctor-nurse" conflicts and traditional role perceptions, some analysts believe that PAs have somewhat clearer identities, greater mobility, and willingness—by role, definition, and name—to serve as physician associates than are NPs. Their roles are more flexible because of this willing dependence (Salmon 1985).

Many of the barriers to full utilization for NPs and PAs are common to both. These

Table 10-3 *Comparison of PAs and NPs, 1992*

CHARACTERISTIC	RESPONSE CATEGORY	PAs	NPs
Estimated practicing clinicians		21,633	27,500
Total graduates		25,333	49,500
Sampled		11,300	1,738
Gender (%)	Female	42.4	96.1
	Male	57.6	3.1
Race/ethnicity (%)	Unknown	0.0	0.7
	White, non-Hispanic	90.3	91.3
	Black, non-Hispanic	4.1	3.7
	Hispanic	3.1	1.2
	American Indian/Alaskan Native	0.7	0.0
	Asian/Pacific Islander	1.8	1.0
Age group (%)	Unknown	0.0	2.8
	<25 years	2.6	0.1
	25–34	33.0	11.3
	35–44	47.4	46.2
	45–54	14.9	25.7
	55–64	2.0	12.0
	>64	0.1	2.6
Region (%)	Northeast	32.2	26.4
	Midwest	20.5	16.7
	South	29.9	34.0
	West	17.4	22.8
	Canada	0.0	0.2
Years working (%)	<5 years	43.9	29.1
	6–10	31.8	27.3
	11–15	12.8	27.9
	16–20	9.1	11.4
	>20	2.4	1.5
	Unknown		2.8
Average work week (%)	Full-time (>32 hours)	90.8	75.3
	Part-time (<32 hours)	9.2	24.7
Gross annual income (%)	<$20,000	0.3	6.4
	$20K–29,999	3.1	11.3
	$30K–39,999	25.4	21.5
	$40K–49,999	35.1	30.2
	$50K–74,999	30.1	23.3
	>$75K	6.0	20.0
	Unknown		5.2
Independent practice legislation	Number of states	0	6
Primary care		48%	90%

(Data from American Academy of Physician Assistants General Census, 1993; Washington Consulting Group, Survey of Certified Nurse Practitioners and Clinical Nurse Specialists: December 1992.)

include physician dependence, institutional "job" dependence, limited power when compared to physicians, legal status less than optimal, partial reimbursement, and variance on qualifications and training (Bullough 1975; Eastaugh 1981).

The barriers unique for NPs include time control needs and a relative lack of professional organization. PAs, on the other hand, may be limited by the social/political license afforded NPs because of their lack of a homogeneous professional base. Nursing is the common denominator for all NPs, and the nursing lobby is a powerful voice. Nurses believe they have one foot up the rung of professional acceptance because of their nursing background. PAs, on the other hand, began their profession as former corpsmen, but have chosen to seek diversification in their students and now have a wide profession base. These attributes that facilitate or inhibit full expression of a profession are called *enablers* and *barriers* (Table 10-4).

Unlike PAs, who have a single national academy that consolidates all PA efforts (the AAPA), no single organization represents all NPs. The American Academy of Nurse Practitioners, the American College of Nurse Practitioners, the American Nurse Association, and the National Alliance of Nurse Practitioners all claim some representation and have their advocates and critics. Other organizations represent different specialties of nurse practitioners nationally such as the National Association of Pediatric Nurse Associates & Practitioners (NAP NAP), Association of Women's Health, Obstetrics, and Neonatal Nurses (AWHONN), and the National Association of Nurse Practitioners in Reproductive Health. Four NP certification boards exist for credentialing NPs, depending on specialty and preference. The American Nursing Association, a powerful special interest group, acts on NP behalf from time to time. Because of this splintering of NP factions the likelihood of developing any alliances with NPs on the national level remains limited.

Nurse practitioner education is provided in 202 universities and other institutions with 527

Table 10-4 *PA and NP enablers and barriers to future roles in health care*

ENABLERS — NPs	ENABLERS — PAs
Professional base	Role flexibility
Independence of physicians	Willingness to assume dependent posture with physicians
Cost savings potential	Cost savings potential
Interchangeability with PAs	Interchangeability with NPs
Social appeal	Relatively greater mobility than NPs
Nursing numbers offer wide political potential to influence legislation	Professional organization
Large number of training programs granting graduate degrees.	Relatively clear identify

BARRIERS — NPs	BARRIERS — PAs
Physician independence	Physician dependence
Limited relative power	Limited relative power
Reduced reimbursable functions	Reduced reimbursable functions
Limited power (absolute)	Limited power (absolute)
Limited mobility compared to PAs	Lack of homogeneous professional base such as nursing
Specialized training	Variable qualifications/ training
Predominantly female with inherent time control needs (part-time, day shift, child dependence, etc.)	Small number of training programs. Range from junior colleges to graduate programs in academic medical centers
Professional disorganization	

programs or clinical tracks (Table 10-5). At least 75 nursing institutions have plans to add Master's degrees or post-Master's degree NP programs to their curricula by 1997 (Harper 1996).

Currently, a standardized measuring stick of what an NP should know and what the educational program should cover is nonexistent. Efforts are underway to develop more cohesive professional bodies and uniform standards so that information may be gathered that measures the NP roles more accurately.

Table 10-5 *Number and curriculum focus of NP programs* [a]

NURSE PRACTITIONER PROGRAM SPECIALTY	NUMBER	PERCENT
Family	143	77.7
Pediatric	64	34.8
Gerontologic/geriatric	51	27.7
Adult	49	26.6
Obstetric-gynecologic/ women's health	47	25.5
Neonatal	33	17.9
Adult psychiatric/mental health	23	12.5
Acute care (adult)	22	11.9
Oncology	9	4.9
Occupational health	8	4.3
School	6	3.3
Child and adolescent psychiatric/ mental health	5	2.7
Perinatal	5	2.7
Other (includes dual track options)	18	9.8
Total programs	483	100.0

[a] Only Master's-level programs.

(Data from American Association of the Colleges of Nursing, 1996.)

In many ways, tension between PAs and NPs is probably healthy because society is best served when both providers strive to improve their image and delivery of care. Both the public and the respective professions benefit when each is compared alongside each other as well as with physicians. Delivering quality care at affordable cost and providing choice in types of providers can only enhance the image of American medicine.

MANAGED CARE ORGANIZATIONS

Key health care reform policy goals are to lower medical care access barriers, cost-containment, and incorporating to a greater extent, new organizational structures ("managed competition") in health services delivery. In effect, this direction likely means a greater reliance on health maintenance organizations (HMOs) and other types of prepaid and managed health care delivery systems. The clinical staffing mix of future HMOs will be based in large part on the capabilities and efficiency of employed health care professionals, both physician as well as nonphysician, to provide the required range, access, and quality of medical diagnostic, therapeutic, and preventive care services in a manner acceptable to enrollees.

Many believe these efforts will result in improved levels of health care service access, promote grater effectiveness in medical care resource allocation, and place less emphasis on ability to pay as a criterion for American citizens seeking health care insurance coverage. A likely outcome of health system reform is the reconfiguration of America's health delivery system built on HMOs and other managed care plans. Such a change, as we have noted, will continue to have significant effects on the workforce. As these delivery systems become the principal locus of provision of primary care services for many individuals, it is likely that there will be an increased demand for both physician and nonphysician primary care providers.

In a recent analysis, Weiner (1996) assessed the requirements for physicians, both primary care and specialty, within managed care system through the year 2000. Projected estimates were developed using clinical performance data and setting requirement standards based on available information obtained from multiple segments of the health system, and applying these derived standards to the proportion of Americans assumed to be receiving medical care services within each sector. A particular focus was placed on HMO staffing levels under the likelihood that market share will increase with health reform. Requirement estimates were then compared to projections of physician supply performed by the Bureau of Health Professions through the year 2000. Supply estimates were developed under two alternative physician workforce training scenarios, one assuming that 20% of medical school graduates will enter primary care practice areas between 1993 and

2000, and the other assuming a 50% entry to primary care. An important conclusion of the analysis is that, under either scenario, the supply of physicians in the workforce will significantly outstrip the expected requirements for these physicians. Specifically, there will be a surplus of approximately 125,000 physicians (45 physicians/100,000 population), or nearly a quarter of all patient care physicians expected to be in active practice in the year 2000. Under the first physician workforce scenario, Weiner estimates that there will be a shortage of about 6,000 primary care physicians and an excess of 131,000 specialists. Under the second scenario, the marked imbalance is narrowed somewhat with the supply of physicians in primary care estimated to be about 13,000 more than estimated requirements; the surplus of specialists would number 113,000.

Analysts frequently use HMO staffing patterns to estimate national clinical workforce requirements. Based on a national survey of group and staff-model HMOs, they found that two-thirds employ a PA and/or NP. A correlation analysis also found that the HMOs that had the lowest ratio of primary care physicians to members also had the highest percentage of PA/NPs as employees (Dial 1995). This implies that PAs and NPs are being used in high ratios to substitute for physician services in these settings.

GOVERNMENT AND FINANCING ISSUES

The federal government provides substantial amounts in support of health professions education. Physicians receive a large share of the $4.9 billion Medicare subsidy of GME through direct medical education (DME) and indirect medical education assistance (IMEA) payments. These funds go to teaching hospitals to support the clinical education of physicians and include training assistance for a number of other health professionals. Currently, they do not include PAs or advanced practice nurses (clinical nurse specialists, NPs, or CNMs) as

eligible for support through the Medicare channel. In the past, federal dollars supporting PA and NP training have been administered through grant awards programs, a mechanism that in a number of instances has borne positive results. Current incentives/rewards for teaching hospitals sponsoring GME programs are driven more by institutional needs than by societal needs. Changing the structure and financing policies of Medicare DME and IMEA to better emphasize the training of generalist physicians is a strategy to modify GME. Making health professions' educational programs receiving federal support more accountable to the public in terms of graduate outcomes (i.e., patterns of specialty and practice location) is now an increasingly accepted premise.

Medicare policy has been slow to respond to shifting patterns of physician educational and practice. It has long been advocated that generalist physician numbers could be promoted by shifting the locus of GME training experiences to increase residents' time in outpatient/ambulatory care clinics, yet Medicare does not allow funding support in these settings. Policy changes in the financing of health professions education is a key part of health care reform. The Clinton administration's proposed bill, the Health Security Act, contained an extensive array of changes affecting GME size and funding. While this was not enacted, a major reform policy goal remains in place and is aimed to produce a 55% level of primary care physicians in the workforce. To help attain these goals, the development of a new IMEA fund to support the cost of academic health center functions beyond the usual provision of patient health care services, establishment of an institute for health care workforce development, a series of initiatives to augment Title VII and VIII funding above the current level, and a GME funding pool of $200 million for advanced practice nursing. This later proposal should be modified to include PAs in the likelihood that they will be utilized at the same level or higher than NPs and other advanced practice nurses in reform-restructured inpatient staffing. Incremental changes are anticipated in Congress that may eventually achieve this goal. Until then, PA education will have to rely on limited support through the Bureau of Health Professions.

PHARMACISTS

The last remaining barrier for full utilization of PAs is in the area of prescribing. On an individual level, where a PA works with a pharmacist, usually within an institution, there is wide acceptance of PAs and the way they prescribe (Hooker 1993). Anecdotally, some pharmacists have opposed the ability of PAs to prescribe. These attitudes are not based on science since there is a dearth of literature on either side of the issue. For the most part, pharmacists reports suggest that they do not seem concerned about PAs from a safety issue.

One study that examined PA views of drug information sources showed that PAs rated pharmacists as being the best sources of drug information. Next in descending order of drug information reliability were journal articles, physicians, detail persons, and other PAs. This study also found that PAs viewed pharmacists with increasing regard the more they came in contact with them (Fincham 1986).

When PAs were given the authority to prescribe in Wisconsin, a survey of pharmacists indicated that PAs were utilizing the privilege, and that the technical quality of their prescribing was appropriate. However, they were not sure whether it was appropriate for them to prescribe (Huntington 1987).

As pharmacists move into the role of limited prescriber in some states, the expansion of the PA role is likely to continue as pharmacists confront the same barriers that PAs once encountered. Alliances are likely to continue in this area.

PATIENTS

The patient's viewpoint is generally viewed as the most important element in the appraisal of PA acceptance in American society. While relationships with physicians and nurses are placed high on the list of importance, the relationship with the patients is the reasons why PAs have been able to thrive in such a competitive environment. If patient acceptance and satisfaction were low, it is doubtful PAs would still be in existence.

The first study on patient acceptance of PAs was conducted within a few years after the first class of PAs graduated. This study, anticipating that PAs would be dispersed throughout different socioeconomic classes, sought to determine PA acceptance by all classes. The results showed that the upper middle class community was more readily accepting of PAs (and NPs) than lower middle class communities (Conant 1971).

In 1972, a study was conducted in Los Angeles to assess patient acceptance and attitudes with regard to the use of PAs in different roles. Acceptance was highest among nonmarried middle-class respondents who had some exposure to college. As the perceived complexity of procedures a PA might perform was increased, approval decreased; 91% of all respondents approved of most procedures such as injections administered by PAs. This approval rating diminished to 34% in the case of first examination of a patient with a head injury by a PA (Strunk 1973). In another 1972 study, patients rated PAs highly in terms of technical competence (89%), professional manner (86%), and reported improvement in the quality of care (71%) and access to services (79%) (Nelson 1974a). Other studies helped reinforce these findings that PAs were generally well received by the patients they serve regardless of rural or urban setting, or social status (Storms & Fox 1979; Smith 1981; Oliver 1986).

To address a charge by some that physicians treat patients of higher socioeconomic status and PAs treat those of lower status, a study was undertaken in three primary care centers in Florida. Data showed no consistent or substantively significant relationships between the patients' social status and the type of provider (Crandall 1986). Another study using a random survey of all households in Kentucky found a substantial proportion of households come in contact with PAs and NPs and that satisfaction is quite high (Mainous 1992).

Blessing and Elizondo examined patient expectations of PAs in dealing with a series of personal, social, psychological, and health-related items. Results indicated that patients expect the PA to be involved with these problems, but did not expect the PA to be an expert (Elizondo 1990). In a follow-up survey a few years later, the subject groups were PAs, supervising physicians, and PA educators. The results were compared with the previous study, and the findings indicated a high level of confidence in the abilities of PAs (Blessing 1990).

Studies of patient satisfaction involving PAs, NPs, and physicians who work alongside each other are few. The impact of provider attitudes has an impact on the outcome of select disorders. The confidence and attitudes of 3 primary care PAs and 18 physicians were assessed 3 weeks after a clinic visit for low back pain in a large HMO. Patients of more confident providers were significantly more satisfied with the information they received than patients of less confident providers. Differences could not be explained by years in practice, length of visit, patient demographics, or the type of providers (Bush 1993).

In another HMO study, Kaiser Permanente members in the Pacific Northwest rated the "technical competence, skill, and ability" of physicians, PAs, and NPs as "satisfied or very satisfied" more than 75% of the time (Freeborn 1994). Hooker analyzed the same data spanning an 18-month period in the early 1990s with regard to how members view physicians, PAs, and NPs (Fig. 10-2). A 57-item questionnaire specifically asks about satisfaction with a particular medical office visit and a specific provider. Samples are drawn randomly from the automated appointment system and sent within 1 week after a patient's medical office visit. When members were asked how satisfied they were with their latest encounter, adult practice PAs and NPs scored within 1% to 2% of physicians (between 88% and 90% favorable). The technical skill of PAs and NPs rated within 3%

to 4% of physicians. As for overall satisfaction, members regarded adult medicine PAs and NPs almost the same and statistically indistinguishable from each other. In this study, pediatricians were viewed approximately 10% more favorably than pediatric PAs and NPs for reasons not clear in this study (Hooker 1993).

It appears that PAs are held high regardless of the patient's socioeconomic status, condition, and setting. These views seem to be held as a result of confidence in the PA's ability to take care of their medical conditions. Further studies are needed to determine whether these attitudes hold up when similar patients with similar conditions are seen by physicians, NPs, and PAs in the same setting.

PARENTS

Parents of children are listed here because of their reaction to the concept of pediatric PAs and child health associates. In a few years preceding full deployment of child health associates (CHAs), three separate studies reported favorable parent acceptance of pediatric-trained assistants on alternate pediatrician patient visits at approximately one-half the usual pediatric fee (Skinner 1968; Austin 1968). In structured interviews in the homes of 145 mothers in the Seattle area, roughly one-half of the group had regular pediatric care from private pediatricians, one-third from an HMO, and the rest from public health clinics. Approximately 75% of the mothers approved of the pediatric assistant for well-child care, and 94% indicated they would be willing to use the assistant if the physician and assistant were well trained and capable (Patterson 1969). A third study found that the pediatrician's time could be better spent delegating at least 50% of the workload to PAs (Anderson 1970).

Silver reported that 94% of the parents expressed satisfaction with the joint services they received from a pediatrician and a CHA team and with their opportunity to maintain adequate communication with the physician (Silver 1973). Half the parents of children seen

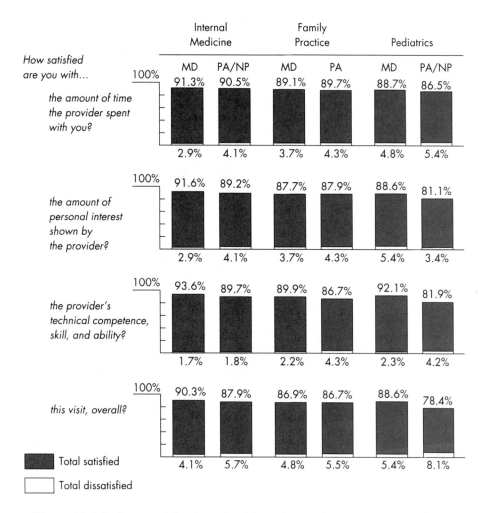

Figure 10-2 Patient sastisfaction, physicians, PAs, and NPs in an HMO. (Data from Hooker 1993.)

in this setting thought that joint care was better than care they received from a physician alone.

INTERNATIONAL MEDICAL GRADUATES

International medical graduates (IMGs) (formerly known as foreign medical graduates) have filled gaps in American medical services during most of the twentieth century. There are an estimated 100,000 unlicensed IMGs in the United

States, most of whom are foreign-born and foreign-trained. Unfortunately, not all can meet the requirements for medical licensure. Recognizing this population as a potential source of medical providers, some state medical boards have used various approaches to assist IMGs who have failed to meet requirements such as remedial activities to correct deficiencies in knowledge and skills, or limited licensure that allows IMGs to practice as physicians in certain settings and/or under supervision. As barriers to medical licensure have increased, many have sought ways to enter health care in lieu of completing the lengthy and expensive medical licensure process. Some IMGs have sought access to PA licensure as a permanent career change, others as an interim step toward licensure as physicians. Unlicensed IMGs have organized to promote state laws to make it easier for them to train or practice as PAs. These attempts to recast these IMGs as PAs have been criticized as creating a double standard for PA qualification, jeopardizing public safety, and creating a regulatory bureaucracy that would be prohibitively expensive (Fasser 1992b; Fowkes 1996).

The AAPA Professional Practice Council maintains that entry to the PA profession should require graduation from an accredited PA educational program and passage of the National Certifying Examination. The AAPA asserts that "passage of an examination by itself is inadequate to define the knowledge needed to practice as a PA." Part of the knowledge required is the socialization to the PA role and understanding of the physician-PA relationship, both taught and experienced as a PA student. Having states develop or administer their own examinations as an alternative entry mechanism would compromise the uniformity of a national PA qualifying standard and possibly discourage reciprocity between states. Moreover, there is evidence that IMGs lack the knowledge and skills necessary to practice as PAs or to validate fast-track or abbreviated educational programs as appropriate solutions (AAPA 1993c).

In California, surveys in 1980, 1993, and 1994 collected information about the interest and preparedness among IMGs seeking PA certification. These surveys revealed that few of the IMGs were interested in becoming PAs as a permanent career, and few could show a commitment to primary care of the underserved. Of the 50 IMGs accepted into California's PA programs in recent years, 62% had academic or personal difficulties. Only 34 IMGs became certified. The City University of New York/Harlem Hospital PA program developed an accelerated program for IMGs in 1992. None of the IMGs who took the same clinical competency examination developed for PA students could pass.

Some states including Maryland, Florida, Michigan, and Washington have used different approaches to alternative pathways to PA licensure for IMGs (Cawley 1994; Bottom 1994). Additional preparatory programs in California that have assessed the readiness of unlicensed IMGs to enter PA programs have shown that the participants did not demonstrate knowledge or clinical skills equivalent to those expected of licensed PAs (Cawley 1994; Fowkes 1996).

IMGs are not likely to be granted certified PA status without attending a formal PA preparatory program. Those who have done so however seem to have adopted to this new career well and do not see conflict with their medical degree and PA certification.

REGISTERED CARE TECHNOLOGISTS

In 1988, the American Medical Association proposed the creation of a registered care technologist (RCT). The proposal called for basic RCT training of 9 months, during which routine patient care duties such as bathing and bedpan and linen changing would be taught. Assisting the nurse in administering bedside medications and more complex nursing duties would require an 18-month training period and would be at a level of an advanced RCT.

The American Nurses Association (ANA) and other nursing groups were vehemently opposed to the creation of the RCT. Nursing leaders expressed their opposition to the proposal as the AMA's desires to strengthen medicine's control over nursing, to weaken their own control of nursing personnel, and to undermine nursing's efforts to standardize their education and credentialing.

In the RCT debate, the AMA delegates stressed the essential value of quality bedside patient care and the way in which the RCT would address this immediate need under nursing supervision. The AMA also argued that RCTs could form a new source of nursing applicants and thus be part of the long-term solution to alleviating the nursing shortage.

Six hospitals were recruited to undertake RCT pilot projects, but nursing opposition was so adamant that only one completed a study and no other was started. The official PA position was never condensed. On one hand, the profession espouses the values of quality patient care and the social good of relieving human suffering. On the other hand, there is little interest in weakening nursing's control of their education and credentialing process (Chavez 1989). In the end, the effort died a natural death and the profession was spared taking sides.

THE AMERICAN ACADEMY OF PHYSICIAN ASSISTANTS

Shortly after the second PA class graduated, it became apparent that some form of communication among all PAs was needed. The Medex program was developing in Seattle, and Alderson Broddus was launching its program. The early graduates of Duke decided that an organization was needed to reach out to all PAs, both students and graduates alike (Stanhope 1992). Out of this effort the American Academy of Physician Assistants (AAPA) was born in April 1968, and the first newsletter representing the nascent profession was sent to all graduates in 1969. From a group of 15 PAs that started an organization in a rented trailer, it now numbers over 24,000 members (Fig. 10-3). Dues are $200 for fellows and $40 for students.

This first foray into professional organization was not a direct lineage, and there was competition for an institution that could represent all PAs. Ballweg (1994) writes that:

> At least three other organizations also positioned themselves to speak for the new profession. These were a proprietary credentialing association, the American Association of Physician Assistants (a group representing U.S. Public Health Service PAs at Staten Island), the National Association of Physician Assistants, and the American College of Physician Assistants from the Cincinnati Technical College PA Program.

In the early 1970s, these four organizations vied for the opportunity to represent all PAs. Newly graduated PAs were asked to join or support one or another organization. Eventually most PAs selected the American Academy of Physician Assistants, probably because of strong leadership both by the elected president, Paul Moson, PA, and the newly hired Executive Director, Donald Fisher, PhD (Ballweg 1994).

The AAPA is the only national professional society for all PAs and is headquartered in Alexandria, Virginia. According to the by-laws of the Academy, the AAPA exists to enhance the role and utilization of physician assistants; to promote the PA profession to the public; assure the competency of physician assistants through active involvement in continuing education and certification processes; to conduct research on the PA profession. The Academy's mission, reaffirmed by the 1992 House of Delegates, is to promote quality, cost-effective, and accessible health care, and to promote the professional and personal development of physician assistants.

Chapter Structure

The Academy is a federated structure of 57 chartered constituent chapters representing the interests of PAs in 50 states, the District of Columbia, Guam, the Air Force, Navy, Army, Public Health Service/Coast Guard, and Veterans Affairs Department. PA educational programs have formed student societies that make up the Student Academy of the American Academy of Physician Assistants (SAAPA).

Purposes and Objectives

Since its founding, the AAPA has defined its purposes to include the following:

- Encourage its membership to render quality service to the public
- Develop, sponsor, and evaluate continuing medical or medically-related education programs for the PA

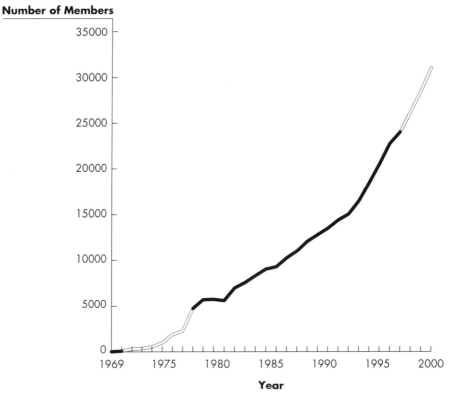

Number of Members

Estimated data based on incomplete records and projections.

Figure 10-3 Membership of the American Academy of Physician Assistants. Based on number of members at 31 January 1996. Estimated data based on incomplete records and projections. (Personal communication, M. Fitzgerald, American Academy of Physician Assistants, 1996.)

- Assist in the role definition for the PA
- Participate in the development of criteria leading to certification
- Develop, coordinate, and participate in studies having an impact directly or indirectly on the PA profession
- Serve as a public information center to membership, health professions, and the public
- Participate in certification of PAs

The objectives of the Academy include:

- Establishing moral and ethical guidelines for the assurance of continuity in the quality of health care delivery by its members

- Developing continuing medical education
- Providing services for members

Governing Bodies

The House of Delegates meets annually to adopt legislation and policy proposed by eight standing committees, three councils, the constituent chapters, the Board of Directors, the Student Academy, the Association of PA Programs, the Surgical Congress, and the Medical Congress. The Academy's fellow members elect 11 members of the Board of Directors. Other bodies of the AAPA include the Physician Assistant Foundation, which grants scholarships to deserving PA students and funds a small grants program, and a

Political Action Committee, which supports federal candidates supportive of the PA profession.

The development of the PA profession and the AAPA was virtually synonymous. It is organized with annually elected PAs as leaders. The leadership of the AAPA consists of a President, Vice President, Secretary, Treasurer, Speaker of the House of Delegates, and a Board of Directors. The president and Speaker of the House are the most visible of the elected executive board (Table 10-6).

The permanent staff is organized under an executive vice president (Table 10-7), a vice president for member programs, a vice president for government and professional affairs, a vice president for information and research services, and a vice president for finance and administrative services. Within this framework are 56 professional staff members who deliver a wide variety of services.

The AAPA has been fortunate to have had capable leadership and organization since its inception. This is accomplished by a remarkably low staff member ratio when compared to other organizations (Table 10-8).

Governmental and Professional Assistance

The AAPA is the only voice in Washington working on behalf of the PA profession. Representing the interests of PAs to public and private policy makers is a vital function of the Academy. It is the profession's advocate before federal courts and the US Congress. The staff of the AAPA provide assistance for policy makers about professional affairs, interpret proposed or enacted laws or regulations, and help identify the right official to contact for specific problems.

The Academy has worked aggressively to improve the regulations of PAs at the state level as well. Through the Academy's State Government Affairs Program and its resources it assists chapters that need help with projects that seek to improve PAs' scope of practice through changes in laws or regulations.

Table 10-6 Leadership of the AAPA

PRESIDENT	SPEAKER OF THE HOUSE
1997–1998 Libby Coyte	William Kolhepp
1996–1997 Sherri McNeely	William Kolhepp
1995–1996 Lynn Caton	William Kolhepp
1994–1995 Debi Atherton Gerbert	M. Randolph Bundschu
1993–1995 Ann L. Elderkin	M. Randolph Bundschu
1992–1993 William H. Marquardt	Debi Atherton Gerbert
1991–1992 Sherri L. Stuart	Debi Atherton Gerbert
1990–1991 Bruce C. Fischandler	Suzanne Reich
1989–1990 Paul Lombardo	Sherri L. Stuart
1988–1989 Marshall R. Sinback, Jr.	Sherri L. Stuart
1987–1988 Ron L. Nelson	Bruce C. Fischandler
1986–1987 R. Scott Chavez	Bruce C. Fischandler
1985–1986 Glen E. Combs	Bruce C. Fischandler
1984–1985 Judith B. Willis	Bruce C. Fischandler
1983–1984 Charles G. Huntington	Burdeen M. Camp
1982–1983 Ron L. Fisher	R. Scott Chavez
1981–1982 Jarrett M. Wise	Charles G. Huntington
1980–1981 C. Emil Fasser	Charles G. Huntington
1979–1980 Ron Rosenberg	John Weed
1978–1979 James E. Konopa	Elaine E. Grant
1977–1978 Dan P. Fox	William Hughes
1976–1977 Roger G. Whittaker	*
1975–1976 Thomas R. Godkins	*
1974–1975 C. Emil Fasser	*
1973–1974 Paul F. Moson	*
1972–1973 John A. Braun	*
1971–1972 Thomas R. Godkins	*
1970–1971 John J. McQueary	*
1969–1970 William D. Stanhope	*
1968–1969 William D. Stanhope	*

*House of Delegates not established until 1977.

(Data from American Academy of Physician Assistants, 1996.)

Table 10-7 Executive Vice President and Staff: AAPA

NAME	TENURE	NUMBER OF EMPLOYEES
Stephen Crane, PhD	1993–present	56
Harry A. Bradley	1992–1993	46
F. Lynn May	1984–1992	19
Peter D. Rosenstein	1981–1984	5
Donald W. Fisher, PhD	1973–1981	3

(Data from American Academy of Physician Assistants, 1996.)

Table 10-8 *Ratio of staff to members in various organizations*

American Academy of Physician Assistants	1 to 420
American College of Physicians	1 to 316
American Occupational Therapy Association	1 to 294
American Academy of Family Physicians	1 to 263
American College of Obstetrics and Gynecology	1 to 189
American College of Cardiology	1 to 169
American Physical Therapy Association	1 to 135

(Data from personal communications, M. Fitzgerald, American Academy of Physician Assistants, 1996.)

Although it would be impossible to list all of the accomplishments of the AAPA, one example may suffice. As the health care reform debate was in the spotlight for much of 1994, the AAPA's officers and lobbyists worked at educating legislators about the role PAs play on the health care team. The AAPA testified repeatedly, reaching every major committee involved in the health care reform debate. Members of the AAPA were invited to the White House for briefings on health care, and First Lady Hillary Rodham Clinton confirmed the rising importance of PAs in her address to the AAPA's national convention.

Under the Academy's Government and Professional Affairs Department, the AAPA continues to push for Medicare coverage of PA services in all practice settings. In response to the AAPA's prodding, the Medicare Carriers Manual was revised to expand the scope of medical services that PAs can provide. In 1994, the Academy won a major victory when the Senate Finance Committee voted for an amendment expanding Medicare coverage for PA services to all outpatient settings at 85% of the physician's reimbursement rate.

State activity has always been at the heart of enabling legislation for PAs, and this activity has increased as state legislatures tackle health care reform. To ensure that the PA point of view is heard and understood, the AAPA has staff that work exclusively on state issues. One result of this effort has been that PAs can prescribe in 39 states, the District of Columbia, and Guam. In addition, California PAs may write transmit-

tal orders for prescription drugs. A model legislative act for states to enable PAs to function as economically as possible is contained in Appendix 1. Other services the Academy provides include consultation and grants for chapters struggling with improving legislation. Reference materials include *Physician Assistants: State Laws and Regulations,* and the monthly *Legislative Watch.* Other services are a handbook on reimbursement policies and rationales of both private insurers and Medicare.

Publications

Several publications are produced by the Academy both for members and inquiries.

The *Journal of the American Academy of Physician Assistants* is the official clinical journal of the Academy. Published monthly by Medical Economics publishing house, it provides news reports, clinical review articles, research reports, a review of research on the PA profession, and other subjects of general interest for the profession. It is sent to all PA graduates, regardless of membership.

The *Membership Directory* is a list of all current members. It also contains publications, bylaws, AAPA annual calendar, and constituent chapter leadership information.

AAPA News is published biweekly. It is intended to keep members up-to-date on issues affecting PAs. Information includes updates on legislative and professional affairs, listings of employment, educational programs, data and survey results, and job opportunities.

Research Division

The Research Division performs a number of functions from internally initiated data collection and analyses, to sponsored projects (Table 10-9). The demand for data from the members, leaders, vendors, and government policy analysts is keen because of the high reliability and remarkably complete databases.

Three annual surveys are conducted by the research division—the membership census, the student census, and the conference survey—and

---

Table 10-9 *AAPA research division studies*

Internally sponsored or initiated data collection, analysis, and
   reporting projects
   Member Census (1996)
   Census of PA Students (1995)
   Survey of Conference Pre-registrants (1966)
   Survey of PA Programs about Applicants (1995)
   Annual Conference Evaluation (1995)
   Market Research (1995)
Externally initiated and/or sponsored projects
   Breast & Cervical Cancer Study (1993–current)
   Prospective Survey of PA Student's Specialty Decision
     (1995)
   Survey of Demand for Advance Trauma Life Support
     (1995)
   Pathway II Evaluation (1995)
Prospective research projects for the coming year
   Survey to determine number of practicing PAs
   Survey of employment benefits
   Surveys regarding member wants, needs, and preferences
Other activities
   Activities to promote and facilitate research by PAs
     (ongoing)
   Data book (historical data on AAPA members)
   Other studies under development

(Data from AAPA Research Division, 1996.)

---

are reported in the various AAPA publications. Individual salary profiles are available to show the compensation range and average of PAs in different areas and different specialties. Outcomes from these studies have improved management capability for the Academy, improved revenue, helped promote the profession, helped form strategic alliances, and improved benefit negotiations for PAs.

In 1993 the AAPA was awarded a cooperative agreement for Breast and Cervical Cancer Patient Education by the Centers for Disease Control and Prevention. This on-going study has added considerable knowledge about the types of patients managed by PAs.

Education

The Annual Physician Assistant Conference is held in late spring in a major city and is attended by more than 5,000 PAs. While the main focus is more than 200 hours of continuing medical education, other events include workshops, technical exhibits, interactive computers, and general sessions featuring nationally renowned speakers and Academy leaders. The semiannual APAP conference is held at this time as well.

The first conference was held in 1973 at Sheppard Air Force Base in San Antonio, Texas. It was attended by a small number of PAs. Since then, the annual attendance has continued to climb (Table 10-10). For many PAs, this is the one major conference they attend each year.

The Constituent Chapter Officers Workshop is organized by the AAPA and held in Washington, DC, every fall. This event helps chapter leaders develop leadership skills, chapter organization, and programming. Leaders also get a chance to meet with their US representatives and senators and national health leaders.

Five regional meetings are held nationwide throughout the year to provide chapter leaders opportunities to network and to meet with leaders of the AAPA.

Clinical and Scientific Affairs

Recognizing the importance of the scientific basis for the clinical practice of PAs and the need to provide more emphasis in Academy activities to this issue area, the Academy created two new departments in 1995: The Department of Clinical Affairs and Education and a Clinical and Scientific Affairs Council. The Council will identify and monitor clinical practice and scientific developments related to the practice of medicine by PAs. Responsibilities include developing reports, issuing papers, and selecting educational documents for the Academy.

Education and Continuing Medical Education

The AAPA's Education Council monitors trends in medical education, assesses PA continuing education needs, develops methods to address

Table 10-10 *List of AAPA national conferences and attendance*

YEAR	PLACE	ATTENDANCE
2001	Anaheim, CA	
2000	Chicago, IL	
1999	Atlanta, GA	
1998	Salt Lake City, UT	
1997	Minneapolis, MN	
1996	New York, NY	6,471
1995	Las Vegas, NV	6,817
1994	San Antonio, TX	5,349
1993	Miami, FL	4,346
1992	Nashville, TN	4,086
1991	San Francisco, CA	3,881
1990	New Orleans, LA	4,447
1989	Washington, DC	4,513
1988	Los Angeles, CA	3,490
1987	Cincinnati, OH	2,814
1986	Boston, MA	3,813
1985	San Antonio, TX	2,864
1984	Denver, CO	2,680
1983	St. Louis, MO	2,179
1982	Washington, DC	2,802
1981	San Diego, CA	1,877
1980	New Orleans, LA	2,205
1979	Fort Lauderdale, FL	1,955
1978	Las Vegas, NV	1,940
1977	Houston, TX	1,525
1976	Atlanta, GA	1,465
1975	St. Louis, MO	765
1974	New Orleans, LA	525
1973	Sheppard Air Force Base, TX	235

(Data from American Academy of Physician Assistants, 1996.)

those needs, develops reports and issues papers regarding educational concerns, and works with the Association of Physician Assistant Programs on educational issues.

The AAPA's CME Logging and Reporting Service helps members track CME hours. A report is sent annually with current CME totals to AAPA members. If a member is certified by the National Commission on Certification of Physician Assistants (NCCPA), the AAPA notifies the NCCPA when 100 hours of CME are completed.

Recertification

The AAPA and NCCPA have worked together to develop Pathway II, an alternative to the proctored Recertification examination. In June 1996, NCCPA assumed complete administrative responsibilities associated with Pathway II.

Public Education

The Public Education program helps spread information about PAs. Articles about PAs have appeared in major papers and on national television networks. Every month, *PA in the News* updates press coverage of the PA profession. Other media that spread the message about PAs are traveling displays, slide shows, and videotapes.

On National PA Day, celebrated each year on October 6th, public education activities are spotlighted. Some of these activities include blood drives, food collection and medical education for the homeless, helping people living with AIDS/HIV infection, and fund raising for local charities. Decals, lapel pins, balloons, brochures, and posters are available.

Project Access is an outreach program designed and conducted each year by the Minority Affairs Committee and its PA volunteers. This effort brings PAs and students together during the annual conference to encourage the pursuit of PA careers.

For Chapter activities, the Academy produces *Fitting in the Pieces*, a public education how-to handbook, distributed to all constituent chapters.

Professional Recognition

The AAPA Academy Awards are the profession's top honors. Awards are given annually to PAs in recognition of the following categories:

- National Humanitarian
- International Humanitarian
- Rural PA of the Year

- Inner City PA of the Year
- Outstanding PA of the Year
- Public Education Achievement Award
- Educator of the Year

Other awards recognize excellence in publishing, public education, and a special honorary membership for important contributions to the profession.

Professional Practice Council

The Professional Practice Council monitors health policy developments in the public and private sectors and writes papers on issues that affect the PA professional practice. The Council has evaluated and written about the following:

- Needle/syringe exchange programs for the prevention of HIV transmission
- Immunization in children and adults
- Hospital privileges and credentialing
- Unlicensed medical graduates
- End-of-life decision making
- Rural health care
- Telemedicine
- Substance abuse disorders
- PAs as Medicaid Managed Care Providers

Most agree that the AAPA has done a credible job of facilitating and promoting the profession. The PA profession enjoys a relationship with other professional medical organizations that is envied and will undoubtedly grow. It has succeeded in winning commission status in all the uniformed services. Medicare reimbursement has been largely won and continues to improve. Thanks to the efforts of the AAPA, Medicaid reimbursement continues to improve in different states. These efforts have been driven by a sense of what is good for the public and what is good for the profession.

Some believe that with these accomplishments, it is now time for the Academy to turn to the first part of the mission statement— "... to promote quality, cost-effective, and accessible health care ..." (Fichandler 1989).

The Physician Assistant Foundation

The PA Foundation seeks to foster the goals and objectives of the Academy by supporting the educational and research needs of the profession. Founded in 1980 as the Education and Research Foundation, and later changed to its present name, it is the philanthropic arm of the AAPA.

Since 1989, the PA Foundation has supported PA education by awarding over $500,000 in scholarships to AAPA student members through its Annual Scholarship Program. In addition, the Foundation has supported research on the profession by awarding over $80,000 in small research grants. The PA Foundation also serves as a position of leadership for the profession (Table 10-11).

Table 10-11 *PA Foundation president*

1996–1997	Paul Lombardo
1995–1996	Paul Lombardo
1994–1995	Lorraine S. Atkinson
1993–1995	Lorraine S. Atkinson
1992–1993	Lorraine S. Atkinson
1991–1992	Lorraine S. Atkinson
1990–1991	J. Jeffrey Heinrich
1989–1990	J. Jeffrey Heinrich
1988–1989	J. Jeffrey Heinrich
1987–1988	James F. Cawley
1986–1987	James F. Cawley
1985–1986	James E. Konopa
1984–1985	Jarrett M. Wise
1983–1984	Jarrett M. Wise
1982–1983	James E. Konopa
1981–1982	James E. Konopa
1980–1981	Noel McFarlane
1979–1980	Donald W. Fisher

(Data from American Academy of Physician Assistants, 1996b.)

PA Day

Every October 6 is PA Day. This date was established in 1987, to acknowledge the work of physician assistants around the country. This date was chosen because it was the day that the first formally trained PAs graduated from Duke University 20 years earlier.

CONCLUSION

No profession stands alone; all are built on relationships with other players in the same arena. The relationship between physicians and PAs began as a strong one and continues today. The evidence is overwhelming that physicians accept PAs in their many and varied roles, and this is not likely to change in the near future as long as PAs avoid seeking independent practice. The relationships with other populations such as nurses, NPs, pharmacists, organized medicine, and patients are stronger today than they have ever been.

Finally, the AAPA is the single body that represents PAs. Activities undertaken by this professional society are unparalleled for any health profession organization and may be the single most important reason for the success of PAs today.

11

Legal Aspects

THE LEGAL BASIS OF THE PA PROFESSION

Medical licensure laws to regulate physicians were enacted in the United States in approximately their present form during the late nineteenth and early twentieth centuries as a matter of public necessity. Protection of the public against quackery, commercial exploitation, deception, and professional incompetence required legally enforceable standards for entrance into and continuation in the medical profession. The State medical practice acts, therefore, specify both ethical and educational requirements for physicians relating to personal character, scientific education, and practical training or experience.

Unlike medical licensure laws, state licensure statutes for physician assistants (PAs), allied and auxiliary health personnel, and nurses were not enacted to correct such abuses of independent, entrepreneurial practice. Instead, the latter statutes have usually been "friendly" regulations enacted with the cooperation of the professions and occupations themselves, and designed to protect both the regulated personnel and the public from unqualified and unethical practitioners. The forms of licensure, however, are generally similar to medical practice acts, except that, in some states for PAs, licensure is permissive rather than mandatory. Accordingly, the statutes define the practice of the various professions and occupations and prescribe the personal, educational, and certification of professional competence qualifications required for such practice.

The most significant and contemporary issues regarding licensure of PAs concern the effect of licensure provisions on the distribution of tasks and duties. For physicians, with unlimited licenses to perform all functions, the critical questions are what functions they may delegate, and under what conditions such delegations may be made. For PAs, the problems are more numerous and complex. First, because their licenses may be limited to a particular segment of health service, it is sometimes necessary to determine those functions which they may not legally perform under ordinary circumstances. These determinations require interpretation of the scope of permissible practice as defined by the relevant licensure statute, and the scope of exclusive practice as defined by licensure statutes. Thus, for example, a PA in a urology practice may be violating his or her scope of practice if a patient has a wart removed from his or her foot. In Missouri, an early licensure stipulated that PAs could not refract and fit patients with prescription lenses.

Functions within the scope of practice for a PA may be either "independent" of, or "dependent" on, receiving orders, direction, or supervision from a physician. Obviously, many variables are involved in determining whether a given function is dependent, and if so, the nature and degree of supervision required for its performance. The same complexity characterizes another problem related to the scope-of-practice, the delegability of functions. Unlike some allied health personnel such as physical therapists and occupational therapists who have unique skills not likely to be duplicated by a physician, the PA has the same skills, more or less, than that of a physician. Therefore, delegation is not one of authorizing personnel to use their exclusive professional skills, but instead one of dividing what the physician would normally have to do.

In general, scope-of-practice issues are the most clouded areas in the legal regulation of PAs, since they have not been adequately addressed by the licensure statutes or related court decisions. After 30 years of experience with delegation of physician tasks to PAs, that so few cases have come under the legal spotlight reflects some confidence that PAs are practicing within their legal jurisdiction.

History

The early licensure statutes reflected the recommendations of the Flexner report on medical education, published in 1910, which initiated efforts to raise standards of medical school admission, instruction, and curriculum to place these schools under the jurisdiction of universities and to provide full-time faculty and adequate facilities for teaching and clinical experience (Starr 1982). The incorporation in medical licensure laws of requirements that proprietary schools could not meet resulted in the closing of medical doctor diploma mills, as the inadequate medical schools of the time were called. Standards of ethics and competency provided in the early licensure laws were derived from the view of leaders of the medical profession that medicine should be based on an educational system that was responsive to the needs and the social and scientific status of the country at that time.

Although vast changes have taken place in the social and scientific status of the country since the original enactment of the medical practice acts, no fundamental changes have been made in the statutory standards of professional competence and ethical behavior. In investigating the adequacy of current licensure laws to meet modern scientific and social conditions, this section turns to the important question of authority for delegation of functions.

Licensing, Certification, and Registration

Thirty years after graduation of the first PA, the legal status of the PA lacks geographic uniformity (Pohutsky 1982). Different states provide specific requirements for licensing, certification, and/or registration. Generally, physicians and attorneys are licensed. These are licenses to act independently and without supervision other than peers. As such, PAs tend to be either certified or registered in a state. Requirements in most states include graduation from an accredited PA program, national certification, and some sort of screening questionnaire about involvement with the law for any sort of felony or malpractice.

Most state laws specifically prohibit physicians from delegating professional responsibilities to an individual the physician knows, or has reason to know, is not qualified by training, experience, or licensure to perform the delegated duties. Physician employers have a responsibility to check regularly to ensure that supervised personnel have kept their licenses, certification, and registrations current and have met all requirements of continuing education necessary for renewal. Establishing an annual review of records may be the best way to ensure that nothing is overlooked by either the PA, employer, or supervising physician.

Supervision

Various state statutes require that a physician supervise a PA. Supervision is defined by law as "responsible control." Control implies both the establishment of overall limits and policies to be met by the supervised professional and the day-to-day supervision of care. Direct supervision requires the physician be in the facility and, occasionally, in the same room as the individual performing the duty. Direct supervision further implies that the physician will be immediately available if the need arises.

More often, supervision is indirect and may be implied or explicitly stated but usually requires the availability of the physician for consultation. This is often interpreted to be by telephone or some other electronic means in a timely or consistent manner (McKinney 1990).

> Supervision shall be continuous but shall not be construed as necessarily requiring the physical presence of the supervising physician at the time and place where such services are performed (N.Y. [Educ.] Law 6542[3]).

Availability need not necessarily be physical presence. Carrying a beeper and telephone access may be appropriate, depending on the circumstances of the patient and the rules imposed by the boards responsible for licensure. The degree usually depends on the complexity of the task, risk to the patient, training of the PA, setting in which care is rendered, necessity for immediate medical attention, and number of other professionals the physician supervises. Generally, the more complex the task and the greater the potential risk to the patient, the more direct and explicit the supervision. Backup should be made available if for some reason the usual methods of contact fail or the supervising physician is out of town.

Review implies the physician will regularly examine the notes and see the work the PA is doing. This process may consist of a review of medical record progress notes made by the PA, or some other predetermined means of ensuring supervision. Generally, the physician should be able to demonstrate that the supervised PA is performing at the expected skill level and is compliant with any protocols and procedures that may be in place to ensure quality of care. This should be done with some regularity (Harty-Golder 1995). How this is done and with what frequency are generally left up to the supervising physician and the PA.

Delegation of Functions

The most significant contemporary questions arising from mandatory licensure for the practice of medicine concerns the delegation of functions by physicians to PAs. As previously noted, the statutory definitions of medical practice give physicians an unlimited license to perform all functions of health service, even those for which other health personnel may also be licensed (or even better suited). However, the concomitant licensing of other health personnel indicates that the statutes do not contemplate all health service to be conducted by physicians. Most health administrators and authorities generally agree that the serious shortage of physicians can be overcome only by allocating certain tasks to PAs, nurse practitioners, and other specialized personnel with less education. The need for such expansion of the professional productivity of physicians seems certain to continue, and even increase, over time.

What is the legal basis for the expansion of PA activity? For example, does the medical and the PA practice act permit a PA to insert a pacemaker in a patient suffering severe bradycardia? For most jurisdictions, there can be no certain answers to such questions because legal authorities have not had to deal with the underlying issues. In a few states, however, the answers have begun to emerge from court decisions, attorney general opinions, or legislative enactment. As a practical matter, delegation of health service functions is predominantly governed by prevailing custom and practice. In the few relevant court decisions, however, it has been held that professional custom is no defense for a contravention of licensure laws.

One case in particular is important to illustrate, not only because of the court's handling of elements of licensure, custom, and supervision in deciding the delegation question, but because of its influence on the development of the PA profession. The case *People v. Whittaker* (No. 35307, Justice Court of Redding Judicial District, Shasta County, Calif [December 1966]), involved the right of a neurosurgeon to use a trained surgical assistant to assist in brain surgery. The assistant was charged with practicing medicine without a license, although he was always within sight and under direct supervision of the surgeon, because he operated a cranial drill and Giegle saw, positioned by the surgeon, to bore holes and excise skull flaps during neurosurgical operations. The surgeon was charged with aiding and abetting an unlicensed person to practice medicine. The jury of a Justice of the Peace Court found both parties guilty of the charges in one instance in which the surgeon had sufficient time to call another physician to assist him but did not try to do so. As a standard for judging the physician's use of an unlicensed trained assistant, working under direct supervision, the following instruction was given to the jury:

> In determining whether acts in this case, if any, performed under the direct supervision and control of a duly licensed physician, were legal or illegal, you may consider evidence of custom and usage of the medical practice in California as shown by the evidence in this case.

The *Whittaker* judgment has since been appealed because of its importance as a test of the right of a physician or surgeon to use an extra pair of hands under conditions not constituting a medical emergency. The case is significant for its allowance of prevailing "custom and usage of the medical practice" in the state to determine the propriety of a physician's delegation and supervision of patently medical, but essentially mechanical, functions.

The interesting footnote to this case is that Roger Whittaker, the defendant, was a Vietnam veteran, a Navy trained corpsman, and a first assistant to the neurosurgeon for over 125 similar cases. Eugene Stead, MD, the founder of the PA program at Duke University was called to serve as an expert witness in this case. In the course of the legal proceedings, Dr. Stead had the opportunity to meet with Whitaker and told him about the new educational program that had been inaugurated at Duke. Whitaker became a member of the third PA class at Duke (Condit 1993).

The key issue in the licensure of PAs is the scope of functions that may be delegated to them and the educational and certification qualifications to permit such delegation safely. The short-

age of PAs, along with other skilled health personnel, new scientific and technologic developments, and new methods of organizing health services have made the question of delegation all the more important. It appears that licensure laws are in the process of being amended to authorize broader scope of functions for qualified PAs. It also appears that PAs have used their delegated role without much malpractice or criminal judgments against them.

State Practice Acts

State practice acts vary tremendously, both in regulatory approach and in the scope of practice they authorize. They may influence the formal prescriptive authority and the administrative protocols organizations develop. Within each organization, however, PAs often have wide latitude for prescribing and carrying out protocols. Although practice acts are intended to ensure quality of care, these organizations, from small physician offices to large medical centers, and institutions such as HMOs, and Veterans Administration programs, often provide their own controls on quality, rather than relying on state practice acts to set the standards.

Although state practice acts may provide a weak mechanism for guiding actual practices within a state, they play an important role in defining professions and restricting what PAs can do. In some instances, they can even define the amount of care a physician can delegate. For example, in Virginia the regulations about PA management state that the supervising physician shall see and evaluate any patient who presents with the same complaint twice in a single episode of care and has failed to improve significantly.

Since these acts may present a threat of litigation for PAs and physicians when practicing within a state, they cannot be simply ignored. The development of model PA state practice acts, as outlined in Appendix 1, can give states an alternative that, if developed with input from all affected groups, would represent a national consensus (PPRC 1994).

Barriers to Practice

Barriers to PA practice, along with nurse practitioners (NPs) and nurse midwives, are those policies and constraints that inhibit full use of professionals (Henderson 1994). These include federal and state regulations, pressures about cost-effectiveness, prescribing privileges, acceptance by patients, acceptance by health professionals, reimbursement, and demand for additional medical providers (Dehn 1995). Numerous studies have investigated the impact of these barriers on the practice of medicine by PAs (Cawley 1985a; Cook 1986; Fenn 1987; Willis 1993b; Dehn 1995). These barriers have been the subject of study and research by Sekscenski and colleagues at the Office of Health Professions at the Bureau of Health Professions, Health Resources and Services Administration. After a review of the literature and consultation with researchers, legal scholars, and select experts, three main categories of information were identified that inhibit the full utilization of nonphysician providers by the state: legal authority, reimbursement, and prescriptive authority (Sekscenski 1994).

The data were quantified primarily according to 1992 data from the AAPA (AAPA State Laws and Regulations 1992), and supplemented by 1993 findings of the Prospective Payment Review Commission (PPRC) concerning Medicaid reimbursement (PPRC 1993). In the legal authority area, states earned five points if they licensed PAs, an additional five points depending on the extent to which statutes and regulations limited their scope of practice, and another 10 points depending on the mandated degree of supervision. Fewest points were given to states requiring direct, on-site supervision. States automatically received 40 points for reimbursement unless their Medicaid reimbursement was more restrictive than the PAs' scope of practice, in which case they received 30 points. Medicare reimbursement, consistent across states, was excluded from reimbursement scoring for PAs. In the category of prescriptive authority, states received 20 points if they had any prescriptive author-

ity, and an additional 1 to 20 points depending on the restrictions placed on that authority (Table 11-1).

Reimbursement

Reimbursement has been a source of struggle for PAs, especially in regard to compensation from third-party payers, Medicare and Medicaid, which usually reimburse at a percentage of a physician's fee (Dehn 1995). Private insurers generally cover PA services when they are

Table 11-1 *Provider practice scores for PAs, NPs, and CNMs by state, 1992*

STATE	PAS	NPS	CNMS
Alabama	39	33	32
Alaska	90	93	84
Arizona	99	86	76
Arkansas	54	48	35
California	58	30	80
Colorado	80	59	50
Connecticut	87	58	93
Delaware	55	60	60
District of Columbia	92	53	60
Florida	48	68	98
Georgia	59	32	70
Hawaii	38	27	42
Idaho	89	46	54
Illinois	59	14	31
Indiana	37	34	25
Iowa	99	73	55
Kansas	87	52	68
Kentucky	42	78	68
Louisiana	37	20	37
Maine	94	42	90
Maryland	49	93	69
Massachusetts	83	68	57
Michigan	89	45	70
Minnesota	83	68	100
Mississippi	0	72	59
Missouri	39	63	27
Montana	98	98	98
Nebraska	93	46	50
Nevada	98	73	30

(Continues)

Table 11-1 (Continued)

STATE	PAs	NPs	CNMs
New Hampshire	95	95	70
New Jersey	37	65	54
New Mexico	94	62	78
New York	98	93	67
North Carolina	92	43	90
North Dakota	87	98	55
Ohio	51	14	60
Oklahoma	46	40	54
Oregon	99	100	80
Pennsylvania	86	66	34
Rhode Island	93	50	84
South Carolina	37	41	59
South Dakota	94	65	70
Tennessee	42	27	56
Texas	77	42	54
Utah	93	91	73
Vermont	86	68	57
Virginia	42	38	47
Washington	100	90	70
West Virginia	96	89	47
Wisconsin	95	67	62
Wyoming	97	94	80
Mean	72.5	60.2	62.1
Median	86.0	62.0	60.0
Standard Deviation	25.3	23.8	19.2

(Data from Sekscenski 1994.)

included as part of the physician's bill or as part of a global fee for surgery (Finerfrock 1991).

As the visibility of the PA profession improves, third-party payers have been more willing to reimburse their services. The American Medical Association recommends that

> ... reimbursement for services of a physician assistant be made directly to the employing physician. In instances where the PA is providing services in the physician's office and in conjunction with the physician, the cost of such services would appropriately be a part of the physician's charge, as is now the case with other personnel he employs. When the PA provides physician-like services to a patient under the direction of, but in a

location physically remote from the employing physician, the AMA has recommended that the physician bill for such services on the basis of the usual, customary and reasonable charges concept ... (Mastrangelo 1994).

On the other hand, CHAMPUS (Civilian Health and Medical Program of the Uniformed Services) covers all medically necessary services provided by a PA, provided that the supervising physician is an authorized CHAMPUS provider. PAs are paid a rate of 85% of the allowable charge for comparable services by a physician. The rate for assisting in surgery is 65% of that charged by a physician.

Forty-one states cover PA services under Medicaid. The rate, paid to the employing practice, is either equal to or slightly lower than that paid to physicians. At least five states specifically exclude Medicaid coverage for PAs assisting in surgery.

The biggest struggle with reimbursement is with Medicare part B. The Medicare policy for PAs is as follows: Those in skilled nursing and nursing facilities are reimbursed at a rate equal to 85% of a physician's rate. Those in rural sites also receive 85%, while those in federally designated rural sites receive cost-based reimbursement. Medicare requires that there be a physician on site when PAs provide services. Medicare supervisory guidelines are problematic since they may be interpreted differently from one setting to another. Another problem is the companies that administer Medicare tend to interpret PA reimbursement irregularly.

PA MALPRACTICE LIABILITY AND LITIGATION

Although there have been malpractice lawsuits involving allegations of negligence by PAs, very few have resulted in reported cases that can be cited as precedent. Nevertheless, a study of the suits filed reveals certain patterns of liability. The following section is modified from a paper authored by James G. Zimmerly, MD, JD, MPH, and Jane Carol Norman, JD (Zimmerly 1985).

Negligence

A claimant who brings a medical negligence action against any health care provider must prove that four elements exist: duty, breach of duty, proximate cause, and damages.

DUTY

The claimant first must show that the health care provider had a duty to provide medical care. For example, in all states but Vermont, health care providers are not required to stop and render care in a roadside emergency (Vt Stat Ann tit 12 519). Therefore, they could not be found negligent for failure to provide care. On the other hand, some courts have ruled that a physician on call in an emergency department has a duty to render medical assistance to any emergency patient whether or not the person is eligible for treatment at that facility (*Guerrero v Copper Queen Hospital*, 537 P2d 1329). In most circumstances, the duty to treat is activated when medical treatment is begun, and continues until the patient has recovered from the condition or has released the health care provider from the continuing duty to treat.

BREACH OF DUTY

Breach of duty is predicated on provision of the standard of care of a reasonably prudent physician practicing under the same or similar circumstances. This is an *objective* standard, and an expert witness in a medical negligence trial is not asked what he or she personally would have done in the situation, but what an average, reasonably prudent health care provider in the community would have done. This standard of care was spelled out in a case heard in 1988 (*Pike v Honsinger*, 155 NY 201, 49 NE 760 [1988]).

A physician and a surgeon, by taking charge of the case, impliedly possessing that reasonable degree of learning and skill that is ordinarily possessed by physicians and surgeons in the locality in which he practices, and which is ordinarily regarded by those conversant with the employment as necessary to qualify him to engage in the business of practicing medicine and surgery. Upon consenting to treat a patient, it becomes his duty to use reasonable care and diligence in the exercise of his skill and the application of his learning to accomplish the purpose for which he was employed ... there must be a want of ordinary and reasonable care, leading to a bad result.

So, breach of duty necessitates a lack of *reasonable* care under the circumstances.

PROXIMATE CAUSE

In addition to the duty to treat and a breach of that duty, negligence involves proof that the breach was the actual cause of the claimant's injury. For example, a health care provider may have been negligent, even grossly negligent, in a case of wrongful death. But if the health care provider can show that the patient would have died regardless of the treatment rendered, the negligence cannot be held to be the proximate cause of death.

DAMAGES

A claimant also must have sustained some damage to prosecute a medical negligence suit successfully. For example, medication errors frequently are made in hospitals; too much, too little, or the wrong type of medication is given, or it is administered via the wrong route. Many of these errors can be blamed on negligence, but the vast majority result in little or no damage. Medical negligence suits routinely cost more than $20,000 to prosecute, and it is unlikely that an experienced malpractice attorney would accept a case with estimated damages less than $50,000.

Standard of Care

Of the four requisite elements in negligence cases, the most difficult to prove is breach of duty. As previously mentioned, in a medical negligence action involving a physician, the duty is breached only when the physician has not performed as a reasonable and prudent physician would have performed under the same or similar circumstances. But to what standard of care should a PA or other health care extender be held? To that of a reasonably prudent PA or of a reasonably prudent physician? Two federal court opinions involving physician extenders illustrate the confusion in this area.

In the case of *Haire v United States* (*Haire v US*, No. 75-55-ORL-CIV-R, 1976), the mother of a 23-month-old girl took her to the pediatric clinic at a military medical center in Florida, where she was seen by a medical technician. This technician had worked as a medic in Vietnam for 2 years and had received inservice training, primarily observation of the supervising pediatrician, before being assigned to the clinic. The medical technician examined the child and recorded that she had a runny nose due to an upper respiratory infection. He prescribed a decongestant and discharged her. Over the next 10 days, the child's appetite diminished and her runny nose persisted. On the tenth day, her temperature was noticeably elevated. The next day, her mother brought her back to the clinic, where she again was seen by the medical technician. He examined the child's ears and throat and listened to her chest. He told the mother that the patient's tonsils were causing her distress, and then discharged the child without referring her to a physician. The next day, the patient's mother noted "twitching" of her daughter's hands, and a temperature of 103° F. She rushed the child to a local emergency room, where a physician performed a lumbar puncture and diagnosed *Haemophilus influenzae* meningitis. Despite the rapid institution of appropriate treatment, the child died 3 days later.

The child's family sued the medical center, claiming that the "physician extender" failed to diagnose or test for meningitis, and that the child should have been referred to a physician on her second clinic visit. At the trial, a board-certified pediatrician testified on behalf of the family that if the child had been seen by a pediatrician on the second visit, the physician would have suspected meningitis and conducted ophthalmic and neurologic examinations to confirm the diagnosis. The court held the technician to the standard of care of a board-certified pediatrician, and since he had not performed the neurologic and ophthalmic examinations that a board-certified pediatrician would have performed, the court found him negligent. The parents were awarded $15,000 each for emotional suffering.

In the case of *Polischeck v United States* (*Polischeck v US*, 535 F Supp 1261 [ED Pa 1982]), another federal court took a different approach. A 44-year-old woman experienced a headache associated with nausea, vomiting, and fever. She complained to her husband of pressure behind her eyes and the feeling that the "top of her head was blowing off." The next day, she went to the emergency room of a government medical center and was evaluated by a PA. Her temperature was 100.4°F and her blood pressure was 144/90 mmHg. The PA questioned the patient about her illness and recorded that she had experienced "sudden onset of headache 4 days ago with malaise, nausea, and ocular myalgia." A brief neurologic examination revealed photophobia but no nuchal rigidity. A complete blood count demonstrated a slightly elevated white blood cell count. The PA diagnosed flu syndrome, prescribed an analgesic/anxiolytic/muscle relaxant, and instructed the patient to return to the emergency room if her symptoms became worse. This medical center allowed PAs to use their discretion in deciding whether to consult a physician and did not require supervising physicians to review the charts of patients seen by PAs, so the patient was not seen by a physician, and her chart was not reviewed or countersigned by a physician.

Two days later, on a Friday, the patient returned to the emergency room when her condition had not improved. She again was seen by the PA, who referred her to the emergency room physician. The physician examined the patient, diagnosed "headaches, etiology unknown" and advised the patient to go to the internal medicine clinic the following Monday if her headaches persisted, or sooner if they became worse. That evening the patient's husband could not rouse her. He took her back to the emergency room, where the same physician examined her and diagnosed intracerebral hemorrhage. Because the medical center was not equipped to handle this type of patient, she was transferred to another hospital, where an arteriogram demonstrated a large subdural hematoma and a right posterior communicating artery aneurysm. A frontoparietal craniotomy was performed. However, the patient never regained consciousness and she died 3 days later.

The patient's husband filed suit in federal court, claiming that the medical center was negligent in not having his wife seen by a physician on her first visit. He also claimed that the physician was negligent in treating the patient on her second visit. At the trial, the plaintiff's expert medical witnesses testified that the standard of care in the community required that patients not be discharged from emergency rooms until they had been seen, or at least their charts had been reviewed, by a licensed physician. The court reasoned that the PA himself was not negligent in failing to diagnose the patient's subarachnoid hemorrhage on her first visit.

Indeed, it hardly seems reasonable to expect a person with only two years of general medical training to be able to recognize a medical condition when it is presented in a patient possessing only some of the condition's textbook symptoms.

Therefore, the court held the PA to the same standard of care as other PAs in the community with similar training; compared with these peers, he was not negligent. However, the court did find the medical center negligent for failure either to have the patient seen, or her records reviewed, by a physician on her first visit, as was standard in the community.

These two decisions disagree about the standard of practice that a PA must meet. Decisions in other cases involving health care extenders may be helpful in clarifying this issue.

Thompson v Brent: In removing a cast from a patient's leg with a Stryker saw, a nurse accidentally cut the patient's leg, leaving a scar. The court held her to the standard of care of a physician and ruled that she had been negligent (*Thompson v Brent,* 245 S2d 751 [La 1971]).

Barber v Reinking: A practical nurse administered an injection that caused injury to a patient. In that state, only registered nurses were authorized by law to administer injections. The court held the practical nurse to the standard of care of a registered nurse and ruled that she had been negligent (*Barber v Reinking,* 411 P2d 861 [Wash 1966]).

Thompson v United States: A practical nurse in a Veterans Administration hospital told a drugged, disoriented patient to go to the laboratory by himself. On the way, the patient fell and injured his finger, which ultimately had to be amputated. The nurse was held to the standard of care of a nurse, not a physician (*Thompson v US* 368 F Supp 466 [WD La 1973]).

Whitney v Day: A nurse anesthetist working in a hospital was held to the same standard of care as other nurse anesthetists in the community, not to the standard of an anesthesiologist (*Whitney v Day,* 300 NW2d 380 [1980]).

It would appear from these cases that PAs who are practicing in a state where they are recognized and allowed to practice, and are performing procedures that they legally or traditionally can perform in the community, should be held to the standard of a PA. However, PAs who are practicing in a state that does not recognize them and are performing procedures that only physicians or nurses are licensed to perform in that community probably should be held to the standard of a physician or a nurse.

Evidence of Standard of Care

How is the standard of care proved in a medical negligence suit? In addition to hiring an expert witness, the plaintiff's attorneys most likely will subpoena all hospital or clinic manuals, regula-

---

Table 11-2 *PA legal references*

Vt Stat Ann tit 12 519.
Guerrero v Copper Queen Hospital, 537 P2d 1329.
Pike v Honsinger, 155 NY 201, 49 NE 760 (1898).
Haire v US, No. 75-55-ORL-CIV-R, 1976.
Polischeck v US, 535 F Supp 1261 (ED Pa 1982).
Thompson v Brent, 245 S2d 751 (La 1971).
Barber v Reinking, 411 P2d 861 (Wash 1966).
Thompson v US 368 F Supp 466 (WD La 1973).
Whitney v Day, 300 NW2d 380 (1980).

This is an incomplete list and does not represent the range of legal cases or literature on litigation involving PAs. The reader is referred to the legal literature for recent cases.

---

tions, and protocols referring to PAs. These usually are admissible evidence of the applicable standard of care. If a PA has failed to follow a hospital's protocol or other applicable regulation, there will be strong, although not necessarily conclusive, evidence that the standard of care was not met. Violation of a state law regarding the duties of PAs also is strong evidence of a breach of the standard of care (Table 11-2).

In addition to hospital or clinic protocols and regulations, the courts also may consult guidelines issued by professional organizations, including standards used by the Joint Commission on the Accreditation of Hospitals. Therefore, it is important that PAs also be aware of the guidelines issued by these organizations.

Although data are limited, current evidence indicates that the increase in the number of malpractice claims, size of awards, and rate increases physicians have been undergoing in the 1980s has not been the PA experience (DHHS 1988).

✕ PRESCRIBING

Richard E. Johnson, PhD, Senior Investigator at the Kaiser Permanente Center for Health Research, Northwest Region, contributed to this section.

As a result of legal statutes, PAs are sanctioned to perform a wide variety of services in all the states (except Mississippi), the District of Columbia, Guam, and in various federal agencies (Army, Navy, Air Force, Coast Guard, Public Health Service, federal and state correction systems) (Gara 1988). These statutes allow physicians to delegate authority to PAs to diagnose, test, treat, and follow-up the patients they manage. A substantial amount of evidence indicates that physicians have successfully delegated a great deal of such authority (Schafft 1987a).

One major aspect of treatment that has had limited sanction is drug prescribing. When legally authorized, the privilege of prescribing is usually restricted. Since the use of medication is the most frequently performed treatment in medical care, the absence of this privilege limits the scope of medical practice. It restricts where and how PAs can practice. Consequently, the issue of prescribing privilege is a significant concern of the PA profession. It is also an issue among managers, administrators, and policy makers in the larger health care community since PAs appear to be less costly substitutes for physicians in a variety of clinical situations.

Legal Status of PA Prescribing

PAs were first authorized limited prescribing privileges in Colorado in 1969 (Silver 1971b). Child Health Associates (pediatric PAs and NPs) could order drug treatments without consulting their supervising physicians as long as the latter reviewed and approved the order. New York authorized prescribing privilege to PAs in 1972; Maine, New Mexico, and North Carolina followed in 1973. By 1979, PAs had prescribing privileges in 11 states (Weston 1980). As of 1996, PAs are authorized by statute or regulation to prescribe in 40 states, the District of Columbia, and in most federal facilities including the military and the Veterans Administration.

The underlying principle in these jurisdictions is one of dependent prescribing by PAs to whom supervising physicians have delegated this authority. With few exceptions—such as dentists and veterinarians, and in some states podiatrists, optometrists, and nurse practitioners—the legal right to prescribe is still largely the exclusive domain of the physician.

The authorization to prescribe applies almost completely to the outpatient setting. Inpatient medications are generally considered orders and usually come under a different review process. Most states where PAs are legally authorized to prescribe have constraints on their prescribing. Such constraints include the following:

- Requiring the supervising physician to co-sign each prescription order written by a PA

- Prescribing from a drug formulary, and/or limiting prescribing to select classes or schedules of drugs defined by the Controlled Substances Act of 1970 as having the potential of abuse

- Prescribing by drug treatment protocols

- Limiting the quantities of certain drugs that PAs may prescribe (Gara 1990).

The Controlled Substances Act defines five schedules of drugs, each with drug preparations that have differing potential for abuse by users. Schedule I drugs have the greatest potential for abuse and Schedule V the least. Not included in the Act are drug preparations that have no potential for abuse by users but whose use requires a written order from a licensed prescriber. These drug preparations, referred to as *prescription legend* drugs can be prescribed by PAs with prescribing privilege. PAs may also prescribe over-the-counter medications, drug preparations that do not, by law, require the written order of a licensed prescriber.

Among the states with prescribing regulations in place, only a few grant PAs prescribing privileges for Schedule II through Schedule V drugs in addition to "prescription legend" drug preparations. Schedule I drugs are not relevant to this discussion, as it is illegal for licensed practitioners in the United States to prescribe these drugs. The prescribing privilege for Schedule II drugs is limited to half a dozen states. In the other states, the prescribing privilege applies to Schedule III through Schedule V

drugs including prescription legend drugs, with some restrictions by various states on prescribing Schedule III drugs.

Current Extent of PA Prescribing

Although PAs prescribe in a wide variety of settings, little empirical data are available about how and when PAs prescribe. The restrictions on prescribing privileges have undoubtedly limited the interest of researchers in examining PA prescribing. Some market surveys and a few published research studies have shown interest with PAs who prescribe. A 1990 survey, administered in the states that had some form of prescribing authority for PAs, found that 90% of a selected sample of PAs prescribe when provided the authority (Willis 1990). Sixty percent or more of the PAs reported prescribing urinary/vaginal agents, upper respiratory medications, gastrointestinal agents, antiarthritic/antigout agents, and analgesics (Willis 1990a). Among these PAs, the mean number of prescriptions written per week was 50. It was estimated from the survey that PAs write a total of 35.5 million new prescriptions each year (1990). When extrapolated to 1996 and when refill prescriptions are included, the total is about 75 million. In 1996, the 40 states with prescribing privileges for PAs have more than three-fourths of all the PAs in the United States and contain approximately 75% of the total US population.

At an annual conference in 1987, PAs participated in a survey representing 17% of the PAs attending the conference. Questions concerning prescribing were answered by 144 PAs (approximately 6% of all attendees). This survey indicated that PAs wrote an average of 24 prescriptions per day and an average of 50 new prescriptions per week. They reported that they were free to prescribe their drug of choice for 88% of their routine prescriptions. Furthermore, they reported prescribing muscle relaxants, antiinflammatory drugs, potassium supplements, and beta-blockers, as well as recommending infant formulas, fish oil products, and calcium supplements (Mittman 1993).

Rubin surveyed 466 PAs by a national convenience sample and reported that 96% of them ordered at least one prescription per day and that almost one-half ordered 20 or more prescriptions per day (Rubin 1977). Seventy-eight percent of the surveyed PAs were in primary care. About 50% reported that their supervising physician never rescinded a prescription order they initiated, while 2% indicated their prescription orders were rescinded more than 10% of the time. The most frequently prescribed classes of drugs were non-narcotic analgesics, antibiotics, antihistamines, antihypertensives, and cough and cold preparations (Rubin 1977).

In 1984, a survey of 170 randomly selected PAs in New York state returned questions on prescribing, with a 67% response rate (Mittman 1984). New York permits physicians to delegate prescribing privilege to the PAs they supervise; outpatient prescribing is restricted to nonscheduled drugs. All respondents reported that the most frequently prescribed types of drugs, in order of frequency, were oral antibiotics, antihistamine/decongestants, topical antibiotics, pain/fever medications, and otic/ophthalmic preparations. They also reported recommending over-the-counter preparations an average of nine times a day. Aspirin and other pain medications, cold and allergy products, cough preparations, and antacids were the most frequently recommended. Those in non-hospital-based settings, about one-half of the respondents, reported writing an average of 17 outpatient prescriptions per day (Mittman 1984). They also attempted to provide some insight into attitudes that could affect PA prescribing. Eighty-eight percent of PAs agreed with the statement that "the average patient does not feel treated without getting a prescription." Seventy-one percent agreed with the statement that "the pharmaceutical companies that regularly call on PAs are the ones whose products the PA will tend to prescribe." Pharmaceutical sales representatives were mentioned by PAs as one of the five factors that most influenced their selection of drug products (Mittman 1984).

The findings of these studies begin to show the extent and nature of PA prescribing when delegated, but come from small market surveys and nonrepresentative samples of PAs that signal caution in interpreting the findings. The reports consistently show that PAs prescribing fits the types of drugs commonly associated with primary care.

Reasons for Restrictions

Several reasons have been advanced as to why state regulatory agencies have limited the prescribing privilege to PAs. One early reason is that PAs are not sufficiently trained to be competent prescribers. Further, since the agencies regulating PA practice have historically been largely comprised of physicians, a second reason, related to the first, is the potential of increased legal liability of supervising physicians because of PAs' perceived lack of prescribing competence. Physician reluctance can also come from cultural and/or economic reasons. Another possible reason for these agencies limiting or denying prescribing privileges to PAs is the opposition of other health professionals (namely nurses and pharmacists).

Concerns about patient safety and physician liability have had some historical validity given the substantial amount of variation that has characterized the evolution of PA training and educational programs. The pharmacology and therapeutics component of the PAs' educational experience had been singled out as a major area of concern (Camp 1984). At one time, the pharmacology preparation varied widely among PA programs and ranged from one semester (covering such topics as basic mechanisms of drug action, enzyme induction, drug absorption, distribution, metabolism, excretions, and various families of drugs) to minimal exposure in practical therapeutics. Not mentioned in these observations was that students gained instruction in pharmacology during clinical rotations as part of their patient management experience under physician supervision. Moreover, during this time, no clear definition existed across programs of what drug families the student should know and what specific disease problems the student should learn to manage (Heller 1978). Pharmacology and medical therapeutics are a part of the core requirements of every PA program. Of 55 PA programs surveyed in 1990, 49 averaged 66 hours of instruction in pharmacology, with a range of from 28 to 128 hours (Oliver 1993a). A model clinical therapeutics curriculum has been developed that is expected to be used by most programs beginning in 1996 (Wilson 1995).

Another potentially powerful reason is that the medical profession may not wish to share the act of prescribing. The act of prescribing has been described as "the most common and overt expression of the physicians' power" (Pellegrino 1976). Much of this power is ascribed to the symbolism associated with prescribing. Throughout history, the ingestion of substances has been associated with magical, mystical, and religious elements that transcends any pharmacologic effects. When coupled with the ingrained urge to "take something" for an illness, this historical association gives extraordinary power to the person who has the exclusive right to provide the "something" (Pelligrino 1976).

The act of prescribing manifests the physician's power in a variety of ways. It gives the physician the authority to define the clinical situation as medical, it establishes that the patient is "really ill," and it implicitly reinforces the physician's ability to handle the illness. The act of prescribing maintains the physician's power by providing the physician time for the illness to unfold when a diagnosis is uncertain or a condition is obscure. The act of prescribing maintains the physician's control of the situation even though scientific observation may indicate no medication is needed. Sharing prescribing with PAs removes physicians as the only source of such power.

The symbolic weight of prescribing has other practical implications for the physician. For one thing, prescribing a drug notifies the patient that the physician is concerned and is trying to help. Prescribing a drug can take the place of communicating with the patient. Finally, prescribing can be used to both guide and to end the office visit, as well as to provide a link with the patient for continuing visits (Pellegrino 1976; Smith 1980). Thus, delegating prescribing authority to PAs also empowers them in their relationships with patients and may be perceived as reducing the power of the physician.

Another possible reason to limit the prescribing privilege is an economic one. The initial purpose of the creation of PAs was to alleviate a shortage of physician services. In more recent years, however, given the more abundant supply of physician services, the distinction of whether PAs complement physician services or are alternatives for physician services is less clear. The latter situation implies PAs are currently in competition with physicians for patients.

Opposition to prescribing privileges for PAs from other health professions, such as pharmacists, is another possible reason. The opposition, however, is basically confined to attempting to influence regulatory agencies and state legislatures through testimony and lobbying efforts. Such efforts may delay the granting of prescribing privileges in some states but have not been sufficient to prevent them.

Medical Justification for PA Prescribing

Although the data to assess the safety and effectiveness of PA prescribing are sparse, there is ample empirical evidence that PAs prescribe effectively and safely. Safety, in this context, refers to the prescribing that minimizes the risk of an adverse consequence from the drug prescribed, and effectiveness refers to the contribution of the drug to the outcome of treatment. Such data from outpatient primary care settings would be of particular importance since the largest share of PAs are employed in these settings (Schafft 1987a). Some data are available that compare physician and PA patterns of practice include prescribing as one of the criteria to assess the quality or appropriateness of the diagnostic and treatment processes, or the outcomes of care.

Goldberg and colleagues evaluated the quality of care provided by 23 PAs in Air Force primary medicine clinics, where PAs assumed a considerable portion of the care formerly provided by physicians (Goldberg 1981). Quality of care judgments were based on diagnostic, therapeutic, and disposition criteria. Therapeutic criteria included desirable actions (e.g., prescribing the appropriate class of antibiotic for infectious otitis media at the first visit), and undesirable actions (e.g., prescribing an antibiotic for viral syndrome with gastroenteritis). On five of six such criteria identifying desirable therapeutic action, PAs performed as well as physicians. For all eight criteria identifying undesirable action, PAs performed as well as or better than physicians (Goldberg 1981).

Kane and colleagues compared the quality of care performance of PAs to that of their supervising physicians, one criterion being whether medication was ordered for specific diagnoses (Kane 1976). They found PAs were less likely than physicians to use antibiotics for fevers of undetermined origin and for upper respiratory tract infections, and somewhat less likely to use systemic steroids for contact dermatitis and asthma. These data indicated that PA prescribing decisions for these morbidities were as good or better than those of physicians (Kane 1976).

Duttera and Harlan evaluated the appropriateness of care provided by PAs in 14 rural primary care settings (Duttera 1978). They concluded that PAs were competent, both in diagnostic and therapeutic skills, for the three following practice patterns: (1) when all patients were initially seen by the PA and then by the physician, (2) when patients (not preselected) were managed concurrently by physicians and PAs, and (3) when patients with specific problems were assigned to PAs (Duttera 1978).

Kane and colleagues also compared functional outcomes, patient satisfaction with care and outcome, and mean costs per acute episode of care for family practice residents, faculty, and Medex-trained PAs at two family practice centers associated with a university family practice training program. PAs performed as good as or better than the others in each of the measures (Kane 1978b).

Record compared the performance of PAs and physicians in a large HMO in handling episodes of four specific morbidities: strep throat, upper respiratory infection, bursitis, and bronchitis. One outcome criterion was safety, in terms of the rate of adverse effects from antibiotics and other drugs provided in the treatment of upper respiratory infection. They found no differences in the rates between PAs and physicians (Record 1978).

Tompkins investigated how physicians and PAs at two different clinics medically managed patients with acute respiratory illnesses. The PAs used clinical algorithms to guide their choices of diagnostic tests and treatment. The findings showed that the PAs did not prescribe antibiotics needlessly or more than internists for conditions not generally requiring an antibiotic, and prescribed antibiotics similarly for treatable bacterial conditions. Internists had the highest medical care costs per patient. The authors concluded that the care provided by the PAs was as effective as, and less costly than, the care provided by physicians (Tompkins 1977).

A study in Iowa reported that 95% of physicians and 93% of PAs believed that PAs were qualified to prescribe medication with little or no supervision by the physician (Ekwo 1979). Similarly, all 29 Montana physicians who responded to a survey expressed confidence in the ability of the PAs they were supervising to prescribe most therapeutic agents, and 40% had no reservations at all about them prescribing any agent (Willis 1990a).

In another study, a stratified sample of 19.6% of Wisconsin pharmacists were surveyed about their attitudes toward PA prescribing (Huntington 1987). The survey was conducted 8 months after PAs were authorized to prescribe nonschedule prescription drugs with the physician supervisor required to co-sign the patient's medical record. Slightly over one-half of the 329 pharmacist respondents (47% response rate), reported dispensing prescriptions written by PAs. At the time of the survey, Wisconsin PAs were prescribing an average of 27 prescriptions per month, or about 1 per day. The findings indicated that pharmacists found PAs' prescriptions "completed appropriately and legibly prepared." They were confident in "filling a prescription from a PA." Nevertheless, Wisconsin pharmacists expressed little support for expanded prescribing authority for PAs (Huntington 1987). Reasons for this conclusion were not mentioned in the analysis.

Hooker examined prescribing by quantity and found that adult primary care PAs and NPs prescribed 15% of the prescriptions in the department of Internal Medicine and Family Practice while staffing the departments at 20% full-time equivalent personnel (Hooker 1993).

Finally, personal communication was made with the legislative office of the American Academy of Physician Assistants to ascertain whether they were aware of any malpractice claims that had been brought against PAs as a result of their prescribing. The office indicated no evidence of a claim having found its way through the courts.

Summary and Conclusions

The findings from reports that describe prescribing by PAs and that medically justify prescribing privileges for PAs are limited in number and in rigor. Much of the information about what and how much PAs' prescribe has come from market surveys and various reports that have used convenience or otherwise unrepresentative samples of PAs. The findings applicable to medically justify PA prescribing have been compiled from studies that have one or more common methodologic problems. One problem has been the small sample sizes of physicians and PAs in comparative studies. Another problem has been the types of sites of comparative studies, such as military installa-

tions, rural practices, university teaching hospitals, and clinics. These settings are not representative of the main stream of primary care and where the majority of PAs practice (Kane 1976; Record 1978; Kane 1978a; Duttera 1978; Goldberg 1981). In addition, patient populations have been nonrandomized, and measures of quality and appropriateness have been process measures. Finally, medical care record data have not been standardized and in some instances have been incomplete (Sox 1979; OTA 1986). Nevertheless, a consistent finding appears to be that when PAs are delegated the prescribing decision or provided protocols to guide them in specified clinical situations, they do at least as well as physicians in writing prescriptions, ordering drug treatment, and producing "good" processes of care. Although the evidence is not sufficient to generalize to all PA prescribing, it does appear sufficient to predict adequate performance of PAs when they are delegated the handling, including the drug treatment, of acute episodes of illness in office-based primary care. Liability insurance premiums have not increased and the remarkably few malpractice claims have not centered on prescribing as an issue of safety.

Although progress has been made and continues to be made in achieving prescribing authority for PAs, it has taken more than 30 years to gain such privilege, albeit generally limited, in 40 states (Table 11-3).

While the body of evidence is limited, there is good reason to believe that PAs prescribe safely and effectively. If they were not doing so, an abundance of reports would be available to identify the problem. For prescribing privilege to be less restricted, rigorous research assessing the effectiveness of PAs is needed. It would be particularly useful for health planners, managers, and policy makers to know more definitively how cost-effective PAs are as alternatives to physicians when delegated the handling, including the drug treatment, of conditions common to primary care, and in different settings. Since many PAs are specialized, it would be useful to know whether PAs are more cost-effective than the physicians they work with.

Table 11-3 *Prescriptive privileges for PA*

STATES	PRESCRIPTIVE AUTHORITY	RESTRICTIONS	CONTROLLED SUBSTANCES
AL	X	Noncontrolled from board formulary	
AK	X	Physician name and DEA number required on prescription	Schedule III–V
AZ	X	No refills: DEA registration required	Schedule II and III limited to 72-hr supply; Schedules IV and V, 34-day supply
AR			
CA	X	Must have patient-specific order from MD	
CO	X	Written protocol on case-by-case and per-patient-visit basis required: MD countersign on charts required within 3 days	Controlled
CT	X		Schedule IV and V
DE	X	Therapeutics approved by physician and board	
D.C.	X	Noncontrolled only	
FL	X	Board formulary	
GA	X	Delegation by physician	Schedule III–V; limited to 30-day supply: maintenance drugs limited to 90-day supply
HI			
ID	X	Board formulary	
IL			
IN			
IA	X	Must be ordered by physician in written protocol, or in an emergency	Schedule III–V orally; Schedule II orally in emergency
KY			
LA			
ME	X	DEA registration	Schedule III–V
MD			
MA	X		Schedule II–V
MI	X	Noncontrolled only	
MN	X	NCCPA-certified required	Excludes anesthetics, other than local ones
MS			
MO	X		
MT		Delegation by physician	Schedule II–V; limited Schedule II to 34-day supply
NE	X	Physician authorization required	Medications including 72-hour supply of Schedule II
NV	X	Board approval and pharmacy registration required	Controlled; limited to supervising physician's prescriptive authority
NH	X	Pharmacy law examination required	Controlled
NJ			
NM	X	Board formulary	Schedule II–V
NY	X	Noncontrolled only	
NC	X	Pharmacy board approval required	Schedule II–V; Schedules II and III limited to 7-day supply
ND	X		Schedule III–V

(Continues)

Table 11-3 (Continued)

STATES	PRESCRIPTIVE AUTHORITY	RESTRICTIONS	CONTROLLED SUBSTANCES
OH			
OK	X	Noncontrolled on board formulary	
OR	X	Physician and board approval and DEA registration required	Schedule III–V
PA	X		Formulary drugs except Schedules I and II and parenterals (except insulin and allergy kits)
RI	X	State drug control office and DEA registration required	Schedule V
SC	X		Schedule V
SD	X		Schedule II–V; Schedule II limited to 48-hour supply
TN	X	Noncontrolled only	
TX	X	Limited to underserved areas, practices with high rates of indigent patients, physician's primary practice site, hospital, or other site	Individually determined dangerous drugs prescriptions limited to physician's primary practice site
UT	X		Schedule IV and V (7-day supply)
VT	X	Physician authorization required	Individually determined
VA	X	Noncontrolled on board formulary	
WA	X	DEA number required	Schedule II–V
WV	X	2 years of experience, board approved pharmacology course, and NCCPA. Board formulary. DEA required	Schedule III–V
WI	X	With written protocols and consultation with physician	Controlled
WY	X	DEA number required	Schedule III–V
Total	41		30

(Data from the American Academy of Physician Assistants and the Intergovernmental Health Policy Project, The George Washington University, 1995.)

Rigorous research is indicated to show if PAs with prescribing privilege are as effective, that is, can they provide the same or better outcomes of treatment for the same or less costs than physicians in conditions where drug treatment is indicated. Effectiveness refers to expected favorable health- and psychosocial-related outcomes of treatment, whereas cost-effectiveness refers to lesser total costs generated to produce similar health- and psychosocial-related outcomes. Favorable health-related outcomes, for example, would be the absence of therapeutic failures (drug retreatment or refills), complications from undertreatment or overtreatment including the adverse effects of drugs. Favorable psychosocial outcomes include, as examples, maintenance of functioning and social roles and satisfaction with the treatment provided. A summary of controlled substances is presented in Table 11-4.

DRUG ENFORCEMENT ADMINISTRATION

Every provider who administers, prescribes, or dispenses any controlled substance, other than as a direct agent of another registrant, must be registered with the Drug Enforcement Administration (DEA). A PA who is required to register must submit a completed Form DEA-224 to the Drug Enforcement Administration, Registration Unit, PO Box 28083, Central Station, Washington, DC 20005. Before 1994, PAs, NPs, and certified nurse midwives (CNMs) were registered similar to physicians with a registration number beginning with the letter A or B, followed by a letter corresponding to the first letter of their last name. In 1994, the DEA chose to reclassify nonphysician providers under the term *mid-level practitioners*, and require new registration num-

---

Table 11-4 *Controlled Substance Act*

Schedule I are those with no accepted medical use in the United States and have a high abuse potential. Some examples are heroin, marijuana, LSD, peyote, mescaline, psilocybin, etc.

Schedule II are drugs with a high abuse potential with severe psychic or physical dependence liability.

Schedule II controlled substances consist of certain narcotic, stimulant, and depressant drugs. Examples of narcotics are opium, morphine, codeine, methadone, and meperidine. Examples of the stimulants are amphetamine and methamphetamine. Examples of the depressants are amobarbital, pentobarbital, secobarbital, and methaqualone.

Schedule III drugs have an abuse potential less than those in Schedule I and II, and include compounds containing limited quantities of certain narcotic drugs and nonnarcotic drugs such as paregoric and barbituric acid derivatives not included in another schedule.

Schedule IV drugs have an abuse potential less than those listed in Schedule II and include such drugs as phenobarbital, chloral hydrate, meprobamate, chlordiazepoxide, diazepam, and dextropropoxyphene.

Schedule V drugs have an abuse potential less than those listed in Schedule IV and consist of preparations containing limited amounts of certain narcotic drugs generally for antitussive and antidiarrheal purposes.

---

bers beginning with the M (for "mid-level") and the first letter of the last name, followed by a computer-generated sequence of seven numbers.

The registration must be renewed every 3 years. The cost of the registration for a PA in 1996 was $150. The certificate of registration must be maintained at the registered location and kept available for official inspection. Every prescriber registered with the DEA receives a re-registration application approximately 60 days before the expiration date of their registration. If more than one practice location is used from which he or she dispenses controlled substance from personal supplies, then each location must be independently registered. A move to a new location requires a request for modification of registration in writing to the DEA office.

There are some exceptions to this process, such as being in the Armed Forces or other government agencies such as the Public Health Service and the Veterans Administration. Other

administrative details such as recordkeeping requirements, inventory, prescription orders, control and reporting of substance theft or loss, and guidelines for prescribers of controlled substances can be found in the 1993 *Mid-Level Practitioner's Manual : An Informational Outline of the Controlled Substances Act of 1970* (obtained from the DEA at the preceding address).

POLITICS

No chapter on legal aspects of PAs is complete without a discussion of the political ramifications of an expanding workforce that includes PAs. David Mechanic (1974) writes:

It is becoming fashionable to think of health politics as the process of federal policy making. But the character of health care is molded, equally, by the clash of interests at the community level, the organization and promotion of particular structures of professional organization, and the continuing decisions made at the level of operating agencies of all sorts. Decisions about the character of health care are made at many points and by many individuals. This characteristic, particularly, gives the health context its complex diversity and uneven response to change.

In the article "The Politics of Ambulatory Care" Bellin (1982) has approached this subject by discussing the players who deliver ambulatory care.*

It is logical first to consider the politics of health care practitioners themselves. Government refers to them generically as "providers."

In delivering ambulatory care, not only physicians but a variety of health professionals and allied health professionals strive for legitimacy. Functional lines of demarcation are increasingly blurred. Territories once the exclusive domain of the [physician] have been challenged, sometimes de jure by

---

*From Bellin, 1982, with permission.

legal and legislative means, often de facto by gradual changes in customary practice. A partial list of combatants includes:

- Orthopedists vs. podiatrist
- Ophthalmologist vs. optometrist
- Psychiatrist vs. clinical psychologist vs. psychiatric social worker
- Primary care physician vs. nurse practitioner vs. physician assistant

The medical professional lays historic claim to the entire human body, including the feet, the eyes, the psyche, and the right to make preliminary assessment of a patient's health status. Nevertheless there appears to be an inexorable and irreversible process at work, periodically made manifest in quarrels among professionals over anatomic and physiologic. Although the physician possesses extraordinary prestige, there has been, during the past few decades, a progressive demysticization of the [physician's] knowledge and skills, in part as a result of the increasing formal education and sophistication of the lay public. Demysticization has facilitated the trickling down of certain functions and procedures of [physicians] to the "limited-licensed" health care practitioners, such as the podiatrist, the optometrist, the clinical psychologist, and now those primary care professionals called nurse practitioners and physician assistants. [Physicians] have been disinclined to do certain tasks deemed routine or disagreeable or of low status and have allowed some of these tasks to go by default to others eager to fill the functional vacuum, provide needed service, and enhance their professional status. The podiatrist has been less loathe than the orthopedist to operate on corns and calluses. The ophthalmologist has preferred to perform eye surgery rather than fit glasses, so the optometrist has prescribed and fitted lenses. Local [physician] shortages have provided further encouragement to the limited licensed practitioner to enlarge his professional territory. Cost has

been another factor. Customarily, the limited-licensed practitioner has been less expensive than the [physician] specialist in the same functional domain.

The limited-licensed practitioner has legitimized the acquisition of once [physician]-specific tasks by legislatively expanding the legal scope of licensure and by adding pertinent courses in the curriculum of the professional school. To the orthopedist's annoyance, the modern podiatrist now performs vascular and bone surgery on the feet and prescribes medications with systemic effects. Despite opposition by ophthalmologists, the optometrist has sought and has won the right in an increasing number of states, albeit with curricular safeguards, to prescribe eye drops for diagnostic purposes. Once the limited-licensed practitioners have secured the right to do certain things once hitherto performed only by MDs, they never give up that right. [physician] hostility has retarded but failed to halt this process.

In ambulatory care delivery the latest political controversy relates to what is to be the ultimate role of physician assistant (PA) and nurse practitioner (NP), each having come into being originally to alleviate the impact of the critical shortage of primary care physicians. The NP resents ever being placed in a hierarchical or reimbursement position lower than or subordinate to the nonnurse PA. To avoid friction between the PA and the NP, it is sometimes prudent to assign them to different departments or agencies. Yet they have certain political goals in common. Both the PA and NP prefer to attenuate if not eliminate altogether the supervisory role of the [physician] vis-à-vis their own work. Both would like to prescribe, being independent of the [physician's] overview. Although not unanimously held, these views reflect PA and NP expansionist tendencies that characterize all limited-licensed professionals today in ambulatory care delivery. In contrast, the [physician] champions the principle of [physician] supervision of PA and NP, who would remain, of course, nonautonomous. In the [physician]-approved model, the PA and NP would handle routinizable situations according to an unambiguous protocol. There are also pecuniary considerations. Subordinate to the [physician], the PA or NP would cost the [physician] less than another [physician] as employee or partner but could generate income to supplement the physician's.

The contemporary PA is striving for legitimacy in an era of political change. While this is being played out on a number of fronts, the political/policymaking arena is probably the most important. Since the physician no longer has control of this process, it is likely that policy makers will continue to recognize the attributes of PAs based on outcome and economical data, and not the soft social values that some exhort that all health care should be controlled by the physician.

NATIONAL PRACTITIONER DATA BANK

The National Practitioner Data Bank (NPDB) is a federal repository for any state board actions or malpractice actions against physicians, dentists, PAs, NPs, and other licensed health professionals. It was established to restrict the ability of incompetent practitioners to move from state to state without discovery of previous substandard performance or unprofessional conduct. All PAs applying for privileges to a hospital or medical center must submit information that is then forwarded to the NPDB (Gara 1990). As of 1996, no study has examined PAs or the rate of litigation that has been brought to the attention of the NPDB.

THE NATIONAL COMMISSION ON CERTIFICATION OF PHYSICIAN ASSISTANTS

The educational process of PA training relies heavily on a quantifiable product. For most this means not only graduation, but passing a national examination of certification. The National Commission on Certification of Physician Assistants (NCCPA) is the major overseeing agency entrusted to ensure that qualifications of the profession are being met. Its most important charge is to help assure the public of the entry level and continued competency of PAs. This is accomplished through various mechanisms such as written examination, evaluating how the PA approaches a patient under various scenarios, certificate registration based on acquisition of continuing medical education (CME), and periodic recertification examinations. While individual states retain the authority concerning who may and may not practice as PAs, the NCCPA advises states concerning PA enabling legislation. Currently, the majority of states require that a PA be board certified or board eligible before he or she may practice in that state. The intent of this entry restriction is seen as competency assurance in the public interest.

The history of the NCCPA arose because of the need for evaluation of the graduate of PA programs. It was acknowledged that, since program accreditation is not an infallible science, some means of assuring entry-level practitioner competence was necessary to ensure that a quality control system was in place for the public. In 1971, the National Board of Medical Examiners (NBME) was funded by the Division of Associated Health Professions of the US Department of Health, Education and Welfare (DAHP/DHEW) and the Kellogg Foundation to develop a certifying examination, which came to be known as the National Certifying Examination for the Assistant to the Primary Care Physician.

Specifically, the NCCPA has responsibility for the following functions:

- Determine eligibility criteria for the National Certifying Examination

- Review applications to take the examination and register candidates

- Administer the examination under subcontract to the National Board of Medical Examiners

- Determine pass/fail standards for the certifying examination for PAs
- Issue and verify certificates
- Periodically recertify PAs through the continued demonstration of competency
- Publish lists by state of PAs certified each year

History

With the proliferation of PA training programs in the early 1970s, it became clear that a mechanism was necessary to accredit programs to ensure the quality of the educational process. The result was the advent of what is now known as the Joint Review Committee on Educational Programs for Physician Assistants in collaboration with the American Medical Association (AMA) Council on Medical Education. This committee, however, only reviewed the educational process and not the product of the programs. Simultaneously, PA graduates began to develop their professional organizations into what are now the American Academy of Physician Assistants (AAPA) and the Association of Physician Assistant Programs (APAP).

The next step, under the auspices of the federal government, the AMA, and the Kellogg Foundation, with the blessing of the AAPA and APAP, was to develop a mechanism to evaluate the product of the training programs. Thus, the National Board of Medical Examiners (NBME) Certifying Examination for Assistants to the Primary Care Physician was developed and first administered in December 1973. At the same time, nurse practitioner, nurse clinician, and child health associate programs were gaining momentum; graduates of these programs were also eligible to take the examination. Additionally, there was an unknown number of PAs who had not graduated from a formal program. It was decided that the 1974 examination would be open to informally trained PAs who met certain eligibility criteria to be determined by a committee of NBME. A Standard Setting Committee under the NBME was also established to determine pass/fail levels.

These were new and uncomfortable roles for the NBME whose traditional charge had been confined to the developing, administering, and scoring of examinations for physicians. With this in mind, the AMA and the NBME worked to bring together representatives of 12 other professional groups in late 1973 to form a free-standing, independent commission to assure the PA profession, employers, state boards, and most important, patients, of the competency of this type of health professional. In February 1975, after being formally structured and organized, NCCPA opened a national office in Atlanta, Georgia (Glazer 1977). David Glazer, the executive director of the NCCPA from 1973 to 1996, was selected at that time and played a pivotal role in helping the NCCPA become the excellent organization it is today.

In an effort to ensure career-long accountability, NCCPA developed a two-part program, consisting of certificate re-registration every 2 years, based on continuing medical education, and recertification by examination every 6 years. NCCPA administered the entry-level examination for recertification from 1981 through 1983. The major purpose of this administration was to attempt to identify any content areas that penalize people working in specialty practices to help identify the "core" area to be tested by a separate recertifying examination. That new examination was developed in 1984 and has been administered ever since. Currently, the only sanction resulting from failure is the requirement for reexamination within the next 2 years. NCCPA established a policy that recertification must be accomplished within 7 years following the most recent NCCPA examination. Those people out of the NCCPA system longer than 7 years must take and pass the Physician Assistant National Certifying Examination (PANCE) to resecure NCCPA certification, unless the recertification requirement is waived in the eighth or ninth year by successful appeal. No appeals are considered past the ninth year. The NCCPA appeal process has been extended to cover individuals wishing to challenge other potentially adverse NCCPA actions or decisions.

NCCPA Examination

The NCCPA examination emphasizes clinical practice. While many test items require knowledge or basic pathophysiology of disease processes, only a relatively few questions deal directly with basic health sciences such as biochemistry of a human cell. Both the PANCE and the PANRE (Physician Assistant National Recertification Examination) have been designed to assess essential knowledge and skills of PAs in conducting a variety of health care functions normally encountered in practice. The emphasis of the examinations is on general functions and those extended core functions specific to either primary care or surgery. General functions have been identified as those that PAs should be skilled in performing irrespective of specialty training or practice; primary care and surgical extended core functions have been identified as those important to the appropriate extended core practice.

The PANCE is separated into two sections (the General Examination and the Extended Core Examination[s]), consisting of three separate components. To qualify for certification, all candidates must pass both parts of the General Examination, as well as at least one extended core examination component. The General Examination is composed of two sections: a written and practical examination:

1. A 25-question multiple-choice examination designed to assess the candidate's knowledge related to clinical material presented in printed and pictorial form
2. Clinical Skill Problems: A 1-hour assessment in which candidates are presented three clinical vignettes and are evaluated on the basis of selecting and performing the appropriate physical examination steps

Two extended core examinations are offered, one in primary care and one in surgery. In addition to the General Examination, all candidates must take at least one extended core component but may elect to take both for an additional fee.

1. Primary Care: A 150-question multiple-choice examination designed to assess the candidate's knowledge related to clinical material specific to PA practice in primary care
2. Surgery: A 150-question multiple choice examination designed to assess the candidate's knowledge related to clinical material specific to PA practice in surgery

Examinations are developed by independent test committees. Membership includes physicians and PAs employed in both academic and clinical settings. Many medical specialties and subspecialties are represented, including family practice, surgery, obstetrics/gynecology, pediatrics, geriatrics, general medicine and psychiatry (Table 11-5).

Test committees (with the exception of the Clinical Skill Problems committee) meet twice annually to develop each examination. Ten committees review the previous year's examination performance, finalize the current examination blueprint, make assignments for and prepare new test items, and meet again to present and defend test items. Once test items have gone through final selection, they are categorized and edited as necessary. After initial printing, test committee chairs meet to review and edit the final draft (NCCPA 1995).

The representative diseases with which PA students are expected to be familiar with are listed in Table 11-6. The Disease List is prepared from empirical data drawn from several sources, including the National Ambulatory Medical Care Survey and the National Hospital Discharge Survey. Although the Disease List is not complete, it does serve as a primary reference for identifying the clinical problems the PA should be prepared to encounter in the PANCE and PANRE.

Recertifying

One of the unique features of the PA profession is the voluntary recertification process. Studies have shown that the half-life of medical knowledge is about 7 years. It was decided in 1980 that every 6 years was an appropriate time to

Table 11-5 *PA National Certifying Examination content outline*

History and physical
Diagnostic studies
Diagnosis
Prognosis
Managing patients
   Health maintenance
   Clinical intervention
   Clinical therapeutics
   Legal and ethical issues
Applying scientific concepts

(Data from NCCPA Content Outline for PANCE and PANRE, 1995.)

retest individuals on their basic medical knowledge. The intent was to ensure the public that PAs are keeping abreast of the core knowledge to practice medicine.

The PANRE is comprised of 300 multiple choice questions arranged into two separate test booklets. It is usually administered twice a year, with one examination site at the national convention every May.

Controversies

At least one study has suggested that the NCCPA examination may need some reevaluation since students without degrees and those with associate degrees complete the PA program and pass the NCCPA examination at a higher percentage than those with baccalaureate and graduate degrees (Lary 1991). This finding is in direct conflict with one of the current methods used for student selection.

Lary also found wide discrepancy for non-Caucasian students, between program completion rate (89%) and NCCPA pass rate (56%). This discrepancy might indicate a cultural bias in the NCCPA examination (Lary 1991).

In 1995, the number of certifying examinations totaled 2,913, with 2,272 attaining certification. The failure rate was 22%, with 641 candidates unsuccessful in reaching the

pass/fail score level of 410. A total of 700 PAs were awarded recognition in primary care, 152 in surgery, and 1,204 in both. In all, 137 examinees failed on the basis of not achieving a minimum score of 300 on the clinical evaluation.

The recertifying examination in 1995 was taken by 2,792 examinees, with 494 PAs taking the examination 1 year early (fifth year of cycle) and 139 taking it late (seventh year of the cycle). A total of 2,689 examinees passed the examination (103 failures) for an overall pass rate of 96%.

In an era of quality assurance and public accountability, the need for medical education update is continuous. For a fast growing, young profession like the PA, an attitude toward maintenance of quality with periodic recertification seems imperative even if it is a frustrating and time-consuming requirement (Hill 1996).

Conclusion

Statutory changes permitting physicians to utilize PAs in an innovative manner have been dif-

Table 11-6 *Disease list of clinical problems for PA National Certifying Examination*

Disease/disorders of the central nervous system
Disease/disorders of the eye
Disease/disorders of the ear, nose, mouth, throat
Disease/disorders of the respiratory system
Disease/disorders of the circulatory system
Disease/disorders of the digestive system
Behavioral and emotional problems
Disease/disorders of the musculoskeletal system
Disease/disorders of the skin and subcutaneous tissue
Disease/disorders of endocrine, nutrition, and metabolism
Disease/disorders of the kidneys and urinary tract
Disease/disorders of the male/female reproductive systems
Disease/disorders of the blood/blood-forming organs
Pregnancy/childbirth/neonates
Infectious/parasitic diseases
Injuries/wounds/toxic effects/burns
Health maintenance
Presentation of ill-defined symptom complex

(Data from NCCPA Content Outline for PANCE and PANRE, 1995.)

ficult to achieve, and there is a fair amount of discrepancy in state laws among the states. These laws usually indicate the educational qualifications and the dependent nature of the practice. All states indicate the number of PAs who can work at one time under supervision with a physician.

Registration of PAs also varies widely. Some use a registration process, others a credentialing or licensing process. In some states, the process is flexible and general; in other states the description must be rigidly inclusive of the activities the PA will perform.

Prescribing is a contentious area for some states despite the limited data on safety. Forty states now authorize PAs to prescribe in some form, and others are considering prescribing laws. In states that allow prescribing by PAs, reports of prescribing violations or problems are almost nonexistent (D. Gray, personal communication, 1996). The empirical evidence suggests that PAs do it frequently and do it well.

12
Future Directions

Why physician assistants (PAs) and not some other type of provider? Why did PAs succeed when they could have failed? The answers to these question are important because if PAs are to understand what the future might hold for them, they need to understand their past including their successes and failures. Reflecting on why PAs have succeeded, Fowkes writes:

In the early part of this century the Flexner report changed the emphasis in our medical schools from a practical approach to a biomedical emphasis as the priority in education. This made medical schools slow to respond to the changing social environment, and less responsive to health care needs. In the 1960s primary care was a new concept. There was a recognized need for these services, a maldistribution of physicians and types of services, and questions about who should do it. A discipline of family medicine was emerging but was not large enough to have much influence. It takes medical schools (and nursing schools for that matter) an enormous amount of time to make critical changes. One of the critical features of the physician assistant movement has been its flexibility and resourcefulness. One only has to look to the way the training programs responded to the early awareness of AIDs, homelessness, drug abuse, and domestic violence by incorporating these conditions in their curriculum. The physician assistant is the only flexible category of health professionals. Both PA programs and PA practitioners have demonstrated their abilities to quickly modify elements of education and practice in response to social need (Fowkes 1996).

Other major social forces which influenced the PA movement may have been:

- The changing lifestyles of the population, which grew out of the 1960s. Physicians may have realized they did not want to work as hard as their predecessors and needed help
- Women entered the workforce in a major way, many seeking a return to a new career in health care
- The commitment to be a dependent profession, closely associated with physicians
- The early establishment of specific skills and competencies expected of PAs through program accreditation and a national board which allows for state reciprocity
- The national emphasis on training primary care generalists, with PAs assuming diverse roles after obtaining a set of core competencies

We may not know all the reasons why PAs have succeeded as well as they have, but there is a fair amount of understanding of what PAs are and how they arrived at their present status after being introduced to Americans only 30 years ago. It has been, and continues to be, one of the most exciting careers that have developed in the twentieth century. However, important issues must be addressed in the future.

One of the nagging issues facing the profession is the appropriate number of PAs to train.

There are two sides to this question. One side believes that as many PAs should be trained as the market will bear. Others believe that it is unrealistic to expect that physicians in any appreciable numbers will by themselves reverse the trend of professional specialization. If this notion holds true, doctors will continue to avoid primary care practices, and it remains doubtful that established specialist physicians will convert to generalist roles in any appreciable numbers. The continuing decline in interest among young physicians in primary care careers and generalist practices has not yet been reversed, and it will take decades, even if the number of medical graduates choosing primary care significantly increases, before adjustments in graduate medical education outcomes will have an impact on service delivery. This prospect raises the question of which type of health care personnel will provide primary care now and in the near future. As physicians become increasingly specialized, moving further away from primary care, PAs are likely to assume a greater profile in delivering primary care services. This is particularly true in settings such as health maintenance organizations (HMOs), other types of managed care systems, and organized health care systems such as Veterans Affairs (VA), state and federal correctional systems, and the military. Some believe that physicians are really no longer in the primary care business and that PAs, working with physician "managers," may be the best providers to meet future primary care needs. They recommend increasing PA educational output and utilization in primary care roles (Meikle 1992).

The future for PAs and other nonphysician health professions is likely to be determined by political, economic, and legal factors that affect the evolution of their roles in relation to those of physicians (Jones 1995). As our health care system changes from one encompassing a disease-oriented and economically open-ended structure to one stressing a more preventive, patient-centered, and cost-conscious direction, nonphysicians will assume a higher profile. The further evolution of the professional roles of PAs and other nonphysicians in US health care will be determined by changing trends in the division of medical labor, more accountable public perceptions of levels of physician responsiveness to societal health care problems, population-based needs, and patient satisfaction and outcome. In the future, the interdisciplinary team approach to health care will become a standard, and Americans will demand increasing accountability from its health professionals. This new accountability will require adjustments in the educational preparation of medical and health care providers, approaches extending the biomedical model to encompass both the population-based and behavioral sciences. The PA concept in American medicine has emerged as a creative and effective health workforce approach to augment clinical service gaps in multiple areas. PAs are well integrated into medical practices and have demonstrated clinical competency and versatility. Expansion of PA utilization will likely continue in several sectors of the health system.

FUTURE DEMAND FOR PAs

Medical marketplace demand for primary care PAs is anticipated to grow. One estimate of primary care needs suggests that a primary care physician can cover the needs of 1,600 to 1,800 persons annually in a managed care practice setting (Hummel 1994b). Given these figures, the United States will need 150,000 primary care physicians for a population of approximately 250 million. However, only 88,000 primary care physicians under age 55 are in active practice. With the addition of a PA to the practice, the patient panel for a PA-physician primary care team could increase to at least 2,400 (a conservative one-third increase in practice productivity). "This increase in total practice productivity suggests that work force requirements for primary care physicians could be reduced if more physicians were able to utilize PAs" (AGPAW 1995).

The demand for PAs in hospitals is expected to increase as well. The 1993 survey by the Association of American Medical College Council of Teaching Hospital members revealed that in a majority of institutions, residency program directors indicated that they were already using PAs and/or NPs or were planning to employ them in the future. Directors of these programs also indicated that these PA/NPs were utilized on clinical services to replace the service of physicians (AGPAW 1995). The American Hospital Association survey of 3,184 hospitals reported that the vacancy rate for PAs rose from 10.1% in 1991 to 12.3% in 1992 and were expected to climb higher yet in 1993. The 1992 vacancy rate for PAs was the second highest of the 25 health occupations reported in the AHA survey (AHA 1992). Other indicators of increased demand for PAs include:

- The US Department of Labor projects a 36% increase in the number of PA jobs from 1992 to 2005 (AGPAW 1995

- The Bureau of Labor Statistics career outlook projections for health care professionals indicate increased demand for PA services

- Estimates of the Bureau of Health Professions project future demand for nonphysician providers

- State survey data of practicing PAs suggest increasing market demand for PAs (Von Seggen 1993)

In response to their charge from the Committee on Graduate Medical Education (COGME), Advisory Group of Physician Assistants and the Workforce (AGPAW) developed a list of recommendations addressing PA education, PA practice characteristics, practice obstacles, and current and anticipated demand. The advisory group has called for:

- Expanding the output of PA educational programs from the current level of more than 1,700 graduates a year to 4,000 a year by the year 2000

- Increasing federal support for PA educational programs to expand the supply of PA graduates

- Increasing National Health Service Corps scholarships and loan repayment programs supporting PA students

- Developing federal policy to support and encourage increased representation from racial and ethnic minorities in the PA profession

- Including PAs in national and state health work force planning activities

- Encouraging states to provide a more uniform regulatory climate for PAs

The Pew Health Professions Commission predicts that by the end of the century, a number of forces will interact to produce an American health care system that will be different than the one we are used to. The more obvious changes in health care will be:

- More managed care with better integration of services and financing

- More accountability to those who purchase and use health services

- More awareness of and responsiveness to the needs of enrolled populations

- Ability to use fewer resources more effectively

- More innovation and diversity in providing health care

- Less focus on treatment and more concern about education, prevention, and care management

- Orientation to improving the health of the entire population

- Reliance on outcomes data and evidence (Pew 1995)

This demand-driven system in health care and health professional practice will create difficult realities for many health professionals and great opportunities for others. Some of these realities will be:

- Closure of as many as half of the nation's hospitals and loss of perhaps 60% of hospital beds
- Massive expansion of primary care in ambulatory and community settings
- A surplus of 100,000 to 150,000 physicians (mostly nonprimary care specialties), as the demand for specialty care shrinks; a surplus of 200,000 to 300,000 nurses generated as hospitals close; a surplus of 40,000 pharmacists as the dispensing function for drugs is automated and centralized
- Consolidation of many of the more than 200 allied health professions into multiskilled professions as hospitals re-engineer their service delivery programs
- Demands for public health professionals to meet the needs of the market-driven health care system
- Fundamental alteration of the health professional schools and the ways in which they organize, structure, and frame their programs of education, research, and patient care (Pew 1995)

THE CASE FOR DOWNSIZING PA PROGRAMS

The other side of the PA supply coin is that health care continues to be a labor intensive enterprise. Since the cost of this labor is expensive, the outcomes of different types of labor will be scrutinized and compared. This bodes well for the profession in the short run. Managers will increasingly recognize the value added of a PA instead of a physician in increasingly more ways. Demand will continue for a while, a rapid rise in programs will continue, and within a few years the supply of PAs will double, perhaps as early as 2004. This expansion will be welcomed by many, but the greatest threat to the PA profession is the marketplace because as salaries increase, the cost-effectiveness of PAs (and nurse practitioners [NPs]) will

diminish under this invisible hand—the pricing oneself out of the market. "If PA income continues to increase at the levels we have seen recently, then cost, value, and productivity differentials will influence hiring decisions" (Jones 1995). Eventually there will be more PAs than opportunities, and relationships with physicians may suffer.

The dependence of PAs on physicians will probably continue to serve the profession for a while as it continues to reach out to organized medicine for professional guardianship (Huntington 1989). By demonstrating competence to the physician, the PA's clinical role in practice is ultimately established through a process of ongoing negotiation. Professional autonomy is determined through performance of delegated and negotiated tasks and exists within the practice limits of the supervising physician (Cawley 1984).

Significant increases in the role of PA and NP utilization in HMOs will be augmented by the degree to which physicians can be persuaded to hire them, and to use them once hired is less predictable (Robyn 1980). This uncertainty confirms the need to develop PA programs gradually and underlines the necessity for an administrative structure able to fine tune and monitor this development.

Because the future of the shape of the US health care workforce is so uncertain, the answers to the fundamental question of how many PAs are enough remains perplexing.

INCREASING DEMAND FOR PAS

The ability of PAs to effectively identify, attract, and efficiently serve the varieties of consumers will largely determine their professional survival. Both organization and financing services will be key variables in these efforts. This will require understanding both the microeconomics and macroeconomics, as well as the health care changes to maintain their demand. Some of these strategies are outlined in Table 12-1.

Demand-side innovation, which addresses both old and new markets, requires increasing marketing sophistication and awareness. Strategies toward this goal include creation of new opportunities in the form of new specialties and subspecialties. Among emerging new roles for PAs are wellness/disease prevention; clinical, biological, and health services research; legal; genetics; toxicology; and medical administration. Expanded roles will be in geriatrics, oncology, molecular biology, genetics, and chronic disease management (Dieter 1989). A major challenge to society and to the health care system is to provide effective, humane, and economical care to the millions of individuals with chronic disease. PAs and NPs are probably in a better position to do this than physicians because patients will increasingly be absorbed by managed care organizations, and their medical care will require intensive efforts to contain costs through innovative forms of labor.

Many of the restrictions on NPs in both mobility and time are likely to affect PAs as well. NPs, and nurses in general, have evidence of increasing need for part-time employment and ability to determine work time. As the composition of PAs shifts to be younger and female, these restrictions will affect PA (and physicians) even more than they do now.

SELF-ACTUALIZATION

Responsibility for administering the profession belongs to the profession itself. When PAs emerged in the late 1960s, the laws governing the

practice of medicine were amended to recognize the physician's ability to delegate tasks to supervised individuals (Fasser 1984). Most of these laws have been modified and expanded, but the power to regulate PAs has remained, with only a few exceptions, in the hands of the licensing boards that tend to be predominantly controlled by physicians (Gara 1988). If PAs are going to seek their own destiny, they must overcome these shortcomings in self-actualization and begin seeking avenues to educate their regulators.

Gara reminds us that formal participation of PAs in the regulatory process is a worthy goal but not a panacea for problems that may exist between physician licensing boards and PAs. Once a PA becomes a board member or sits on a citizen committee, he or she assumes the role of protector of the public health and safety. The responsibilities of that person are to the citizens of the state, not to the profession. Advocacy of professional concerns still rests with state PA associations (Gara 1988).

LESSONS FROM OTHER SYSTEMS

In projecting the future for PAs in the US health care system, it is useful to consider the experiences of similar types of health practitioners in the medical systems of other countries. Practitioners similar to PAs have been utilized in a number of other nations. Examples include the feldsher in Russia, the barefoot doctor in China,

---

Table 12-1 *PA Areas to Increase Demand*

MACRO (ON THE PROFESSIONAL ORGANIZATIONAL LEVEL)	MICRO (ON THE INDIVIDUAL LEVEL)
Aggressive, creative marketing	Aggressive, creative individual marketing
Research on economic utilization	Creative self or group employment
Creative organization and financing	Expansion of client areas and contact
Expansion of client areas and contact (scope of practice)	Utilization of advanced technologies
Utilization of advanced technologies	Inclusion in policy making
Other	Administrative rank high enough to effect change

(Data from Salmon 1985.)

the assistant medical officer in parts of Africa (Pereira 1996), and a wide range of the variously named health providers working primarily in developing countries throughout the world.

The natural history and pertinent experiences of these practitioners have been examined, and when compared to the American experience with nonphysician providers, it is clear that only a few parallels exist (Cawley 1983a). Experience with nonphysician clinicians and their successful or unsuccessful integration into a country's health delivery system are based primarily on how these providers fit into the medical, economic, and cultural systems of the nations that employ them. Rarely are experiences with these types of providers exportable to other countries (Celentano 1982). Each nation that has created and utilized nonphysician providers has fashioned them and their roles to meet specific needs and requirements in that country's systems. However, some overriding patterns do exist that are relevant in the assessment of the American PA.

Nonphysician practitioners are created by the existing cadre of medical providers in a country and emerge from specific perceived needs in health care delivery. In nearly all cases, these needs involve a shortage of fully trained physicians to provide adequate medical services to the population. This was in fact the fundamental rationale for the creation of PAs in the United States.

Once nonphysicians enter the delivery system, evolving circumstances and changes in the system affect the roles and perceptions of these providers. As the supply of a country's physician population rises and as experience with these practitioners accumulate, new perceptions of the roles that these providers can assume often develop. In some instances, there is no further need for these providers in the health care system. In others, the role of the nonphysician provider changes and becomes more technically oriented. In still other systems, nonphysician clinicians evolve into well-established members of a health care delivery team, participating with physicians in a wide variety of clinical functions. The broadest generalizations that can be made is that nonphysicians must adjust and adapt to changing forces within the health delivery system in which they work once they outlive the rationale of their initial creation (Cawley 1983a). As we have seen, this is what has occurred with PAs in the United States.

RESEARCH

The research community will continue to evaluate the affects PA employment has on quality, cost, access, and other aspects of health care delivery. Only by carefully documenting the capabilities using acceptable research methodologies will we be able to measure the profession's ability to meet the needs of the medical marketplace. Staffing currently remains a function of physician attitudes instead of administrative rationale (Hooker 1994b). Radical changes in health care staffing will not happen in the near future unless the data proving that PAs can function safely and effectively in almost all health care roles are placed before policy makers and managers.

Undoubtedly, there will be encroachments on the homeostasis of the PA in the area of finances, choice, and professional domain. The girders of physician support of PAs are linked to being less successful and more dependent, regardless of skill and outcome. Relative to PAs, economics are the overwhelming determinant of essential functions.

The PA profession must seek to formulate questions that will guide research in ways not only theoretically fruitful, but historically appropriate.

As part of this process we offer the following questions:

- Will the market forces be sufficient to create a long-term demand for PAs?
- Should the PA profession promote efforts to restrict trainees, or should the profession try to recruit more gifted trainees into the PA profession that might stimulate areas of research?

- Should the American Association of Physician Assistants (AAPA) contribute to funding research by supporting proactive, innovative studies that would enhance health care delivery?

- Should AAPA help educate and nurture institutional leadership within organizations that have sufficient vision to recognize the pivotal role that PAs can play to more cost-effective health care delivery?

- How can the profession document the efficacy, efficiency, and economy of PAs as primary care providers for Americans?

- How can PAs continue to demonstrate innovation, high quality, and technical sophistication in primary care medicine?

CONCLUSION

Growth and opportunity are the catchwords for the PA profession as it moves into the twenty-first century. Numerous changes can be expected, along with stimulating challenges. It is an exciting time to be a PA, and it is hard for a profession to be too concerned about the future when they are riding the crest of a wave where supply cannot keep up with demand. Current focus is on the expansion of the profes-

sion to meet the demand of the changing health care environment that wants more PAs. For the first time, PAs are part of the health policy equation as planners estimate what the health workforce should be like in the years ahead. Like all waves, however, the crest will eventually break and supply will exceed demand. When this wave will break is difficult to predict. An expanding population, an aging population, a greater demand for services, and an uninsured population that needs care create the demand for services. Excessive health care costs, poor access for some citizens, and uneven quality of care bodes well for the profession because they can help meet this demand quickly. However, increased penetration of managed care and efficiency in delivery have begun to dampen physician salaries. If rising PA salaries come close to declining physician salaries, an acceleration of new PA programs and a surge of new graduates may produce the supply side of the equation that may catch up with the demand side sooner than expected.

The quality of American-trained physicians, PAs and of medical care in the United States has never been higher. If PAs want to remain in the great debate about what the composition of the health care workforce should look like, they have to meet the challenge with hard data that they are viable players.

APPENDIX 1

Model State Legislation Regarding Physician Assistants

The following model state legislation was developed by Nicole Gara, Vice President for Government Affairs, American Academy of Physician Assistants.

DEFINITIONS

Physician assistant means a person who has graduated from a physician assistant or surgeon assistant program accredited by the American Medical Association's Committee on Allied Health Education and Accreditation or by its successor agency, and/or a person who has passed the certifying examination administered by the National Commission on Certification of Physician Assistants.

Board means the Medical Licensing Board.

Supervising physician means an MD or DO licensed by the board who supervises physician assistants.

Supervision means overseeing the activities of, and accepting responsibility for, the medical services rendered by a physician assistant. The constant physician presence of the supervising physician is not required so long as the supervising physician and physician assistant are or can be easily in contact with one another by radio, telephone, or other telecommunication device.

QUALIFICATIONS FOR LICENSURE

Except as otherwise provided in this document, an individual shall be licensed by the board before the individual may practice as a physician assistant.

The board may grant a license as a physician assistant to an applicant who

1. Submits an application on forms approved by the board
2. Pays the appropriate fee as determined by the board
3. Has successfully completed an educational program for physician assistants or surgeon assistants accredited by the Committee on Allied Health Education and Accreditation or by its successor agency, and/or has passed the Physician Assistant National Certifying Examination administered by the National Commission on Certification of Physician Assistants
4. Certifies that he or she is mentally and physically able to engage safely in practice as a physician assistant
5. Has no licensure, certification, or registration as a physician assistant under current discipline, revocation, suspension or proba-

tion for cause resulting from the applicant's practice as a physician assistant, unless the board considers such condition and agrees to licensure

6. Is of good moral character
7. Submits to the board any other information the board deems necessary to evaluate the applicant's qualifications
8. Has been approved by the board

TEMPORARY LICENSE

The board may grant a temporary license to an applicant who meets the qualifications for licensure except that the applicant has not yet taken the national certifying examination or the applicant has taken the national certifying examination and is awaiting the results.

A temporary license is valid

1. For 1 year from the date of issuance
2. Until the results of an applicant's examination are available
3. Until the board makes a final decision on the applicant's request for licensure, whichever comes first. The board may extend a temporary license, upon a majority vote of the board members, for a period not to exceed 1 year. Under no circumstances may the board grant more than one extension of a temporary license

A temporary license may be granted to an applicant who meets all the qualifications for licensure but is awaiting the next scheduled meeting of the board.

INACTIVE LICENSE

Any physician assistant who notifies the board in writing on forms prescribed by the board may elect to place his or her license on an inactive status. A physician assistant with an inactive license shall be excused from payment of renewal fees and shall not practice as a physician assistant. Any licensee who engages in practice while his or her license is lapsed or on inactive status shall be considered to be practicing without a license, which shall be grounds for discipline under section __ of this Act. A physician assistant requesting restoration from inactive status shall be required to pay the current renewal fee and shall be required to meet the criteria for renewal as specified in section __ of this Act.

RENEWAL

Each person who holds a license as a physician assistant in this state will, upon notification from the board, renew said license by

1. Submitting the appropriate fee as determined by the board
2. Completing the appropriate forms
3. Meeting any other requirements set forth by the board

EXEMPTION FROM LICENSURE

Nothing herein shall be construed to require licensure under this Act of

1. A physician assistant student enrolled in a physician assistant or surgeon assistant educational program accredited by the Committee on Allied Health Education and Accreditation or by its successor agency
2. A physician assistant employed in the service of the federal government while performing duties incident to that employment
3. Technicians, other assistants or employees of physicians who perform delegated tasks in the office of a physician but who are not rendering services as a physician assistant or identifying themselves as a physician assistant

SCOPE OF PRACTICE — DELEGATORY AUTHORITY — AGENT OF SUPERVISING PHYSICIAN

Physician assistants practice medicine with physician supervision. Physician assistants may perform those duties and responsibilities, including the prescribing and dispensing of drugs and medical devices, that are delegated by their supervising physician(s).

Physician assistants shall be considered the agents of their supervising physicians in the performance of all practice-related activities, including but not limited to, the ordering of diagnostic, therapeutic, and other medical services.

PRESCRIPTIVE AUTHORITY

A physician assistant may prescribe, dispense, and administer drugs and medical devices to the extent delegated by the supervising physician.

Prescribing and dispensing of drugs may include Schedule II through V substances as described in [the state controlled drug act] and all legend drugs.

All dispensing activities of physician assistants shall

1. Comply with appropriate federal and state regulations
2. Occur when pharmacy services are not reasonably available, or when it is in the best interests of the patient, or when it is an emergency

Physician assistants may request, receive, and sign for professional samples and may distribute professional samples to patients.

SUPERVISION

Supervision shall be continuous but shall not be construed as necessarily requiring the physical presence of the supervising physician at the time and place that the services are rendered.

It is the obligation of each team of physician(s) and physician assistant(s) to ensure that the physician assistant's scope of practice is identified; that delegation of medical tasks is appropriate to the physician assistant's level of competence; that the relationship of, and access to, the supervising physician is defined; and that a process for evaluation of the physician assistant's performance is established.

SUPERVISING PHYSICIAN

A physician wishing to supervise a physician assistant must:

1. Be licensed in this state
2. Notify the board of his or her intent to supervise a physician assistant
3. Submit a statement to the board that he or she will exercise supervision over the physician assistant in accordance with any rules adopted by the board and that he or she will retain professional and legal responsibility for the care rendered by the physician assistant

NOTIFICATION OF INTENT TO PRACTICE

A physician assistant licensed in this state, before initiating practice, will submit, on forms approved by the board, notification of such intent. Such notification shall include

1. The name, business address, and telephone number of the supervising physician(s)
2. The name, business address, and telephone number of the physician assistant

A physician assistant will notify the board of any changes or additions in supervising physicians within __ days.

SATELLITE SETTINGS

Nothing contained herein shall be construed to prohibit the rendering of services by a physician assistant in a setting geographically remote from the supervising physician.

EXCLUSIONS OF LIMITATIONS ON EMPLOYMENT

Nothing herein shall be construed to limit the employment arrangement of a physician assistant licensed under this act.

ASSUMPTION OF PROFESSIONAL LIABILITY

If a physician assistant is employed by a physician or group of physicians, the physician assistant shall be supervised by and be the legal responsibility of the employing physician(s). The legal responsibility for the physician assistant's patient care activities shall remain that of the employing physician(s), including when the physician assistant provides care and treatment for patients in health care facilities.

If a physician assistant is employed by a health care facility or other entity, the legal responsibility for the physician assistant's actions or omissions shall be that of the employing facility or entity. Physician assistants employed by such facilities shall be supervised by licensed physicians.

VIOLATIONS

The board may, following the exercise of due process, discipline any physician assistant who

1. Fraudulently or deceptively obtains or attempts to obtain a license
2. Fraudulently or deceptively uses a license

3. Violates any provision of this chapter or any regulations adopted by the board pertaining to this chapter
4. Is convicted of a felony
5. Is a habitual user of intoxicants or drugs to such an extent that he or she is unable to safely perform as a physician assistant
6. Has been adjudicated as mentally incompetent or has a mental condition that renders him or her unable to safely perform as a physician assistant
7. Has committed an act of moral turpitude
8. Represents himself or herself as a physician

DISCIPLINARY AUTHORITY

The board, upon finding that a physician assistant has committed any offense described in section __, may

1. Refuse to grant a license
2. Administer a public or private reprimand
3. Revoke, suspend, limit, or otherwise restrict a license
4. Require a physician assistant to submit to the care or counseling or treatment of a physician or physicians designated by the board
5. Suspend enforcement of its finding thereof and place the physician assistant on probation with the right to vacate the probationary order for noncompliance
6. Restore or reissue, at its discretion, a license and impose any disciplinary or corrective measure which it may have imposed

TITLE AND PRACTICE PROTECTION

Any person not licensed under this act is guilty of a (felony or misdemeanor) and is subject to penalties applicable to the unlicensed practice of medicine if he or she

1. Holds himself or herself out as a physician assistant
2. Uses any combination or abbreviation of the term "physician assistant" to indicate or imply that he or she is a physician assistant
3. Acts as a physician assistant without being licensed by the board

An unlicensed physician shall not be permitted to use the title of "physician assistant" or to practice as a physician assistant unless he or she fulfills the requirements of this (act).

IDENTIFICATION REQUIREMENTS

Physician assistants licensed under this Act shall keep their license available for inspection at their primary place of business and shall, when engaged in their professional activities, wear a name tag identifying themselves as a "physician assistant."

RULE MAKING AUTHORITY

The board shall promulgate, in accordance with the provisions of the (state) Administrative Procedures Act, all rules that are reasonable and necessary for the performance of the various duties imposed upon the board by the provisions of this Act, including but not limited to

1. Setting licensure fees
2. Establishing renewal dates

REPLACEMENT PARTS FOR MODEL LEGISLATION

Supervising Physician — Practice Agreement

Any physician licensed in this state may apply to the board for permission to supervise a physician assistant. The application shall be jointly submitted by the physician and the physician assistant(s) and may be accompanied by a fee as determined by the board.

The joint application shall describe the manner and extent to which the physician assistant will practice and be supervised, including identification of additional licensed physicians who will supervise the physician assistant; and other such information as the board may require. The board may approve, modify, or reject such applications.

Whenever it is determined that a physician or physician assistant is practicing in a manner inconsistent with the approval granted, the board may demand modification of the practice, withdraw approval of the practice agreement or take other disciplinary action as defined in section __ of this Act.

Physician Assistant Scope of Practice

The practice of a physician assistant shall include medical services within the education, training, and experience of the physician assistant that are delegated by the supervising physician.

Medical services rendered by physician assistants may include, but are not limited to

1. Obtaining patient histories and performing physical examinations
2. Ordering and/or performing diagnostic and therapeutic procedures
3. Formulating a diagnosis
4. Developing and implementing a treatment plan
5. Monitoring the effectiveness of therapeutic interventions
6. Assisting at surgery
7. Offering counseling and education to meet patient needs
8. Making appropriate referrals

The activities listed above may be performed in any setting authorized by the supervising physician, including but not limited to: clinics, hospitals; ambulatory surgical centers; patient homes; nursing homes; and other institutional settings.

Locum Tenens Permit

The board may grant a locum tenens permit to any applicant who is licensed in the state. The permit may be granted by an authorized representative of the board. Such applications for locum tenens permits will be reviewed at the next scheduled board meeting. The maximum duration of a locum tenens permit is one year. The permit may be renewed annually on a date set by the board.

Definition: Locum tenens means the temporary provision of services by a substitute provider.

REGULATORY OPTIONS

I. Regulation by the Medical Board

The state board of medical examiners shall administer the provisions of this Act under such procedures as it considers advisable and may adopt rules that are reasonable and necessary to implement the provisions of this Act.

II. Regulation by a Physician Assistant Board

To administer this Act there is hereby established a Board of Physician Assistant Examiners. The board shall consist of five members appointed by the governor, each of whom shall be residents of this state, four of whom shall be physician assistants who meet the criteria for licensure as established by this Act and one of whom shall be a licensed physician experienced in supervising physician assistants.

Initial appointments shall be made as follows

1. Two members shall be appointed for terms of 4 years
2. One member shall be appointed for a term of 3 years
3. One member shall be appointed for a term of 2 years and
4. One member shall be appointed for a term of 1 year

Each regular appointment thereafter shall be for a term of 4 years. Any vacant term shall be filled by the governor for the balance of the unexpired term. No member shall serve more than two consecutive 4-year terms and each member shall serve on the board until his or her successor is appointed.

While engaged in the business of the board, each member shall receive a per diem of $ __ and shall also receive compensation for actual expenses paid in accordance with (other state regulations).

The board shall elect a chairperson and a secretary from among its members at the first meeting of each fiscal year. The board shall meet on a regular basis. A board meeting may be called upon reasonable notice at the discretion of the chairperson and shall be called at any time upon reasonable notice by a petition of three board members to the chairperson.

Powers and duties of the board shall include

1. Promulgation of all rules reasonable and necessary to implement the provisions of this Act
2. Review and approval or rejection of applications for licensure
3. Review and approval or rejection of applications for renewal
4. Issuance of all licenses
5. Denial, suspension, revocation, or other discipline of a licensee
6. Determination of the amount and collection of all fees

III. Regulation by a Medical Board with a Physician Assistant Advisory Committee

There is hereby created a physician assistant committee, which shall review and make recommendations to the board regarding all matters relating to physician assistants that come before the board. Such matters shall include, but not be limited to:

1. Applications for licensure
2. Practice agreements
3. Disciplinary proceedings
4. Renewal requirements
5. Any other issues pertaining to the regulation and practice of physician assistants in this state

COMMITTEE MEMBERSHIP

The committee shall consist of three physician assistants, one physician experienced in supervising assistants, and one member of the board. All committee members must be residents of this state and hold a license in good standing in their respective disciplines.

The chairperson of the committee shall be elected by a majority vote of the committee members.

Committee members shall receive reimbursement for time and travel expenditures (consistent with usual state practices).

APPOINTMENTS

The physician assistant and supervising physician members of the committee shall be appointed by the governor. The board of medical examiners shall designate one member to serve on the board. All appointments shall be made within 60 days of the effective date of this Act. All appointments shall be for 4-year terms, at staggered intervals. Members shall serve no more than two consecutive terms. Reappointments of the physician assistant and supervising physician members of the committee shall be made by the governor.

MEETINGS

The committee shall meet on a regular basis. A committee meeting may be called upon reasonable notice at the discretion of the chairperson and shall be called at any time upon reasonable notice by petition of three committee members to the chairperson.

IV. Adding a Physician Assistant to the Medical Board

To assist in the administration of this Act, the governor shall appoint a licensed physician assistant to the board of medical examiners for a term of __ years [etc., etc., in accordance with existing law]. The physician assistant member will have full voting privileges.

APPENDIX 2

Code of Ethics of the Physician Assistant Profession

The American Academy of Physician Assistants recognizes its responsibility to aid the profession in maintaining high standards in the provision of quality and accessible health care services. The following principles delineate the standards governing the conduct of physician assistants in their professional interactions with patients, colleagues, other health professionals, and the general public. Realizing that no code can encompass all ethical responsibilities of the physician assistant, this enumeration of obligations in the Code of Ethics is not comprehensive and does not constitute a denial of the existence of other obligations, equally imperative, though not specifically mentioned.

- **Physician assistants** shall be committed to providing competent medical care, assuming as their primary responsibility the health, safety, welfare, and dignity of all humans.

- **Physician assistants** shall extend to each patient the full measure of their ability as dedicated, empathetic health care providers and shall assume responsibility for the skillful and proficient transactions for their professional duties.

- **Physician assistants** shall deliver needed health care services to health consumers without regard to sex, age, race, creed, socioeconomic, and political status.

- **Physician assistants** shall adhere to all state and federal laws governing informed consent concerning the patient's health care.

- **Physician assistants** shall seek consultation with their supervising physician, other health providers, or qualified professionals having special skills, knowledge, or experience whenever the welfare of the patient will be safeguarded or advocated by such consultation. Supervision should include ongoing communication between the physician and the physician assistant regarding the care of all patients.

- **Physician assistants** shall take personal responsibility for being familiar with and adhering to all federal/state laws applicable to the practice of their profession.

- **Physician assistants** shall provide only those services for which they are qualified via education and/or experiences and by pertinent legal regulatory process.

- **Physician assistants** shall not misrepresent in any manner, either directly or indirectly, their skills, training, professional credentials, identity, or services.

- **Physician assistants** shall uphold the doctrine of confidentiality regarding privileged patient information, unless required to release such information by law or as such information becomes necessary to protect the welfare of the patient or the community.

- **Physician assistants** shall strive to maintain and increase the quality of individual health care service through individual study and continuing education.

- **Physician assistants** shall have the duty to respect the law, to uphold the dignity of the physician assistant profession, and to accept its ethical principles. The physician assistant shall not participate in or conceal any activity that will bring discredit or dishonor to the physician assistant profession, and shall expose, without fear or favor, any illegal or unethical conduct in the medical profession.

- **Physician assistants,** ever cognizant of the needs of the community, shall use the knowledge and experience acquired as professionals to contribute to an improved community.

- **Physician assistants** shall place service before material gain and must carefully guard against conflicts of professional interest.

- **Physician assistants** shall strive to maintain a spirit of cooperation with their professional organizations and the professional public.

APPENDIX 3

Physician Assistant Programs

The following is a list of Physician Assistant programs with mailing addresses and phone numbers. For further information about the status of a program's accreditation, please contact the program directly.*

ALABAMA

University of Alabama at Birmingham
Surgical Physician Assistant Program
School of Health Related Professions
1714 9th Ave. S., UAB Station
Birmingham, AL 35294-1270
Phone: 205/934-4407
Fax: 205/975-7302

University of South Alabama
College of Allied Health Professions
Department of Physician Assistant Studies
1504 Springhill Avenue, Room 4410
Mobile, AL 36604-3273

ARIZONA

Kirksville College of Osteopathic Medicine
Physician Assistant Program
3210 West Camelback Road
P.O. Box 11037
Phoenix, AZ 85061-1037
Phone: 302/841-4077

CALIFORNIA

Cedars-Sinai Medical Center
Postgraduate Program in Surgery
8700 Beverly Blvd., Room 6215
Los Angeles, CA 90048-1865
Phone: 310/855-3851

Charles Drew University of Medicine
and Science
Physician Assistant Program
School of Allied Health
1621 East 120th Street, MP 42
Los Angeles, CA 90059-3025
Phone: 213/563-5879
Fax: 213/563-4833

Charles R. Drew University of Medicine
and Science
Physician Assistant Graduate Program
in Surgery
12021 S. Wilmington Avenue
Los Angeles, CA 90059
Phone: 310/668-4522

Western University of Health Sciences
Physician Assistant Program
College Plaza
309 East Second Street
Pomona, CA 91766-1889
Phone: 909/469-5378
Fax: 909/629-7255

Los Angeles & University of Southern California
Physician Assistant Pediatric
Residency Program
Physician Assistant Neonatology
Residency Program
Women's and Children Hospital
1240 N. Mission Rd, L919
Los Angeles, CA 90033

---

*Data from Association of Physician Assistant Programs

Morally College of Health Sciences
Physician Assistant Program
4550 La Sierra Avenue
Riverside, CA 92506
Phone: 909/687-4268

University of Southern California
Physician Assistant Program
Department of Family Medicine
1975 Zonal Avenue, KAM B29
Los Angeles, CA 90033-1039
Phone: 213/342-1328
Fax: 213/342-1260

University of California, Davis
Physician Assistant Program
Department of Family Practice
2626 Stockton Blvd., Suite 1025
Sacramento, CA 95817
Phone: 916/734-3550
Fax: 916/452-2112

Stanford University Medical Center
Primary Care Associate Program
School of Medicine
703 Welch Road, Suite G-1
Palo Alto, CA 94304-1760
Phone: 415/723-7043
Fax: 415/723-9692

COLORADO

University of Colorado Health Science Center
Child Health Associate PA Program
4200 E. Ninth Avenue, C 219
Denver, CO 80262-0001
Phone: 303/315-4614
Fax: 303/270-6976

CONNECTICUT

Norwalk Hospital/Yale University
Physician Assistant Surgical Residency Program
Graduate Program in Pediatrics
School of Medicine
Norwalk, CT 06856

Phone: 203/852-2188 (Surgery)
Phone: 203/852-2662 (Pediatrics)

Quinnipiac College
Physician Assistant Program
275 Mt. Carmel Avenue
Hamden, CT 06518
Phone: 203/281-8704
Fax: 203/287-5303

Yale University
Physician Associate Program
School of Medicine
47 College Street, Suite 220
New Haven, CT 06510-3209
Phone: 203/785-2860
Fax: 203/785-3601

DISTRICT OF COLUMBIA

George Washington University, The
Physician Assistant Program
2300 I St., NW
Washington, DC 20037-2337
Phone: 202/994-4034
Fax: 202/994-2124

Howard University
Physician Assistant Program
College of Allied Health Sciences
6th & Bryant Sts. NW
Washington, DC 20059-0001
Phone: 202/806-7536
Fax: 202/806-4476

FLORIDA

Florida College of Physician Assistants
Suite K-1
Miami, FL 33126
Phone: 305/324-9700

Miami-Dade Community College
Physician Assistant Program
Medical Center Campus
950 NW 20th Street
Miami, FL 33127-4693
Phone: 305/238-4744

Nova Southeastern University
Physician Assistant Program
3200 S. University Drive
Ft. Lauderdale, FL 33328
Phone: 954/723-1650
Fax: 954/723-1714

University of Florida
Physician Assistant Program
Box 100176
Gainesville, FL 32610-0176
Phone: 352/395-7955
Fax: 352/395-7966

GEORGIA

Emory University
Physician Assistant Program
1462 Clifton Rd., Suite 280
Atlanta, GA 30322-1063
Phone: 404/727-7825
Fax: 404/727-7836

Medical College of Georgia
Physician Assistant Program
Kelly Administration Bldg. 170
Augusta, GA 30912
Phone: 706/721-2735

Physician Assistant Program
709 Mall Boulevard
Savannah, GA 31406
Phone: 912/352-7900

IDAHO

Idaho State University
Physician Assistant Program
Campus Box 8253
Pocatello, ID 83209-0001
Phone: 208/236-4726
Fax: 208/236-4969

ILLINOIS

Cook County Hospital/Malcolm X College
Physician Assistant Program

1900 West Polk Street
Chicago, IL 60612-3736
Phone: 312/633-8030
Fax: 312/633-5995

Finch University of Health Sciences
Chicago Medical School -
   Physician Assistant Program
3333 Green Bay Road
N. Chicago, IL 60064-3095
Phone: 847/578-3312

Midwestern University
Physician Assistant Program
555 31st Street
Downers Grove, IL 60515-1235
Phone: 630/515-6171
Fax: 630/971-6402

Southern Illinois University at Carbondal
Physician Assistant Program
College of Applied Sciences and Arts
Carbondale, IL 62901-6615
Phone: 618/453-7211

INDIANA

Butler University/Methodist Hospital
Physician Assistant Program
4600 Sunset Avenue
Indianapolis, IN 46206-1367
Phone: 317/940-9471
Fax: 317/940-6172

Lutheran College
Physician Assistant Program
3024 Fairfield Avenue
Fort Wayne, IN 46807-1697
Phone: 219/458-2483
Fax: 219/458-3077

IOWA

University of Iowa
Physician Assistant Program

2333 Steindler Building
Iowa City, IA 52242-1088
Phone: 319/335-8922
Fax: 319/335-8923

University of Osteopathic Medicine
   & Health Sciences
Physician Assistant Program
3200 Grand Avenue
Des Moines, IA 50312-4198
Phone: 515/271-1569
Fax: 515/271-1543

KANSAS

Wichita State University
Physician Assistant Program
1845 Firmount
Wichita, KS 67260-0043
Phone: 316/978-3011
Fax: 316/978-3025

KENTUCKY

University of Kentucky
Physician Assistant Program
103 CAHP Building
121 Washington Avenue
Lexington, KY 40536-0003
Phone: 606/323-1100
Fax: 606/257-2454

LOUISIANA

Louisiana State University Medical Center
Physician Assistant Program
1501 Kings Highway
Shreveport, LA 71130
Phone: 318/675-7317

MAINE

University of New England
Physician Assistant Program
Hills Beach Road

Biddeford, ME 04005
Phone: 207/283-0176, Ext. 2847

MARYLAND

Anne Arundel Community College
Physician Assistant Program
101 College Parkway
Arnold, MD 21012
Phone: 410/315-7310

Essex Community College
Physician Assistant Program
7201 Rossville Boulevard
Baltimore, MD 21237-3855
Phone: 410/780-6159
Fax: 410/780-6405

Sinai Hospital of Baltimore
Physician Assistant Graduate Program
   in Surgery
2401 Belvedere Avenue
Baltimore, MD 21215
Phone: 410/578-9012

MASSACHUSETTS

Northeastern University
Physician Assistant Program
202 Robinson Hall
360 Huntington Avenue
Boston, MA 02115-5005
Phone: 617/373-3195
Fax: 617/373-3338

Springfield College/Baystate Health Systems
Physician Assistant Program
263 Alden Street
Springfield, MA 01109
Phone: 413/788-2420; 800/343-1267

MICHIGAN

Central Michigan University
Physician Assistant Program
Foust 205
Mt. Pleasant, MI 48859

Phone: 517/774-2478
Fax: 517/774-2433

Grand Valley State University
Physician Assistant Program
323 Henry Hall
Allendale, MI 49401-9403
Phone: 616/895-6611
Fax: 616/895-2025

University of Detroit Mercy
Physician Assistant Program
8200 West Outer Drive
PO Box 130 OD
Detroit, MI 48219-0900
Phone: 313/993-6057
Fax: 313/966-1761

Wayne State University
Physician Assistant Program
College of Pharmacy &
   Allied Health Professions
1400 Chrysler Service Drive
Detroit, MI 48202
Phone: 313/577-1368
Fax: 313/577-5400

Western Michigan University
Physician Assistant Program
Kalamazoo, MI 49008-5138
Phone: 616/387-5311
Fax: 616/387-3348

MINNESOTA

Augsburg College
Physician Assistant Program
2211 Riverside Avenue, Box 149
Minneapolis, MN 55455
Phone: 612/330-1039
Fax: 612/330-1757

MISSOURI

Saint Louis University
Physician Assistant Program
School of Allied Health Professions

1504 South Grand Boulevard
St. Louis, MO 63104-1304
Phone: 314/577-8521
Fax: 314/577-8503

MONTANA

Rocky Mountain College
Physician Assistant Program
1511 Poly Drive
Billings, MT 59102
Phone: 406/657-1190
Fax: 406/657-1194

NEBRASKA

Union College
Physician Assistant Program
3800 South 48th Street
Lincoln, NE 68506
Phone: 402/488-2331

University of Nebraska Medical Center
Physician Assistant Program
600 South 42nd Street
Omaha, NE 68198-4300
Phone: 402/559-9495
Fax: 402/559-5356

NEW JERSEY

Rutgers University—University of Medicine
   and Dentistry of New Jersey
Physician Assistant Program
Robert Woods Johnson Medical School
675 Hoes Lane
Piscataway, NJ 08854-5635
Phone: 908/463-4444
Fax: 908/235-4820

Seton Hall University
Physician Assistant Program
65 Bergen Street
University Heights Newark, NJ 07107
Phone: 201/982-5954

NEW MEXICO

University of New Mexico
Physician Assistant Program

Department of Family &
  Community Medicine
400 Tucker NE
Albuquerque, NM 87131
Phone: 505/277-2165

NEW YORK

Albany-Hudson Valley
Physician Assistant Program
Albany Medical College
47 New Scotland Avenue
Albany, NY 12208-3412
Phone: 518/262-5251
Fax: 518/262-6698

Bayley Seton Hospital
Physician Assistant Program
75 Vanderbilt Avenue
Staten Island, NY 10304-3850
Phone: 718/390-5570
Fax: 718/390-5570

Bronx Lebanon Hospital Center
Physician Assistant Program
1650 Selwyn Avenue
Suite 4F
Bronx, NY 10457-7628
Phone: 718/960-1255
Fax: 718/960-1329

The Brooklyn Hospital Center/
  Long Island University
Physician Assistant Program
121 DeKalb Avenue
Brooklyn, NY 11201
Phone: 718/403-8144

Catholic Medical Center
Physician Assistant Training Program
89-15 Woodhaven Boulevard
Woodhaven, NY 11421-2627
Phone: 718/805-7562
Fax: 718/805-7681

City University New York/
  Harlem Hospital Center

Physician Assistant Program
506 Malcolm X Boulevard
WP-Room 619
New York, NY 10037-1889
Phone: 212/939-2525
Fax: 212/939-2529

College of Staten Island
Hospital Physician Assistant Program
Department of Biology
Bldg. 6S, Room 136A
2800 Victory Boulevard
Staten Island, NY 10314
Phone: 718/982-3857

Cornell University Medical College
Physician Assistant Program
1300 New York Avenue
New York, NY 10021-4896
Phone: 212/746-5134
Fax: 212/746-0407

Daemen College
Physician Assistant Program
4380 Main Street
Amherst, NY 14226-3592
Phone: 716/839-8516
Fax: 716/839-8516

D'Youville College
Physician Assistant Program
320 Porter Avenue
Buffalo, NY 14201-1084
Phone: 716/881-7600
Fax: 716/881-7790

LeMoyne College
Physician Assistant Program
Syracuse, NY 13214
Phone: 315/445-4144

Montefiore Medical Center
Surgical Residency Program
Post-graduate Residency in Gynecology/
  Obstetrics for PAs
111 E 210th Street
Bronx, NY 10467

Phone: 718/920-6223 (Surgery)
Phone: 718/920-6311 (Gynecology)

Rochester Institute of Technology
Physician Assistant Program
85 Lomb Memorial Drive
Rochester, NY 14623-5603
Phone: 716/475-2978
Fax: 716/475-5766

St. Johns University
College of Allied Health Professions
800 Utopia Parkway
Jamaica, NY 11439
Phone: 718/990-6275

St. Vincent's Medical Center
Physician Assistant Graduate Program
   in Surgery
355 Bard Avenue
Staten Island, NY 10310

State University of New York at Brooklyn
Physician Assistant Program
Health Science Center
450 Clarkson Avenue, Box 1222
Brooklyn, NY 11203-2012
Phone: 718/270-2324
Fax: 718/270-7751

State University of New York at Stony Brook
Physician Assistant Program
School of Health, Technology,
   & Management
SHTM—HSC
L2, Room 052
Stony Brook, NY 11794-8202
Phone: 516/444-3190
Fax: 516/444-7621

Touro College
Physician Assistant Program
135 Carman Road, Building 14
Dix Hills, NY 11746-5641
Phone: 516/673-3200
Fax: 516/271-7082

Touro College/Coney Island Hospital
   Extension Center

Physician Assistant Program
2601 Ocean Parkway
Brooklyn, NY 11235
Phone: 718/615-4468

Wagner College
Physician Assistant Program
74 Melville Street
Staten Island, NY 10309-4035
Phone: 718/226-2928
Fax: 718/226-2464

NORTH CAROLINA

Bowman Gray School of Medicine
Wake Forest University
Physician Assistant Program
Medical Center Boulevard
Winston Salem, NC 27157-1006
Phone: 910/716-4356
Fax: 910/716-4432

Duke University Medical Center
Physician Assistant Program
Box CFM 2914
Durham, NC 27710-0001
Phone: 919/286-8225
Fax: 919/286-7916

East Carolina University
Department of Physician Assistant Studies
School of Health Sciences
Carol Balk Building
Greenville, NC 27858-4353
Phone: 919/328-4223

Methodist College
Physician Assistant Program
5400 Ramsey Street
Fayetteville, NC 28311-1498
Phone: 910/630-7495
Fax: 910/630-2133

NORTH DAKOTA

University of North Dakota School of Medicine
Physician Assistant Program

Department of Community Medicine
and Rural Health
Grand Forks, ND 58202-9037
Phone: 701/777-2344
Fax: 701/777-2389

OHIO

Cuyahoga Community College (2 programs)
Physician Assistant Program
Surgeon's Assistant Program
11000 Pleasant Valley Road
Parma, OH 44130-5114
Phone: 216/987-5363
Fax: 216/987-5050

Kettering College of Medical Arts
Physician Assistant Program
3737 Southern Boulevard
Kettering, OH 45429-1299
Phone: 513/296-7238; 800/433-5262
Fax: 513/296-4238

Medical College of Ohio
Physician Assistant Program
School of Allied Health
3000 Arlington Avenue
Toledo, OH 43614
Phone: 419/381-5408

OKLAHOMA

University of Oklahoma
Physician Associate Program/
Graduate Occupational Health Program
Health Sciences Center
PO Box 26901
Oklahoma City, OK 73190-0001
Phone: 405/271-2047
Fax: 405/271-3621

OREGON

Oregon Health Sciences University
Physician Assistant Program
3181 Sam Jackson Park Road
Portland, OR 97201-3098

Phone: 503/494-1408
Fax: 503/494-1409

Pacific University
School of Physician Assistant Studies
Forest Grove, OR 97116
Phone: 503/359-2898
Fax: 503/359-2977

PENNSYLVANIA

Allegheny University of Health Sciences
Physician Assistant Program
Broad & Vine Streets, MS 504
Philadelphia, PA 19102
Phone: 215/762-7135
Fax: 215/762-1164

Allentown College
Physician Assistant Program
2755 Station Avenue
Center Valley, PA 18034
Phone: 215/282-1100, Ext. 1237

Beaver College
Physician Assistant Program
450 South Easton Road
Glenside, PA 19035
Phone: 215/572-2910; 800/776-2328

Chatham College
Physician Assistant Program
Woodland Road
Pittsburgh, PA 15232
Phone: 412/365-1405

Duquesne University
Physician Assistant Program
John G. Rangos School of Health Sciences
130 Health Sciences Building
Pittsburgh, PA 15282-0001
Phone: 412/396-5914
Fax: 412/396-5554

Gannon University
Physician Assistant Program
109 University Square
Erie, PA 16541

Phone: 814/871-7407; 800/426-6668
Fax: 814/871-5662

Geisinger Medical Center
Physician Assistant Graduate Program
  in Surgery
100 N Academy Avenue
Danville, PA 17822-1516
Phone: 717/271-6094

Hahnemann University
Physician Assistant Program
School of Health Sciences and Humanities
Broad & Vine Streets/Mail Stop 504
Philadelphia, PA 19102-1192
Phone: 215/762-7135

King's College
Physician Assistant Program
133 North River Street
Wilkes Barre, PA 18711-0851
Phone: 717/826-5853
Fax: 717/825-9049

Lock Haven University
Physician Assistant Program
Lock Haven, PA 17745
Phone: 717/893-2168

Pennsylvania College of Technology
Physician Assistant Program
One College Avenue
Williamsport, PA 17701
Phone: 717/327-4770

Philadelphia College of Science
  and Textiles
Physician Assistant Program
School House Lane & Henry Avenue
Philadelphia, PA 19144
Phone: 215/951-2908

St. Francis College
Physician Assistant Program
PO Box 600
Loretto, PA 15940-0600
Phone: 814/472-3130
Fax: 814/472-3137

SOUTH DAKOTA

University of South Dakota
Physician Assistant Program
414 E Clark Street
Vermillion, SD 57069-2390
Phone: 605/677-5128
Fax: 605/677-6569

TENNESSEE

Trevecca Nazarene College
Physician Assistant Program
333 Murfreesboro Road
Nashville, TN 37210-2834
Phone: 615/248-1225
Fax: 615/248-1622

TEXAS

Baylor College of Medicine
Physician Assistant Program
Department of Community Medicine
One Baylor Plaza, Room 633E
Houston, TX 77030-3411
Phone: 713/798-4619
Fax: 713/798-3644

Interservice Physician Assistant Program
MCCS-HMP PA Branch
3151 Scott Road
Fort Sam Houston, TX 78234-6138
Phone: 210/221-8004; 8765
Fax: 210/221-8493

University of North Texas School
  of Osteopathic Medicine
Physician Assistant Program
Fort Worth, TX 76107
3500 Camp Bowie Boulevard
Phone: 817/735-2301

University of Texas Southwestern
Medical Center
Physician Assistant Program
6011 Harry Hines Boulevard
Dallas, TX 75235-9090
Phone: 214/648-1701
Fax: 214/648-1003

University of Texas Medical Branch-Galveston
Physician Assistant Program
School of Allied Health Services
Galveston, TX 77555-1028
Phone: 409/772-3046
Fax: 409/772-3014

UTAH

University of Utah
Physician Assistant Program
School of Medicine
50 North Medical Drive
Building 528
Salt Lake City, UT 84132-0001
Phone: 801/581-7766
Fax: 801/581-5807

VIRGINIA

College of Health Sciences
Physician Assistant Program
PO Box 13186
920 South Jefferson Street
Roanoke, VA 24031-3186
Phone: 540/985-4029
Fax: 540/985-9773

Eastern Virginia Medical School of the
    Medical College of Hampton Roads
Physician Assistant Program
721 Fairfax Avenue
Norfolk, VA 23501
Phone: 804/446-5805

WASHINGTON

University of Washington
MEDEX Northwest
Physician Assistant Program
4245 Roosevelt Way NE
Seattle, WA 98105-6920
Phone: 206/548-2600
Fax: 206/548-5195

WEST VIRGINIA

Alderson-Broaddus College
Physician Assistant Program
PO Box 578
Philippi, WV 26416
Phone: 304/457-1700, Ext. 283

College of West Virginia
Physician Assistant Program
609 South Kanawah Street
Beckley, WV 25802
Phone: 304/259-7351, Ext. 436

WISCONSIN

University of Wisconsin-LaCross
Physician Assistant Program
241 Cowely Hall
1725 State Street
LaCross, WI 54601
Phone: 608/785-6620

University of Wisconsin/Madison
Physician Assistant Program
Medical Sciences Center
1300 University Avenue
Madison, WI 53706
Phone: 608/263-5620; 800/442-6698
Fax: 608/263-6434

UNIFORMED SERVICES

Interservice Physician Assistant Program
MCCS-HMP PA Branch
3151 Scott Road
Fort Sam Houston, TX 78234-6138
Phone: 210/221-8004; 210/221-8765
Fax: 210/221-8493

Note: The Interservice PA Program includes
members of the Air Force, Army, Coast Guard,
Navy, and the Bureau of Prisons branches of
service.

Bibliography

A

Aaronson WE. The use of physician extenders in nursing homes: a review. Med Care Rev 1991;48(4):411–447.

Aaronson WE. Is there a role for physician extenders in nursing homes? J Long Term Care Adm 1992;20(3):18–22.

Acuna HR. The physician's assistant and extension of health services. Bull Pan Am Health Organ 1977;11(3):189–194.

AGPAW. Advisory Group on Physician Assistants and the Workforce, Final Report submitted to the Council on Graduate Medical Education. Physician Assistants in the Health Workforce 1994. US DHHS, Public Health Service, Health Resources & Services Administration, Bureau of Health Professions, Division of Medicine, 1995.

Alexander BJ, Lipscomb J. Nonphysician practitioners panel report. pp. 421–465. In Lipscomb J, Alexander BJ (eds): Physician Staffing for the VA: Volume II, Supplementary Papers. Institute of Medicine, National Academy Press, Washington, DC, 1992.

Almanac. Chronicle of Higher Education 1992;39:37.

Amann HJ. Physician's assistants: An extension of the physician. US Navy Med 1973;62:36–38.

American Academy of Physician Assistants. The Development of Standards to Ensure the Competency of Physician Assistants, American Academy of Physician Assistants, Arlington, VA, 1979.

American Academy of Physician Assistants. Physician Assistants: State Laws and Regulations. 6th Ed. Alexandria, VA, 1992.

American Academy of Physician Assistants. Information on The Physician Assistant Profession. Physician Assistant Educational Programs. Alexandria, VA, September, 1993a.

American Academy of Physician Assistants. Annual Census Data on Physician Assistants, 1993. American Academy of Physician Assistants, Alexandria, VA, 1993b.

American Academy of Physician Assistants. A challenge for the physician assistant profession: report of the AAPA Task Force on Unlicensed Medical Graduates. J Am Acad Physician Assist 1993c;6:65–73.

American Academy of Physician Assistants. Hospital Privileges Summary: 1993. Alexandria, VA, 1993d.

American Academy of Physician Assistants. Annual Census Data on Physician Assistants, 1993. American Academy of Physician Assistants, Alexandria, VA, 1994a.

American Academy of Physician Assistants Professional Practice Council Report. Naming the profession. J Am Acad Physician Assist 1994b; 7:521–525.

American Academy of Physician Assistants, Council on Professional Practice. Hospital Privileges for Physician Assistants: J Am Acad Physician Assist 1994c;7(3):183–190.

American Academy of Physician Assistants. New Students in PA Programs (1993 and 1994). Alexandria, VA, 1995.

American Academy of Physician Assistants. General Census Data on Physician Assistants: 1995. Alexandria, VA, 1996a.

American Academy of Physician Assistants. 1991–1995 AAPA Membership Census Report. Alexandria, VA, 1996b.

American College of Surgeons. Statement on surgeon's assistants. American College of Surgeons Bulletin, Oct 1973.

American Hospital Association. Job Description Manual: ADA Workbook. Vol. II. American Society for Healthcare Human Resources Administration of the American Hospital Association and The Wyatt Company. American Hospital Association, Chicago, IL, 1992.

American Medical Association Council on Health Manpower. The child health associate: A new training program in Colorado. JAMA 1970; 212(6):1045–1046.

American Medical Association. Socioeconomic Survey of Practicing Physicians, 1991. AMA, Chicago, IL, 1992.

Anderson C, Neham E, Ravenscroft F, Vickery D. A Site Specific Study of Physician Extender Staffed Primary Care Centers. The METREK Division of the MITRE Corporation (MITRE Tech. Rep. MTR-7495), 1977.

Anderson KH, Powers L. The pediatric assistant. North Carolina Med J 1970;31(1):3–8.

Anderson M, Astin A, et al. Why the shortage of black professors? J Blacks Higher Education 1993;1:10.

Association of Physician Assistant Programs. Physician Assistant Programs Directory, 15th Ed., Alexandria, VA, 1996.

Atwater JB. Must local health officers be physicians? Am J Public Health 1980;70(1):11.

Atwater RE. Recruiting relationships: Q & A. PA Career, November 1993, p. 7.

Austin G, Foster W, Richards JD. Pediatric screening examinations in private practice. Pediatrics 1968;41:115–119.

B

Baker JA, Oliver D, Donahue W, Huckabee M. Predicting role satisfaction among practicing physician assistants. J Am Acad Physician Assist 1989;2(6): 461–470.

Ballenger MD, Estes EH. Licensure or responsible delegation? N Engl J Med 1971;284(6):331.

Ballweg RM. The impact of women on the PA profession. J Am Acad Physician Assist 1992;5(9): 655–662.

Ballweg RM. History of the profession. In Ballweg RM, Stolberg S, Sullivan EM (eds): Physician

Assistant: A Guide to Clinical Practice. WB Saunders, Philadelphia, PA,1994.

Barnes W, Magnuson L. An important untapped resource of health manpower for the seventies. Arch Environ Health 1971;23:82–87.

Bednash GD. The Interplay Between the Supply of Physicians and Advanced Practice Nurses. In Osterweis M, McLaughlin CJ, Manasse HR, Hopper (eds): The U.S. Health Workforce: Power, Politics, and Power. Association of Academic Health Centers, Washington, DC, 1996.

Begely B. PA-C: PA-SEE or Passe. J Am Acad Physician Assist 191;4(4):297.

Beinfield MS. Postgraduate surgical education versus on-the-job training. J Am Acad Physician Assistants 1991;4(6):451–452.

Bellin LE. The politics of ambulatory care. pp. 95–109. In Pascarelli E (ed.): Hospital-Based Ambulatory Care. Appleton-Century-Crofts, Norwalk, CT, 1982.

Berg RH. More than a nurse, less than a doctor. Look. 1966;30(18):58–61.

Bergman AB. Physician's assistants belong in the nursing profession. Am J Nurs. 1971;71(5): 975–977.

Berry TR, Dieter PM. Recruitment of physician assistants: implications for the future. J Am Acad Physician Assistants 1989;2(5):383–392.

Blaser L. The business of clinical practice. J Am Acad Physician Assistants 1993;6(6):402–406.

Blendon RS. Can China's health care be transplanted without China's economic policies? N Engl J Med 1979;300:1453–1458.

Blessing JD, Elizondo E. PA involvement in patients' psychological problems: a follow-up survey of PAs, physicians, and educators. Phys Assist 1990;14(10):24–30.

Bliss A, Cohen E (eds). The New Health Professionals—Nurse Practitioners and Physician's Assistants. Germantown, Maryland: Aspen Systems Corporation, 1997.

Bonner S. Auxiliares de enfermeria and feldshers. Phys Assist 1976;1(1):37–40.

Borland B, Williams F, Taylor D. A survey of attitudes of physicians on proper use of physician's assistants. Health Serv Rep 1972;87(5):467–472.

Bottom WD. Physician assistants: current status of the profession. J Family Pract 1987;24(6): 639–644.

Bottom WD. Geriatric medicine in the United States: new roles for physician assistants. J Community Health 1988;13(2):95–103.

Bottom WD. Unlicensed physicians as PAs: policy implications for the profession. J Am Acad Physician Assist 1994;4:97–101.

Borden SL. The Professional Liability Handbook: A Basic Guide for Physician Assistants. American Academy of Physician Assistants, Alexandria, VA, 1990.

Brady GF. Job to career satisfaction spillover among physician's assistants. Med Care 1980;18(10): 1057–1062.

Brandon J. Students come from smaller towns and have more education. AAPA News, April 1993; 10–11.

Breslau N, Novack A. Public attitudes toward some changes in the division of labor in medicine. Med Care 1979;17(8):859–867.

Briggs RM, Schneidman BS, Thorson EN, Deisher RD. Education and integration of midlevel health-care practitioners in obstetrics and gynecology: experience of a training program in Washington State. Am J Obstet Gynecol 1978;132(9):68–77.

Browning EK, Browning JM. Microeconomic Theory and Applications. 4th Ed. Harper Collins, New York, NY, 1992.

Brutsche RL. Utilization of PAs in federal correctional institutions. Physician Assist 1986;10(9): 60–66.

Buchanan JL, Kane RL, Garrard J et al. Results of the Massachusetts Nursing Home Connection Program. RAND Corporation, Santa Monica, RAND/JR-01, 1989.

Bullough B. Barriers to the nurse practitioner movement: problems of women in a woman's field. Int J Health Serv 1975;5(2):210–214.

Bureau of Health Manpower Education. Selected Training Programs for Physician Support Personnel. National Institutes of Health, Department of Health, Education and Welfare, Washington, DC, 1971.

Burnett WH. Building the primary health care team: the state of California approach. Fam Community Health 1980;3(2):49–61.

Bush T, Cherkin D, Barlow W. The impact of physician attitudes on patient satisfaction with care for low back pain. Arch Fam Med 1993;2(3): 301–305.

Byrnes JF. The evolution of surgical PAs. J Am Acad Physician Assist 1991;4(6):449–451.

C

Camp B. PA prescriptive privileges: an ongoing controversy. Physician Assist 1984;8(3):11, 14.

Cardenas AP. Forensic pathology and the PA (letter to the editor). J Am Acad Physician Assist 1993; 6(1):77.

Cargill VA, Conti M, Neuhauser D, et al. Improving the effectiveness of screening colorectal cancer by involving nurse clinicians. Med Care 1991; 29:1–5.

Carter RD, Gifford JF. The Emergence of the Physician Assistant Profession. In Perry HB, Breitner MA (eds): Physician Assistant: Their Contribution to Health Care. Human Sciences Press, New York, NY, 1982.

Carter RD, Oliver DR. An analysis of salaries for clinically active physician assistants. Phys Assist 1983;7:14–27.

Carter RD, Perry HB (eds): Alternatives in Health Care Delivery, Emerging Roles for Physician Assistants. Warren Green Publishers, St. Louis, MO, 1984a.

Carter RD, Gifford JF. The Emergence of the Physician Assistant Profession. In Carter RD, Perry HB (eds): Alternatives in Health Care Delivery. Warren Green Publishers, St. Louis, MO, 1984b.

Carzoli RP, Martinez-Cruz M, Cuevas LL, et al. Comparison of neonatal nurse practitioners, physician assistants, and residents in the neonatal intensive care unit. Arch Pediatr Adolesc Med 1994;148(12):1271–1276.

Cawley JF, Golden AS. Nonphysicians in the United States: manpower policy in primary care. J Public Health Policy 1983a;4(1):69–82.

Cawley JF, Ott JE, DeAtley C. The future for physician assistants. Ann Intern Med 1983b;98(6): 993–997.

Cawley JF, Stein WA. GEMENAC revisited: questionable assumptions and conflicting data. Phys Assist 1983c;7(3):161–162.

Cawley JF. The division of labor in medicine. Phys Assist 1984;8(4):7–8.

Cawley JF. The physician assistant profession: current status and future trends. J Public Health Policy 1985a;6:78–99.

Cawley JF. Medical writing (Editorial). PA Drug Update 1985b;2:10.

Cawley JF. The Cost Effectiveness of Physician Assistants. American Academy of Physician Assistants, Alexandria, VA, 1986a.

Cawley JF, Combs GE, Curry RH. Non-physician providers. Am J Public Health 1986c;76(11): 1360.

Cawley JF, Perry HB. Who is that house officer? The shifting roles of personnel in graduate medical education. J Am Acad Physician Assist 1988; 1(4):255–257.

Cawley JF. Hospital physician assistants: past, present, and future. Hosp Top 1991;69(3):14–19.

Cawley JF. Federal Health Policy and PAs. J Am Acad Physician Assist 1992a;9:679–688.

Cawley JF. Federal Support for PA Education. Presented at the National Primary Care Conference, March 29–31, 1992b.

Cawley JF. IMGs seek to qualify as PAs in Maryland (letter). Fed Bull 1994;81:71–72.

Cawley JF. The evolution of new health professions: a history of physician assistants. The US Health Workforce: Power, Politics, and Policy. In Osterweis M et al (eds): The Association of Academic Health Centers, Washington, DC, 1996a.

Celentano DD. The optimum utilization and appropriate responsibilities of allied health professionals. Soc Sci Med 1982;16:687–698.

Chaffee D. Do PAs have a future in cardiovascular surgery? Phys Assist 1988;12(4):107–108.

Chavez RS. Why PAs should endorse registered care technologist. J Am Acad Physician Assist 1989;2(2):79–81.

Clawson DK, Osterweis M (eds). The Roles of Physician Assistants and Nurse Practitioners in Primary Care. Association of Academic Health Centers, Washington, DC, 1993.

Colwill JM. Where have all the primary care applicants gone? N Engl J Med 1992;326:387–394.

Committee on Allied Health Education and Accreditation. Essentials and Guidelines for an Accredited Educational Program for the Physician Assistant. (Initially adopted 1971; revised in 1978, 1985, and 1990) CAHEA, Chicago, 1990.

Committee on Graduate Medical Education. Fourth Report to Congress and the Department of Health and Human Services: Recommendations to Improve Access to Health Care Through Physician Work Force Reform. Health Resources and Services Administration, Rockville, MD, 1994.

Conant L, Robertson L, Kosa J, Alpert J. Anticipated patient acceptance of new nursing roles and physicians' assistants. Am J Dis Child 1971; 122:202–205.

Condit D. PAs: Russian style. Health Pract Physician Assist 1977;1(1):37–40.

Condit D. PA Opportunities. PA 84 1984;8–10.

Condit D. A quarter century of surgical physician assistants. Phys Assist 1992;15(4):3.

Condit D. Our military heritage. Phys Assist 1993;X:58,61,62,65–67.

Cook JH. The legal status of physician extenders in Iowa: review, speculations, and recommendations. Iowa Law Review 1986;72(1):315–339.

Cooper J, Willig S. Nonphysician for coronary care delivery: are they legal? Am J Cardiol 1971; 28:363–365.

Coryell W, Clininger R, Reich T. Clinical assessment: use of nonphysician interviewers. J Nerv Ment Dis 1978;166(8):599–606.

Council on Graduate Medical Education. Third Report of the Council. Improving Access to Health Care Through Physician Workforce Reform. U.S. Department of Health and Human Services. Health Resources and Services Administration, Rockville, MD, 1992.

Council on Graduate Medical Education. Fourth Report to Congress and Health and Human Services Secretary. Recommendations to Improve Access to Health Care Through Physician Workforce Reform. U.S. Department of Health and Human Services. Health Resources and Services Administration, Rockville, MD, 1994.

Crandall LA, Santulli WP, Radelet ML, et al. Physician assistants in primary care. Med Care 1984; 22(3):268–282.

Crandall LA, Haas WH, Radelet ML. Socioeconomic influences in patient assignment to PA or MD providers. Phys Assist 1986;10(3):164–170.

Crovitz E, Huse MM, Lewis DE. Selection of physician's assistants. J Med Educ 1975;48:551–555.

Curran WJ. Legal responsibilities for actions of physician's assistants. N Engl J Med 1972;5:254.

Currey CJ. Choosing to become a PA: implications for student recruitment. J Am Acad Physician Assist 1990;3(4):287–290.

Currey CJ. National survey of PA attitudes about AIDS care. J Am Acad Physician Assist (abstract) 1992;5(5):360.

Currey R. Medicine for Sale: Commercialism vs Professionalism. The Grand Rounds Press, Knoxville, 1992.

Curry RH. Recruitment and retention of PAs: implications for the future. J Am Acad Physician Assist 1989;2(5):322–324.

Curry RH, Luckie WR. The role of the primary care PA. Phys Assist 1994;8(9):31–34,39,40.

Cyr KA. Physician-PA practice in a military clinic: a statistical comparison of productivity/availability. Phys Assist 1985;10(4):112–113, 119,123–124.

D

Darr K. Credentialing hospital clinicians. Hosp Top 1989;67:4–5.

DeBarth K. Outer Banks PA. Medicine at the edge. Clin Rev 1996;6(7):148–158.

Dehn RW, Asprey DP. A study of PA perceptions: impediments to the practice of medicine in Iowa. J Am Acad Physician Assist 1995;8(1): 49–58.

Demots H, Coombs B, Murphy E, et al. Coronary arteriography performed by physician assistant. Am J Cardiol 1987;60:784–787.

Department of Defense, U.S. Government, Office of Secretary of Defense, Manpower and Research Affairs. Studies of the Effectiveness of Paramedical Personnel Usage in Medical Care Delivery. NPS-54-78-1, November, Arlington, VA, 1977.

Department of Health, Education, and Welfare, U.S. Physicians for a Growing America: Report of the Surgeon General's Consultant Group on Medical Education, 1959.

Department of Health, Education and Welfare, U.S. Public Health Service, Health Resources Administration, National Center for Health Services Research. Research Digest Series. An Evaluation of Physician Assistants in Diagnostic Radiology. DHEW Pub. No. (HRA) 77–3164. March 1977.

Department of Health, Education and Welfare, U.S. Public Health Service, Alcohol, Drug Abuse, and Mental Health Administration. Nurse Practitioners and Physician Assistants in Substance Abuse Programs. DHEW Pub No. (ADM) 79–884. 1979.

Department of Health and Human Services, U.S. Sixth Report to the President & Congress on the Status of Health Personnel in the United States 1988. Chapter 4, Physician Assistants. Public Health Service, Bureau of Health Professions, HRSA, Rockville, MD, HRS-P-OD-88-1 (HRP-0907200), June 1988.

Department of Health and Human Services, U.S. Health Personnel in the United States: Eighth Report to Congress 1991. U.S. Department of Health and Human Services, Public Health Service, Health Resources and Services Administration, Bureau of Health Personnel. DHHS Pub No. HRS-O-OD-92-1. 1992.

Dermatology World. Physician assistants following managed care into dermatology practices. Dermatology World 1996;6(2):13.

DeNicola L, Kleid D, Brink L, et al. Use of pediatric physician extenders in pediatric and neonatal intensive care units. Crit Care Med 1994;22(11): 1856–1862.

D'Ercole A, Skodol AE, Struening E, et al. Diagnosis of physical illness in psychiatric patients using axis III and a standardized medical history (published erratum appears in Hosp Community Psychiatry 1991;42(5):539) Hosp Community Psychiatry 1991;42(5):395–400.

Devore L, Shapiro S. The physician's assistant: a new breed of dental educator. J Dent Educ 1978; 42(10):568–571.

Dial TH, Palsbo SE, Bergsten C, et al. Clinical staffing in staff- and group-model HMOs. Health Affairs 1995;14(2):168–180.

Diekman DJ, Ferguson KJ, Boebbeling BN. Motivation for hepatitis B vaccine acceptance among medical and physician assistant students. J Gen Intern Med 1995a;10:1–6.

Diekman DJ, Schuldt SS, Albanese MA, Boebbeling BN. Universal precautions training of preclinical students: impact on knowledge, attitudes, and compliance. Prev Med 1995b;24(9):580–585.

Dieter PM, Fasser CE. Physician assistants in geriatrics: meeting the demand. J Am Acad Physician Assist 1989;2(1):49–51.

Dobmeyer TW, Sondebegger BA, Lowin A. A report of a 1972 survey of physician assistant's training programs. Med Care 1975;13(4):294–307.

Donaldson M, Yordy K, Vanselow N (eds). Defining Primary Care: An Interim Report. Institute of Medicine: National Academy Press, Washington, DC, 1995.

Donovan P. Vermont physician assistants perform abortions, train residents. Fam Plann Perspect 1992;24(5):225.

Dubaybo BA, Samson MK, Carlson RW. The role of the physician assistant in critical care units. Chest 1991;99:89–91.

Dungy CI. The child health associate: the new image in the nursery. Am J Public Health 1975;65(11):1179–1183.

Duttera M, Harlan W. Evaluation of physician assistants in rural primary care. Arch Intern Med 1978;138:224–228.

Dychtwald K, Zitter M. Changes during the next decade will alter the way elder-care is provided, and financed. Mod Health 1988;18(16):38.

E

Eastaugh SR. Hospital nursing technical efficiency: nurse extenders and enhanced productivity. Hosp Health Serv Adm 1990;35:561–573.

Eastaugh SR. PEs: an efficient solution to primary care maldistribution. Hosp Prog 1981;62(2):32–35.

Ehrenberg R, Smith R. Modern Labor Economics. 3rd Ed. Scott Foresman, Glenview, IL, 1988.

Ekwo E, Daniels M, Oliver D, Fethke C. The physician assistant in rural primary care practices: physician assistant activities and physician supervision at satellite and non-satellite practice sites. Med Care 1979;17(8):787–795.

Elizondo E, Blessing JD. The ability of PAs to solve patient's phychosocial problems. A preliminary report on patient expectations. Physician Asst 1990;14(2):75–76,79–82.

Elliott CH. The physician assistant—newest member of the corporate health care team. Pers Adm 1984:87–92.

Ellis BI. Physician's assistants in radiology: has the time come? Radiology 1991;180(3):880–881.

Emelio J. Barriers to Physician Assistant Practice. Health Personnel in the United States: Ninth Report to Congress, Bureau of Health Professions, Health Resources and Services Administration, Department of Health and Human Services, 1994.

Engel GV. An evaluation of the continued viability of the occupation of the physician's assistant. J Med Educ 1981;56(8):659–662.

Erkert JD. Nurses' attitudes toward PAs. Phys Assist 1985;9(12):41–44.

Estes EH. Advantages and limitations of medical assistants. Geriatrics 1968a;16(10):1083–1087.

Estes EH. The Duke Physician's Assistant Program. Arch Environ Health 1968b;17:690–691.

Estes EH. In McClure WW. How much doctoring by those 'assistant doctors'? Med Econ 1968c;211–27.

Estes EH. Advantages and limitations of medical association. J Am Geriatr Soc 1968d;16:1083–1087.

Estes EH. The critical shortage—physicians and supporting personnel. 1968e;69(3):957–962.

Estes EH, Howard DR. The physician's assistant in the university center. Ann NY Acad Sci 1969;166(3):903–910.

Estes EH. The training of physician's assistants: a new challenge for medical education. Mod Med 1970a;39:90–93.

Estes EH, Howard DR. Potential for new classes of personnel: experiences of the Duke Physician's Assistant Program. J Med Educ 1970b;45(3):149–155.

Estes EH, Howard DR. Paramedical personnel in the distribution of health care. Arch Interm Med 1971;127:70–72.

Estes EH. Training doctors for the future: lessons from 25 years of physician assistant education. In Clawson DC, Osterweis M (eds): The Roles of the Physician Assistants and Nurse Practitioners in Primary Care. Association of Academic Health Centers, Washington, DC, 1993.

Evenhouse S, American Academy of Physician Assistants, oral testimony before the Physician Payment Review Commission, June 19, 1992. Cited in Physician Payment Review Commission, Annual Report to Congress. Chapter 4, Reforming graduate medical education, Washington, DC, 1993.

F

Faircloth KP, Barker HR, Hunt MA. Attitudes toward surgeon's assistants: a survey of health professionals in training and/or utilizing hospital. Ala J Med Sci 1976;13:124–132.

Fasser CE, Andrus P, Smith Q. Certification, registration and licensure of physician assistants. In Carter RD, Perry H (eds): Alternatives in Health Care Delivery: Emerging Roles for Physician Assistants. Warren H. Green, St Louis, MO, 1984.

Fasser CE. Educating Physician Assistants: The Past Ten Years. Phys Assist 1987;11:152–154.

Fasser CE. Historical Perspectives of PA Education. J Am Acad Physician Assist 1992a;5:663–670.

Fasser CE, Smith QW. Foreign medical graduates as physician assistants: solution or threat? J Am Acad Physician Assist 1992b;5(1):47–52.

Feldstein PJ. Health associations and the legislative process. In Litman TJ, Robins LS (eds): Health Politics and Policy. 2nd Ed. Delmar Publishers, Albany, NY, 1991.

Fenn PA. Acceptance of physician assistants in Western North Carolina. Phys Assist 1987;11(5):161–162.

Ferraro KF, Southerland T. Domains of medical practice: physicians' assessment of the role of physician extenders. J Health Soc Behav 1989; 30:192–205.

Fichandler B. Time to develop a social conscience. J Am Acad Physician Assist 1989;xxx:225–226.

Fincham JE. How pharmacists are rated as a source of drug information by physician assistants. Drug Intell Clin Pharm 1986;20(5):379–383.

Fine LL, Machotka P. Role identity development of the child health associate. J Med Edu 1973;48: 670–675.

Fine LL, Scriven S. The child health associate: a non-physician primary care practitioner for children. PA J 1977a;7(3):137–142.

Fine LL. Pediatrician receives more than a helping hand from child health associates. Commitment 1977b;3(1):14–18.

Finerfrock W. Federal programs that affect physician assistant education. J Am Acad Physician Assist 1989;2(3):210–211.

Finerfrock W. Payments for first-assisting at surgery. J Am Acad Physician Assist 1991;4(6):517–520.

Fischer I. Doctors' assistants and what they do in the Netherlands. World Health Forum 1995;15: 269–270.

Fisher DW, Horowitz SM. The physician's assistant: profile of a new health profession. In Bliss A, Cohen E (eds): The New Health Professionals: Nurse Practitioners and Physician's Assistants. Aspen System Corporation, Germantown, Md, 1977.

Fisher LA. I loved our new physician assistant—for 13 days. Med Econ 1995;72(1):75–77.

Ford AS. The Physician Assistant: A National and Local Analysis. Praeger Special Studies in US Economic, Social, and Political Issues. New York: Praeger, 1975.

Ford LC. Nurse practitioner education. In Hamburg J et al (eds): Review of Allied Health Education. The University Press of Kentucky, Lexington, 1979.

Foreman S, President, Montefiore Medical Center, Bronx, New York, oral testimony before the Physician Payment Review Commission, June 19, 1992. Cited in Physician Payment Review Commission, Annual Report to Congress, 1993. Chapter 4, Reforming graduate medical education.

Fottler MD. Physician attitudes toward physician extenders: a comparison of nurse practitioners and physician assistants. Med Care 1979;17(5): 536–549.

Fowkes VK, Hafferty FW, Goldberg HI, Garcia RD. Educational decentralization and deployment of physician's assistants. J Med Educ 1983;58(3): 194–200.

Fowkes VK, McKay D. A profile of California's physician assistants. (Correspondence). The West J Med 1990;153:328–329.

Fowkes VK, Cawley JF, Herlihy N, Cuadrado RR. Evaluating the potential of international medical graduates as physician assistants in primary care. Acad Med 1996;71(8):886–892.

Fox DP, Whittaker RG. PAs in the Veterans Administration: a report of a national survey. Phys Assist 1983;7(2):106–116.

Fox JG, Storms DM. New health professionals and older persons. J Community Health 1980;5(4):254–260.

Frampton J, Wall S. Exploring the use of NPs and PAs in primary care. HMO Practice 1994;8(4):165–170.

Frary T, Professional Practice Council of the AAPA. A new definition of "physician assistant." J Am Acad Physician Assist 1996;9(1):22–27.

Freeborn DK, Pope CR. Promise and Performance in Managed Care: The Prepaid Group Practice Model. The Johns Hopkins University Press. Baltimore, 1994.

Freeborn DK, Hooker RS. Satisfaction of physician assistants and other nonphysician providers in a managed care setting. Public Health Rep 1995;110(6):714–719.

Freedman MA, Jillson DA, Coffin RR, Novick LF. Comparison of complication rates in first trimester abortions performed by physician assistants and physicians. Am J Public Health 1986;76(5):550–554.

Freeman RW, Gollub RE, Wolski M, et al. Planning health services for a city jail: impact of contractural services on men's sick call. Med Care 1981;19(4):410–418.

Frick JE. Physician assistants as house officers: our experience. Phys Assist 1983;7:13–16.

Frick JE. The Urban Health Care Setting: The Harper-Grace Hospital Experience. In Zarbock S, Harbert K (eds): Physician Assistants: Their Present and Future Models of Utilization. Praeger Publishers, New York, NY, 1986.

Friedman MM. A physician's assistant in your ED? Emerg Med Serv 1978;68–70.

Fryer GE. The United States medical profession: an abnormal form of the division of labor. 1991;13:213–230.

Fulop T, Roemer MI. International Development of Health Manpower Policy. Offset Publication #61. World Health Organization, Geneva, 1982.

Fulop T, Roemer MI. Reviewing Health Manpower Development. Public Health Paper #83. World Health Organization, Geneva, 1987.

G

Gambert SR, Rosenkranz WE, Basu SN, et al. Role of the physician extender in the long-term care setting. Wisc Med J 1983;82(9):30–32.

Gara N. Physician assistants' participation in professional regulation. J Am Acad Physician Assist 1988;1(1):48–52.

Gara N. State laws for physician assistants. J Am Acad Physician Assist 1989;2:303–313.

Gara N, Coombs B. The national practitioner data bank: a registry for reporting disciplinary action. J Am Acad Physician Assist 1990;3(8):641–645.

Gara N. AMA adopts guidelines on PA practice. AAPA News 1995;16(7):1,4,20.

General Accounting Office. Health Care Access: Innovative Programs Using Nonphysicians. GAO/HRD-93-128. August 1993.

Genova NJ, Coburn AF, Agger M. The influence of market factors on physician assistant practice settings. Masters Dissertation. Edmund S. Muskie Institute of Public Affairs, University of Southern Maine, Portland, ME, 1995.

Gentile CA. Development of an Emergency Medical Physician's Assistant Program in North Carolina. Emerg Med Serv 1976;5(6):36, 37, 64.

Giardino A, Giardino E. Resident and nurse practitioners: responding to education and patient care needs. Am J Dis Child 1990;144(8):857; 144(9):953–954.

Gifford JF. The development of the physician assistant concept. In Carter RD, Perry HB (eds): Alternatives in Health Care Delivery: Emerging Roles for Physician Assistants. St Louis, Warren H. Green, 1984.

Gifford JF. The fate of America's prototype PA. Phys Assist 1987a;11(7):95–96.

Gifford JF. Prototype PA. North Carolina Med J 1987b;48(11):601–603.

Gittins P. Physician Assistants in plastic and reconstructive surgery. Newsline for Physician Assistants. 1996;5(9):4–7.

Glazer DL. National Commission on Certification of Physician's Assistants: a precedent in collaboration. In Bliss AA, Cohen ED (eds): The New Health Professionals: Nurse Practitioners and Physician's Assistants. Aspen Systems Corporation, Germantown, MD, 1977.

Glazer-Waldman H, Yturri-Byrd K, Hart JP. An assessment of the health beliefs and health behaviors of physician assistants. J Am Acad Physician Assist 1989;2(6):476–482.

Goldberg G, Jolly DM, Hosek S, Chu DS. Physician's extenders performance in air force clinics. Med Care 1981;19:951–965.

Goldberg H. Role of the PA in a prepaid medical care group. Phys Assist 1983;7(1):829–833.

Goldberg HI, Hafferty FW. The effect of decentralized education versus increased supply on practice location. Med Care 1984;22:760–769.

Golden AS, Hagan JL, Carlson D. The Art of Teaching Primary Care. Springer Publishers, New York, 1981.

Golden AS, Cawley JF. A national survey of performance objectives of physician assistant training programs. J Med Educ 1983;58:418–424.

Golden RM, Menchel SM. Physician assistants in forensic pathology. Phys Assist 1986;10(2):101–102.

Goldfrank L, Corso T, Squillacote D. The emergency services physician assistant: results of two years experience. Ann Emerg Med 1980;9(2):96–99.

Golladay FI, Miller M, Smith KR. Allied health manpower strategies: estimates of the potential gains from efficient task delegation. Med Care 1973;11:457–469.

Golladay FL, Smith K, Davenport E, et al. Policy planning for mid-level health workers: economic potentials and barriers to change. Inquiry 1976;13:80–89.

Gonzalez ML. Socioeconomic Characteristics of Medical Practice 1995. American Medical Association, Center for Health Policy Research, Chicago, IL, 1995.

Gould SH, Gould JS. The microsurgical assistant. J Reconstr Microsurg 1984;1(2):113–117.

Government Accounting Office, United States. Health Care Access: Innovative Programs Using Nonphysicians. Report to the Chairman, Special Committee on Aging, U.S. Senate. August 1993. GAO/HRD–93–128.

Grabenkort WR, Ransay JG. Role of physician assistants in critical care units. Chest 1991;99(1):89–91; comments 1992;101(1):293.

Gray J, Fryer GE. Physician assistants as members of social service child protection units. Child Abuse Negl 1991;15(4):415–421.

Gray J, Lacey C, Alexander S, Andresen M. Do PAs use the procedures and skills they learn? J Am Acad Physician Assist 1995;8(2):45–51.

Green BA, Johnson T. Replacing residents with midlevel practitioners: a New York City area analysis. Health Aff 1995;14(2):192–198.7.

Greenfield S, Komaroff AL, Pass TM, et al. Efficiency and cost of primary care by nurses and physician assistants. N Engl J Med 1978;298(6):305–309.

Greenlee R, Levy J, Allen A. Utilization of a physician assistant in a comprehensive community mental health center. PA J 1977;7(3):143–147.

Gunderson CH, Kampen D. Utilization of nurse clinicians and physician assistants by active members and fellows of the American Academy of Neurology. Neurology 1988;38(1):156–160.

H

Hafferty FW, Goldberg HI. Educational strategies for targeted retention of nonphysician health care providers. Health Serv Res 1986;21:107–125.

Hansen C. Access to Rural Health Care: Barriers to Practice for Nonphysician Providers. Bureau of Health Professions, Health Resources and Services Administration (HRSA–240–89–0037). Rockville, MD: DHHS, November, 1992.

Hansen JP, Stinson JA, Herpok FJ. Cost effectiveness of physician extenders as compared to family physicians in a university health clinic. J Am Coll Health Assoc 1980;28:211–214.

Harbert K. PAs and the coke oven industry. Newsl Maryland Acad Physician Assistants. 1978:6–8.

Harbert K. Past becomes future: portraits of PAs in Operation Desert Storm. Phys Assist 1991;15(9):30,33,34,36.

Harbert K, Shipman RA, Conrad W. The utilization of physician extenders: mid-level providers in a large group practice within tertiary health care setting. Med Group Manag J 1994;26,28,49, 50,52,54.

Harper DC, Johnson J. NONPF Workforce Project: Analysis of Nurse Practitioner Educational Programs, 1988–1995. National Organization of Nurse Practitioner Faculty, Washington, DC, 1996.

Harris CM, Evarts, CM. The relationship of physician assistants to an orthopedic residency program. Clin Orthop 1987;252:252–261.

Harty-Golder B. Physician extenders. J Florida Med Assn 1995;82(6):417–420.

Haug Associates, Inc. Attitudes Toward the Physician's Assistant Program Among the Public, Physicians, and Allied Health Professionals. Vol 1. Prepared for the Board of Medical Examiners, State of California, 1973.

Hayden RJ, Salley MA, Brasseur J, et al. Provider-assisted suicide: a survey of PA attitudes. Phys Assist 1995;19(6):73–78.

Hayes E. Is the midlevel provider imaging's friend or foe? Diagn Radiol 1996;2:33–36.

Health Security Act. Workforce Priorities Under Federal Payment. Title III; Subtitle A, Washington, DC, October, 1993.

Heinrich JJ, Fichandler BC, Beinfield MS, et al. The physician's assistant as resident on surgical service—an example of creative problem solving in surgical manpower. Arch Surg 1980;115:310–314.

Heller R. Officers de Santé: the second class doctors of nineteenth century France. Med Hist 1978, 22:25–43.

Henderson T, Chovan T. Removing Practice Barriers of Nonphysician Providers: Efforts by States to Improve Access to Primary Care. Intergovernmental Health Policy Project. The George Washington University, Washington, DC, 1994.

Henry RA. Evaluation of physician's assistants in Golchrist County, Florida. Public Health Rep 1974;89:429–432. (see also PA Journal 1973;3: 12–15).

Herrera J, Gendron BP, Rice MM. Military emergency medicine physician assistants. Mil Med 1994;159(3):241–242.

Hill IK. Responding to recertification (letter to the editor). Clin Rev 1996;6(7):18–19.

Hillman BJ, Fajaro LL, Hunter TB, et al. Mammogram interpretation by physician assistants. AJR 1987;149(5):907–912.

Hoffman C. Medicaid payment for nonphysician practitioners: an access issue. Health Aff 1994;13(4):140–152.

Holmes SE, Fasser CE. Occupational stress among physician assistants. J Am Acad Physician Assist 1993;6:173–178.

Hooker RS, Brown JB. Rheumatology referrals. HMO Pract 1985; 4(2):61–65.

Hooker RS. Medical care utilization. MD-PA/NP comparisons in an HMO. In Zarbock S, Harbert K (eds): Physician Assistants: Their Present and Future Models of Utilization. Praeger Publishers, New York, NY, 1986.

Hooker RS. A comparison of rank and pay structures for military physician assistants. J Am Acad Physician Assist 1989;2(4):293–300.

Hooker RS. The Coast Guard medical service. Navy Med 1991a;82(1)18–21.

Hooker RS. The military physician assistant. Mil Med 1991b;156(12):657–660.

Hooker RS, Freeborn DK. Use of physician assistants in a managed health care system. Public Health Rep 1991c;106(1):90–94.

Hooker RS. Employment specialization in the PA profession. J Am Acad Physician Assist 1992; 5(9):695–704.

Hooker RS. The roles of physician assistants and nurse practitioners in a managed care organization. In Clawson DK, Osterweis M (eds): The Roles of Physician Assistants and Nurse Practitioners in Primary Care. Association of Academic Health, Centers, Washington, DC, 1993.

Hooker RS, Jones PE. Research on the profession: Who is responsible? J Am Acad Physician Assist 1994a;7(9):664–669.

Hooker RS. PAs and NPs in HMOs. HMO Pract 1994b;8(4):148–150.

Hooker RS, Konrad TR, Gupta GC. Rural health training sites for physician assistants. J Am Acad Physician Assist (abstract from poster session) 1994c.

Hooker RS. Job satisfaction: physician assistants versus nurse practitioners (abstract from poster session). J Am Acad Physician Assist 1995a.

Hooker RS, Cawley JF. Staffing HMOs (letter). Health Aff, 1995b;14(3):282.

Hooker RS, McCaig LF. Emergency department uses of physician assistants and nurse practitioners: a national survey. Am J Emerg Med 1996a:14(3): 245–249.

Hooker RS, McCaig LF. Hospital outpatient department uses of physician assistants and nurse practitioners. (Poster Abstract) 24th Annual National Conference on Physician Assistants, New York, NY, 1996b.

Hospital Employee Health. NPs and PAs in the EHS: do they make better managers? Hosp Employee Health 1991;10(7):81–85.

Howard D. The physician's associate in occupational medicine. J Occup Med 1971;13(11):507–510.

Howard DR. The physician's assistant. J Kans Med Soc 1969;70(10):411–416.

Howard R. The physician's assistant and national regulations. Fed Bull 1972;59:90–106.

Hsiao WC. Transformation of health care in China. N Engl J Med 1974;286.

Hsu RC. Can China's health care be transplanted without China's economic policies? New Eng J Med., 1979;291:124–127.

Hudson CL. Expansion of medical professional services with nonprofessional personnel. JAMA 1961;176:839–841.

Hummel J, Cortte R, Ballweg RM, Larson E. Physician assistant training for Native Alaskan Community Health Aides: the MEDEX Northwest experience. Alaska Med. 1994a;36(4):183–188.

Hummel J, Prizada S. Estimating the cost of using non-physician providers in primary care teams in an HMO: where would the savings begin? HMO Pract 1994b;8(4):162–164.

Huntington CG, Ballweg RM, Trimbath J. The future of the PA profession. Phys Assist 1989;13(1):115, 119,120,123,124,126.

Huntington S, Warwick JS. Pharmacists attitudes toward PAs. Results of a Wisconsin study. Phys Assist 1987;11(9):108–114.

I

Inspector General, US Office of the. Enhancing the Utilization of Nonphysician Health Care Providers. Pub No. 0E1–01–90–02070, May 1993.

Institute of Medicine, National Academy of Sciences, Division of Health Manpower and Resources Development. A Manpower Policy for Primary Care. IOM Publication 78–02. May 1978.

Isiadinso O. Physician's assistant in geriatric medicine. New York State J Med 1979;79(7): 1069–1071.

J

Jacobs A, Johnson K, Breet P, Nelson E. Comparison of tasks and activities in physician-Medex practices. Public Health Rep 1974;89(4):339–344.

Jacobson PD, Parker LE, Coulter I. The role of NPs and PAs in organized settings. In Physician Payment Review Commission: Annual Report to Congress, Washington, DC, 1994.

Jarmul DB, Chavez RS. On ethics of PAs work … role in cavity searches within a correctional facility. J Am Acad Physician Assist 1991;4(7):602–1603.

Jarski RW. A research agenda for the physician assistant profession. Phys Assist 1988;12(3): 14,16,23.

Jarski RW. Ten good reasons for initiating your own clinical research project—and why more PAs don't. J Am Acad Physician Assist 1992;5(10): 719–721.

Jekel JF, Dunaye TM, Siker E, Rossetti M. The impact of nonphysician health directors on full-time public health coverage in Connecticut. Am J Public Health 1980;70(1):34.

Johnson R, Driggers DA, Huff CW. PA utilization in a family practice residency program. Physician Assist Health Pract 1983;7(1):68–70.

Johnson RE, Freeborn DK, McCally M. Delegation of office visits in primary care to PAs and NPs: the physicians' view. Phys Assist 1985;9(1):159–160, 165–169.

Johnson RE, Freeborn DK. Comparing HMO physicians' attitudes towards NPs and PAs. Nurse Pract 1986;11(1):39–49.

Johnson RE, Hooker RS, Freeborn DK. The future role of physician assistants in prepaid group practice health maintenance organizations. J Am Acad Physician Assist 1988;1(2):88–90.

Johnson TM. Physician's assistants, their physician employers, and the problem of autonomy: consensus or conflict? J Family Pract 1978;6(3): 621–625.

Joiner C, Harris A. Physician's assistants and rural health care: a study of physician's attitudes. J Med Assoc State Ala 1974;44(5):251–271.

Jones PE, Quimby LZ. A comparison of rural and non-rural family medicine PAs. J Am Acad Physician Assist 1993;6(6):407–411.

Jones PE, Cawley JF. Physician assistants and health system reform. JAMA 1994a;271:1266–1272.

Jones PE. A descriptive study of doctorally-prepared physician assistant (Abstract). American Academy of Physician Assistants National Conference, Nashville, TN,1994b.

Jones PE. Market forces and the shape of primary care to come. J Am Acad Physician Assist 1995;8(6):13–14,17.

Joyner SL, Easley D. Organ donation: who holds the key? Phys Assist 1984;8(11):109–110, 115–116, 119.

K

Kane R, Olsen D, Wilson W, et al. Adding a medex to the medical mix: an evaluation. J Med Care. 1976;14(12):996–1003.

Kane R, Solomon D, Beck J, et al. The future need for geriatric manpower in the United States. N Engl J Med 1980;302(24):1327–1332.

Kane RL, Gardiner J, Wright DD, et al. Differences in the outcomes of acute episodes of care provided by various types of family practitioners. J Family Pract 1978a;6:133–138.

Kane RL, Olson DM, Castle CH. Effects of adding a Medex in practice costs and productivity. J Community Health 1978b;3:216–226.

Kane RL, Garrard J, Buchanan JL, et al. Improving primary care in nursing homes. J Am Geriatr Soc 1991;39(4):359–367.

Kappes TJ. PA-C vs OPA-C (Letter to the Editor). J Am Acad Physician Assist 1992;5(1):70–71.

Katterjohn KR. Dermatologic physician assistants. J Am Acad Dermatol 1982;6(5):950–951.

Katz HP. An innovative physician assistant laceration management program. HMO Pract 1994;8(4):187–190.

Keith C, Milgrom P. Auxillary utilization in dentistry: possibilities for a dental associate. PA J 1974;4(2):14–20.

Kenyon VA. Feldshers and health promotion in the USSR. Phys Assist 1985;9:25–29.

Kierman B, Rosenbaum HD. The impact of a physician assistant in diagnostic radiology [PA-DR] on the delivery of diagnostic radiological clinical services. Invest Radiol 1977;12(1):7–14.

Kletke PR, Marder WD, Silberger AB. The Demographics of Physician Supply: Trends and Projections. AMA Center for Health Policy Research, Chicago, IL, 1987.

Knaus WA. Inside Russian Medicine: An American Doctor's First Hand Report. Everst House, New York, NY, 1981.

Knickman JR, Lipkin M, Finkler SA, et al. The potential for using nonphysicians to compensate for the reduced availability of residents. Acad Med 1992;67(7):429–438.

Kohlhepp W, Fichandler BC, Stasiulewicz C, et al. Connecticut physician assistants: update. Connect Med 1984;48:657–660.

Kole LA. A new incarnation. J Am Acad Physician Assist 1988;1(1):1–2.

Kole LA. Speculating on the specialization of PAs. J Am Acad Physician Assist 1991;4(6):542–543.

Kraak W. Institutional elderly—more than a success in geriatrics. Physician Assist Health Pract 1979;3(10):70–72.

Krasner M, Ramsay D, Weary D, Johnson M. New health practitioners and dermatology manpower planning. Arch Dermatol 1977;113:1280–1282.

Kress LM. Let's look at the PA, a new member of the health team. Quarterly Rev 1971;39(1).

Kristof ND. Chinese grow healthier from cradle to grave. New York Times, April 14, 1991.

L

Labus JB, The Physician Assistant Medical Handbook, W.B. Saunders, Philadelphia, PA, 1995.

Lairson P, Record JC, James JC. Physician assistants at Kaiser: distinctive patterns of practice. Inquiry 1974;11:207–219.

Lapius SK. Physicians and midlevel practitioners: can the conflict be resolved? Postgrad Med 1983;73(3):94–95.

Larson EH, Hart LG, Hummel J. Rural physician assistants: results from a survey of graduates of MEDEX Northwest. Public Health Rep 1994a;109(2):266–274.

Larson PF, Osterweis M (eds): The Roles of Physician Assistants and Nurse Practitioners in Primary

Care. Association of Academic Health Centers, Washington, DC, 1994b.

Lary MJ. A Critical Analysis of Variables that Predict Success in the Physician Assistant Program of Study and on the National Commission on Certification of Physician Assistants Examination. PhD Dissertation, College of Education, Kansas State University, Manhattan, KS, 1991.

Laur WE, Posey RE, Waller JD. The dermatologic physician's assistant: an overview of one year's experience. J Am Acad Dermatol 1981;5(3):367–372.

Lawrence DM. The impact of physician assistants and nurse practitioners on health care access, costs, and quality: a review of the literature. Health Med Care Serv Rev 1974;1:1–12.

Lawrence DM. Two training programs. MEDEX: The education-development interface. J Med Educ 1975a;50(12 pt 2):85–92.

Lawrence DM, Wilson W, Castle C. Employment of Medex graduates and trainees: five-year progress report for the United States. JAMA 1975b;234(2):174–177.

Lawrence DM. Physician assistants and nurse practitioners: their impact on health care access, costs, and quality. Health Med Care Serv Rev 1978;1(2):3–12.

Legler CF. A survey of physician attitudes toward the PA. Phys Assist 1983;7(5):98–113.

Leiken AM. Factors affecting the distribution of physician assistants in New York state: policy implications. J Public Health Policy 1985;9:236–243.

Li LB, Williams SD, Scammon DL. Practicing with the urban underserved: a qualitative analysis of motivations, incentives, and disincentives. Arch Family Med 1995;4:124–133.

Lichter PR. Confusing licensure with education: medicine's slippery slope. Fed Bull 1995;82(1):16–20.

Lieberman DA, Ghormley JM. Physician assistants in gastroenterology: should they perform endoscopy? Am J Gastroenterol 1992;87(8):940–943.

Lindahl J. PA or OPA: what are the differences? PA Careers 1994;2(2):8.

Litman TJ. Public perceptions of the physicians' assistant: a survey of the attitudes and opinions of rural Iowa and Minnesota residents. Am J Public Health 1972;62(3):343–346.

Lohrenz F, Payne R, Intress R, et al. Placement of primary care physician assistants in small rural communities. Wisc Med J 1976;75:320–328.

Lombardo P, James DN. Ethical problems: cases and commentaries—ethical and legal dilemmas of mid-level practitioners. J Prison Jail Health 1982;2(2):116–124.

Lott RJ. The campaign for commissioning continues. J Am Acad Physician Assist 1989;2(4):245–246.

Lowe D. The training and use of physician's assistants in industry. Med Today 1971;5(2):77–81.

Lurie N, Rank B, Parenti C, et al. How do house officers spend their nights? A time study of internal medicine house staff on call. N Engl J Med 1989;320(25):429–438.

Lynch J. Allied health personnel in occupational medicine: report of the long range planning committee. J Occup Med 1971;13(5):232–237.

M

Machotka P, Ott JE, Moon JB, Silver HK. Competence of child health associates: comparison of their basic science and clinical knowledge with that of medical students and pediatric residents. PA J 1973;3(4):36–41.

Machotka P, Ott JE, Moore V, et al. Predictors of clinical performance of child health associates. J Allied Health 1975;4:25–31.

Mainous AG, Bertolino JG, Harrell PL. Physician extenders: who is using them? Fam Med 1992;24(3):201–204.

Mastrangelo R. The name game. Advance PA 1993;1(3):13.

Mastrangelo R. Reimbursement for PA services: a stubborn issue. Advance PA. 1994;2(2):17–18.

Mathew MS, Stevens R. Medical evaluation of CMHC patients by a physician's assistant. Hosp Community Psychiatry. 1982;33(3):224–225.

Mathews WA, Yohe CD. PAs in psychiatry: filling the gap. Physician Assist 1984;8(6):26,28.

Mauney F, Keller C, King L. The physician's assistant to the cardiovascular and thoracic surgeon. PA J 1972;2:148–151.

Maxfield R. Use of physician's assistants in general surgical practice. Am J Surg 1976;131:504–508.

Maxfield RG, Lemire DR, Wansleben TO. Utilization of supervised physician's assistants in emergency room coverage in a small rural community hospital. J Trauma 1975;15(9):795–799.

May FL. It's a fact: PAs and NPs help ensure cost-conscious quality. Provider 1988;14(4):42.

Mayer RP, Solomon RJ, Trimbath J, Rohrs R. Physician assistants as administrators. Opportunities in management. Physician Assist 1988;87–97.

Mayer T, Mayer GG. HMOs: origins and development. N Engl J Med 1985;312:593–598.

Mayes JR. On the pulse. J Am Acad Physician Assist 1988;6(1):414–415.

McCally M. The PA profession and the need for research. Physician Assist 1983;7(10):7–8.

McCibbin R. Cost effectiveness of physician assistants: a review of recent evidence. PA J 1978;8:110–115.

McCowan TC, Goertzen TC, Lieberman RP, et al. Physician's assistants in vascular and interventional radiology. Radiology 1991;180(3):880–881; 1992;184(2):582.

McGill F, Kliener GJ, Vanderbilt C, et al. Postgraduate internship in gynecology and obstetrics for physician assistants: a 4-year experience. Obstet Gynecol 1990;76:1135–1139.

McKelvey PA, Oliver DA, Conboy JE. PA roles in a tertiary medical center. Physician Assist 1986;10:149–159.

Mechanic D. Politics, Medicine, and Social Science. Wiley, New York, 1974.

Medical Group Management Association. Physician Compensation and Production Survey: 1995 Report Based on 1994 Data. Englewood, Colorado, 1995.

Medical World News. PAs branch out into insurance exams on their own. Med World News 1973; 14(30):17–19.

Meikle TH. An Expanded Role for the Physician Assistant. Bellwether. Association of Academic Health Centers, Washington, DC, 1992a.

Meikle TH. President' Statement. Report of the Josiah Macy, Jr. Foundation. Josiah Macy, Jr. Foundation, New York, NY, 1992b.

Mendenhall RC, Repicky P, Neville R. Assessing the utilization and productivity of nurse practitioners and physician's assistants: methodology and findings on productivity. Med Care 1980;18(6): 609–623.

Meyers HC. The Physician's Assistant: A Baccalaureate Curriculum. Alderson-Broaddus College, Philippi, WV, 1978.

Miles DL, Rushing WA. A study of physician's assistants in rural setting. Med Care 1976;14(2): 987–995.

Miller DC. Handbook of Research Design and Social Measurement. 15th Ed. Sage Publication, Newbury Park, CA, 1991;327–429.

Miller JI, Hatcher CR. The physician's assistant in thoracic and cardiovascular surgery in the community hospital. Am Surg 1978a;44:162–164.

Miller JI, Hatcher CR. Physicians assistants on a university cardiothoracic surgical service: a five-year update. J Thorac Cardiovasc Surg 1978b; 76:639–642.

Miller RN. The status of home care training for physician assistants. Caring 1994;13(9):18–19.

Mittman D, Mirotznik J. PA prescribing behavior and attitudes: a profile. Physician Assist 1984;8(3):15, 16,21–24.

Mittman DE, Rodino FJ, Yackeren TF. How sales reps assess the role of the physician assistant. Med Marketing Media 1993;56–62.

Mittman DE. Name recognition. Clin Rev 1995;5(5): 23–24.

Mondy LW, Lutz DB, Heartwell SF, Zetzman MR. Physician extender services in family planning agencies: issues in Medicaid reimbursement. J Public Health Policy 1986;7(2):183–189.

Morgan PP, Cohen L. Should nurse practitioners play a larger role in Canada's health care system? Can Med Assoc J 1992;146:1020–1025.

Morgan WA. Using state board of nursing data to estimate the number of nurse practitioners in the United States. Nurse Pract 1993;18(2): 65–74.

Morian JP Jr. The PA's role in medical research: implications for PA education. Physician Assist 1986;10(3):141–2,146,161.

Morreale J, Chitradon R. A Cost Analysis of the Use of Physician's Assistants Providing Primary Medical Care in a Psychiatric Setting. Western Psychiatric Institute and Clinic and University Center for Urban Research. Project No 1 MB 44170. University of Pittsburgh, Pittsburgh, PA, 1977.

Morris CR, Dean JR. Hospitals provide rules for assistants privileges. JAMA 1975;49:56–57.

Morris SB, Smith DB. The distribution of physician extenders. Med Care 1977;15:1045–1057.

Moses EB. Selected Facts About Nurse Practitioners and Nurse Mid-Wives. Division of Nursing, Bureau of Health Professions, Health Resources and Services Administration, October, 1993.

Mullan F. Missing: a national medical manpower policy. Milbank Qu 1992;70:381–386.

Muus KJ, Geller JM, Ludtke RL, et al. Comparing urban and rural primary care PAs. J Am Acad Physician Assist 1996;9(8):49–60.

N

Nakatani H. Health manpower planning and redistribution of resources: the experience of Japan. World Health Stat Qu 1987;40:326–334.

National Association of Rural Health Clinics. Rural Health Clinics First National Survey, 1994 Summary Report, Washington, DC, 1994.

National Center for Health Services Research. Nurse Practitioner and Physician Assistant Training and Deployment. U.S. Dept Health, Education, and Welfare, Public Health Service, Health Resource Administration, National Center for Health Services Research. DHEW Publication No. (HRA) 77–3173, 1977.

National Commission on Certification of Physician Assistants, Inc. Content Outline. NCCPA, Atlanta, GA, 1995.

National Health Services Corps. Proposed Strategies for Fulfilling Primary Care Professional Needs: Part II: Nurse Practitioners, Physician Assistants, and Certified Nurse Midwives. A policy paper (white paper) prepared for the National Advisory Council, National Health Service Corps, US Public Health Service. Rockville, MD, 1991.

Nelson EC, Jacobs AR, Johnson K. Patients' acceptance of physician's assistants. JAMA 1974a; 228(1):63–67.

Nelson EC, Jacobs AR, Cordner K, Johnson KG. Financial impact of physician assistants on medical practices. N Engl J Med 1974b;293:527–531.

Nelson EC, Jacobs AR, Breer PE, Johnson KG. Impact of physician assistants on patients' visits in ambulatory practices. Ann Intern Med 1975;82:608–612.

Nelson EC, Johnson KG, Jacobs AR. Impact of MEDEX on physician activities: redistribution of time after incorporating a MEDEX into the practice. J Fam Pract 1977;5:607–612.

Nelson LB. New Jersey physician assistant graduates are successful practitioners. J Med Soc NJ 1982;79(11):829–833.

New York State Council on Graduate Medical Education. Fourth Annual Report 1991. New York, 1992.

Nichols LM. Estimating costs of underusing advanced practice nurses. Nurs Econ 1992;10:343–351.

O

Office of Inspector General, Department of Health and Human Services. Enhancing the Utilization of Nonphysician Health Care Providers. May 1993. OEI–01–90–02070

Office of Technology Assessment, U.S. Congress. Nurse Practitioners, Physician Assistants, and Certified Nurse Midwives: A Policy Analysis. Case Study #37, OTA–HCS–37, Government Printing Office, December, Washington, DC, December 1986.

Office of Technology Assessment, U.S. Congress. Health Care in Rural America. (OTA–H–434). Government Printing Office, Washington, DC, 1990.

O'Hara D. Vermont clinic trains physician's assistants to do abortions. Am Med News 1989;32(46)4–5.

O'Hearn CJ. Physician assistants' role in combat medicine. Postgrad Med 1991;89(5):15,16,19; 90(3):48.

Oliver D, Lauber D, Gerstbrein J, Wombacher N. Distribution of primary care physician assistants in the state of Iowa. J Iowa Med Soc 1977;67: 320–325.

Oliver DR, Carter RD, Conboy JE. Medical practice revenue and salaries of physician assistants. Phy Assist 1985;9(5):138,143–4, 149.

Oliver DR, Conboy JE, Donahuye WJ, et al. Patient's satisfaction with physician assistant services. Phys Assist 1986;10(7):51–60.

Oliver DR. Ninth Annual Report on Physician Assistant Educational Programs in the United States, 1992–1993. Association of Physician Assistant Programs, Alexandria, VA, 1993a.

Oliver DR. Physician assistant education: a review of program characteristics by sponsoring institutions. In: Clawson DC, Osterweis M (eds): The

Roles of Physician Assistants and Nurse Practitioners in Primary Care. Association of Academic Health Centers, Washington, DC, 1993b.

Olson JH. Geriatric medicine: a new horizon for the physician's assistant. J Am Geriatr Soc 1983; 31(4):236–237.

O'Rourke RA. The specialized physician assistant: an alternative to the clinical cardiology trainee. Am J Cardiol 1987;60(10):901–902.

Ortiz L. The role of PAs in Alaskan Air Command. Air Force Medical Service Digest 1979;6–7.

Orubuloye IO, Oyeneye OY. Primary care in developing countries: the case of Nigeria, Sri Lanka, and Tanzania. Social Sci Med 1982;16:675–686.

Ostergard D, Gunning J, Marshall J. Training and function of a women's health-care specialist, a physician's assistant, or nurse practitioner in obstetrics and gynecology. Am J Obstet Gynecol 1975;121(8):1029–1037.

Ott JE. A Demonstration Project on the Education and Utilization of Child Health Associates and Their Impact on Medical Practice, Executive Summary. Division of Medicine, CT #231–75–0006, 1979.

Ouslander JG. Medical care in the nursing home. JAMA 1989;262(18):2582–2590; comments in: 1990;263(22):3023–4.

P

Page RR. The Military Physician's Assistant 1975. DoD Health Studies Task Force, Office of the Assistant Secretary of Defense (Health and Environment), Study File 7.4.5 DASD (HA).

Palmer PN. Latest expansion of physician assistant's scope of practice raises questions (editorial). AORN J 1990;51:671–672.

Pantell RH, Reilly T, Liang MH. Analysis of the reasons for the high turnover of clinicians in neighborhood health centers. Public Health Rep 1980;95(4):344–350.

Parker H, McCoy J, Conner R. Delegation of tasks in radiology to allied health personnel. Radiology 1972;103(2):257–261.

Parnes AZ, Greene MG, Friedmann E. Investigating the earnings gap between male and female PAs. J Am Acad Physician Assist 1990;3(4):295–296.

Patterson PK, Bergman AB, Wedgwood RJ. Parent reaction to the concept of pediatric assistants. Pediatrics 1969;44:69–75.

Pelligrino ED. Prescribing and drug ingestion symbols and substances. Drug Intelligence and Clinical Pharmacy. Nov 1976;624–630.

Pereira C, Bugalho A, Bergstrom S, et al. A comparative study of caesarean deliveries by assistant medical officers and obstetricians in Mozambique. Br J Obstet Gynecol 1996;103:508–512.

Perry HB. Physician Assistants: An Empirical Analysis of Their General Characteristics, Job Performance, and Job Satisfaction. NTIS, PB-263 021/8, 1976.

Perry HB. A comparison of military and civilian physician assistants. Mil Med 1978a;Nov(11): 763–767.

Perry HB. The job satisfaction of physician assistants: a causal analysis. Soc Sci Med 1978b; 12:377–385.

Perry HB. An analysis of the effects of personal background and work setting variables upon selected job characteristics of physician assistants. J Community Health 1980;S,5(4):228–243.

Perry HB, Breitner B. Physician Assistants: Their Contributions to Health Care. Human Sciences Press, New York, NY, 1982.

Perry HB, Detmer DE, Redmond EL. The current and future role of surgical physician assistants: report of a national survey of surgical chairmen in large U.S. hospitals. Ann Surg 1983;193:132.

Perry HB, Redmond EL. Career trends and attrition among PAs. Physician Assist 1984;8(6):121–128.

Perry HB. Role satisfaction: an important and neglected subject. J Am Acad Physician Assist 1989;2(6):427–428.

Peterson M. The Institute of Medicine Report. A manpower policy for primary health care: a commentary from the American College of Physicians. Ann Intern Med 1980;92:843–851.

Pew Health Professions Commission. Health Professions Education in the Future: Schools in Service to the Nation. Pew Commission, San Francisco, CA, 1993.

Pew Health Professions Commission. Critical Challenges: Revitalizing the Health Professions for the Twenty-First Century. The Third Report of

The Pew Health Professions Commission, Center for the Health Professions, University of California, San Francisco, CA, 1995.

Pharris JL. Conceptualizing the role of the physician assistant. Physician Assist 1984;8(4):15,16,19.

Physician Payment Review Commission, Annual Report to Congress, 1993. Chapter 16. Medicaid payment policies for nonphysician providers. 1993a;305–321.

Physician Payment Review Commission, Annual Report to Congress, 1993. Chapter 4. Reforming graduate medical education. 1993b;55–85.

Physician Payment Review Commission. Nonphysician Practitioners. Report to Congress, 1994.

Pinckney DS. U.S. hospitals still short of allied health personnel. Am Medical News May 18, 1992, p. 4.

Pohutsky LC. The Origin and Development of Physician's Assistant Programs in the United States (1960–79). Doctoral Dissertation, Teachers College, Columbia University, New York, NY, 1982.

Pondy LR, Jones JM, Braun JA. Utilization and productivity of the Duke Physician's Associate. Socio-Economic Planning Sciences. 1973;7:327–352 (see also w 1974:4).

Poppen CF. Physician assistants in otorhinolaryngology—head and neck surgery. Newsl Physician Assistants 1996;5(9):8.

Power L, Bakker DL, Cooper MI. Diabetes Outpatient Care Through Physician Assistants—A Model for Health Maintenance Organizations. Thomas Publishing, Springfield, IL, 1973.

Price D. PAs in the Persian Gulf. J Am Acad Physician Assist 1991;4(4):19A–22A.

Price D. PAs in rural practice. J Am Acad Physician Assist 1993;6:423–427.

R

Rabin DL, Spector KK. Delegation potential of primary care visits by physician assistants, Medex and Primex. Med Care. 1980;15:1114–1125.

Rada-Sidinger P, Conner P. PAs as primary care providers for poor and underserved children. J Am Acad Physician Assist 1992;5(10):784–789.

Ramos M. Occupational medicine. An overview for physician assistants. Physician Assist 1989;13(2):79–86.

Record JC. PAs in research: levels of involvement and responsibility. Physician Assist J 1976;6(3):138–140.

Record JC. Cost Effectiveness of Physician Assistants in a Maximum-Substitution Model: Phase II of a Two-Phase Study. DHEW Publication No. HRA 78-1, Contract No. 231-76-0601, 1978.

Record JC, McCally M, Schweitzer SO, et al. New health professionals after a decade and a half: delegation, productivity, and costs in primary care. J Health Polit Policy Law 1980;5(3):470–497.

Record JC. Staffing Primary Care in 1990: Physician Replacement and Cost Savings. Springer, New York, NY, 1981a.

Record JC. The productivity of new health practitioners. In Record JC. Staffing Primary Care in 1990: Physician Replacement and Cost Savings. Springer, New York, NY, 1981b.

Regan DM, Harbert K. Measuring the financial productivity of physician assistants. Med Group Manage J 1991;38(6):50–52.

Reinhardt UE. A production function for physician services. Rev Econ Stat 1972;54:55–66.

Reinhardt UE. The economic and moral case for letting the market determine the health workforce. In Osterweis M, McLaughlin CJ, Manasse HR, et al (eds): The U.S. Health Workforce: Power, Politics, and Policy. The Association of Academic Health Centers. Washington, DC, 1996.

Repicky PA, Mendenhall RC, Neville RE. The professional role of physician's assistants in adult ambulatory care practices. Eval Health Prof 1982;5(3):283–301.

Richmond H. Health care delivery in Cummins Engine Company. Arch Environ Health 1974;29:348–350.

Riess J, Lawrence D. New Practitioners in Remote Practices: Summary of a Study of Training, Utilization, Financing and Provider Satisfaction. Final report for contract No. 1-MB-44168 (Washington, DC: Division of Medicine, Bureau of Health Manpower, Department of Health, Education, and Welfare, 1976).

Riportella-Muller R, Libby D, Kindig D. The substitution of physician assistants and nurse practitioners for physician residents in teaching hospitals. Health Aff 1995;14(2):181–191.

Rivo ML, Kindig DA. A report card on the physician work force in the United States. N Engl J Med 1996;334:892–895.

Rivo ML, Jones PE, Hooker RS, Cawley JF, Rohrs RC. Physician Assistant preparation for primary care practice. 1997 (submitted for publication).

Roback G, Randolph L, Seidman B. Physician Characteristics and Distribution in the U.S.: 1993 Edition. American Medical Association, Chicago, 1993.

Robyn D, Hadley J. National health insurance and the new health occupations: nurse practitioners and physicians' assistants. J Health Polit Policy Law 1980;5(3):447–468.

Roemer MI. Primary care and physician extenders in affluent countries. Int J Health Serv 1977;7: 545–555.

Rohrs R. Where have all the PAs gone? Physician Assist 1988;12:192.

Rom W. Medicine re-enters the workplace—a new era in occupational medicine? (Sounding Board). N Engl J Med 1979;300(12):672–673.

Romeis JC, Schey HM, Marion GS, Keith JF. Extending the extenders. Compromise for the geriatric specialization—manpower debate. J Am Geriatr Soc 1985;33(8):559–565.

Romm J, Berkowitz A, Cohen MA, et al. The physician assistant reimbursement experiment J Ambulatory Care Manage 1979;2:1–12.

Roosevelt J, Frankl H. Colorectal cancer screening by nurse practitioners using 60 cm flexible fiberoptic sigmoidoscope. Dig Dis Sci 1984;29:161–163.

Rosen R. The Montefiore Medical Center experience. In Zarbock S, Harbert K (eds) Physician Assistants: Their Present and Future Models of Utilization. Praeger, New York, NY, 1986.

Rothwell W. PAs in cardiovascular surgery. J Am Acad Physician Assist 1993;6(2):150–157.

Rousselot LM, Beard SE, Berrey BH. The evolution of the physician's assistant: brownian movement or coordinated progress. Bull NY Acad Med 1971;47:1473–1500.

Rubin L. Physician assistants and their prescribing practices. Med Marketing Media 1977;12(4): 50–56.

S

Sadler AM, Sadler BL, Bliss AA. The Physician's Assistant: Today and Tomorrow. Yale University Press, New Haven, 1972.

Sadler-Sparks KJ, Stein WA. The pros and cons of endorsing the baccalaureate degree as the minimum degree for PAs. J Am Acad Physician Assist 1988;1(3):177–181.

Safriet B. Health care dollars and regulatory sense: the role of advanced practice nursing. Yale J Regulation 1992;419–486.

Safriet BJ. Health care dollars and regulatory sense: the role of advanced practice nursing. Yale J Regulation 1992;9:417–488.

Salcido R, Fisher SB, Reinstein L, Willis JB. Underutilization of physician assistants in physical medicine and rehabilitation. Arch Phys Med Rehabil 1993;74:826–829.

Salmon MA, Stein J. Distribution of nurse practitioners and physician assistants: are they meeting the need for primary care? N C Med J 1986; 47(3):147–148.

Salmon ME, Culbertson RA. Health manpower oversupply: implications for physicians, nurse practitioners and physician assistants—a model. Hosp Health Serv Admin 1985;30(1):100–115.

Samsot M, Heinlein M. Orthopaedic PA duties: extensive and on the increase. Newsline for PAs 1996;5(4):4–7.

Samuels ME, Shi L. Report of The Survey of Community and Migrant Health Centers Regarding Utilization of Nurse Practitioners, Physician Assistants, and Certified Nurse Midwives. Bureau of Health Professions, Health Resources and Services Administration, Rockville, MD, 1992.

Schafft GE, Cawley JF. The Physician Assistant in a Changing Health Care Environment. Aspen Publishers, Rockville, MD, 1987a.

Schafft GE, Rolling B. Physician Assistants Providing Geriatric Care: Models and Case Studies. U.S. Department of Health and Human Services, Public Health Service, Health Resources and Services Administration. HRP-0907025. 1987b.

Schappert SM. National Ambulatory Medical Care Survey: 1994 summary. Advance data from vital and health statistics; no 273. National Center for Health Statistics, Hyattsville, MD, 1996.

Scheffler RM. The employment utilization, and earnings of physician extenders. Soc Sci Med 1977; 11:785–791.

Scheffler RM. The productivity of new health professionals: physician assistants and Medex. Res Health Econ 1979;1:37–56.

Scheffler RM, Yoder SG, Weisfeld N, Ruby G. Physicians and new health practitioners: issues for the 1980s. Inquiry 1980;16:195–220.

Scheffler RM, Waitzman NJ, Hillman JM. The productivity of physician assistants and nurse practitioners and health work force policy in the era of managed health care. J Allied Health 1996;25(3):207–217.

Schmittou E. Cadaver kidney procurement: a unique role for a physician assistant. Physician Assist J 1977;7(1):23–28.

Schneider DP, Foley WJ. A systems analysis of the impact of physician extenders on medical cost and manpower requirements. Med Care 1977;15(4):277–297.

Schneider J. Manpower problems in obstetrics and gynecology: statistics and possible solutions. Clin Obstet Gynecol 1972;15(2):293–304.

Schneller ES. The Physician's Assistant: Innovation in the Medical Division of Labor. Lexington Books, Lexington, MA, 1978.

Schneller ES. A PA by any other name—J Am Acad Physician Assist 1994;7(10):689–692.

Schroeder SA. Must America look to non-doctors for primary care? Med Econ 1992;69(24):82–93.

Schroy PC, Wiggins T, Winawer SJ, et al. Video endoscopy by nurse practitioners: a model for colorectal cancer screening. Gastrointest Endosc 1988;34:390–394.

Sekscenski ES, Sansom S, Bazell C, et al. State practice environments and the supply of physician assistants, nurse practitioners, and certified nurse midwives. N Engl J Med 1994;331(19):1266–1271.

Sells CJ, Herdener RS. MEDEX: a time-motion study. Pediatrics 1975;56(2):255–261.

Shapero GH. Women in the PA profession. J Am Acad Physician Assist 1992;5(4):229–230.

Shelton SR, Lyons BA, Allen RM, Allensworth DC. A Delphi study to identify future roles for physician assistants. J Med Educ 1984;59(12):962–963.

Shi L, Samuels ME, Konrad TR, et al. The determinants of utilization of nonphysician providers in rural community and migrant health centers. J Rural Health 1993;9:27–39.

Shi L, Samuels ME, Ricketts TC, Konrad TR. A rural-urban comparative study of nonphysician providers in community and migrant health centers. Public Health Rep 1994;109(6):809–815.

Shortell SM. The future of hospitals and health care management. Forum 1995;1(1):1–2.

Sibley JC, Sackett DL, Neufeld V. A randomized trial of continuing medical education. New Engl J Med 1982;306:511–515.

Sidel VW. Feldshers and `Feldsherism': the role and training of Feldshers in the USSR. N Engl J Med 1968:934–940.

Silver HK. The Syniatrist. JAMA 1971a;217(10): 1368–1370.

Silver HK. New allied health professionals: implications of the Colorado Child Health Associate law. N Engl J Med 1971b;284(6):304–307.

Silver HK, Ott JE. The child health associate: a new professional to provide comprehensive health care to children. Physician Assist J 1973;3(2): 21–26.

Silver HK, McAtee PA. On the use of nonphysician "associate residents" in overcrowded specialty training programs. N Engl J Med. 1984;311(5): 326–328.

Silver HK, McAtee PA. Should nurses substitute for house staff? Am J Nurs 1988;88(12):1671–1673.

Simon A, Link M, Miko A. Twelfth Annual Report on Physician Assistant Educational Programs in the United States, 1995–96. Association of Physician Assistant Programs, Alexandria, VA, 1996a.

Simon CJ, Born PH. Physician earnings in a changing managed care environment. Health Aff 1996b;15(3):124–133.

Singer A, Hooker RS. Determinants of specialty choice of physician assistants. Acad Med 1996;71(8):917–919.

Skinner AL. Parental acceptance of delegated pediatric services. Pediatrics 1968;41:1003–1004.

Smith CW. Patient attitudes toward physicians' assistants. J Family Pract 1981;13(2):201–204.

Smith JL. Physicians' assistants doing endoscopy? (Editorial). Am J Gastroenterol 1992;87(8): 937–938.

Smith KR. Health Practitioners: Efficient Utilization and the Cost of Health Care. Madison: Department of Economics, University of Wisconsin, Madison, WI, 1973.

Smith MC. The Relationship Between Pharmacy and Medicine. In Mapes R (ed): Prescribing Practices and Drug Usage. Croom Helm Ltd., London, 1980.

Smith MO. Correctional medicine: An outstanding setting for the PA. Physician Assist 1996;20(7): 103–110.

Smith RA. MEDEX: A demonstration program in primary medical care. Northwest Med 1969;68: 1023–1030.

Smith RA, Bassett GR, Markarian CA, et al. A strategy for health manpower: reflections on an experience called Medex. JAMA 1971;217(1): 1362–1367.

Smith RA. MEDEX—an operational and replicated manpower training program: increasing the delivery of health services (editorial). Am J Public Health 1972;62(12):1563–1565.

Smith RA (ed). Manpower and Primary Health Care: Guidelines for Improving/Expanding Health Service Coverage in Developing Countries. The University Press of Hawaii, Honolulu, HI, 1978.

Sonntag VKH, Steiner S, Stein BM. Neurosurgery and the physician assistant. Surg Neurol 1977;8:207–208.

Sorem KR, Portnoi VA. Decreased rates of polypharmacy, hospitalization and mortality through geriatric medical team involvement in a nursing home. Association of Physician Assistant Programs, Proceedings Eleventh Annual Physician Assistant Conference. St. Louis AAPA, Alexandria, VA, 1983;65–70.

Sowell T. Knowledge and Decisions. Basic Books, New York, 1980; 246–268.

Sox HC Jr, Sox CH, Tompkins RK. The training of physician's assistants. New Engl J Med 1973;288(16):818–824.

Sox HC Jr. Quality of patient care by nurse practitioners and physician assistants: a ten year perspective. Ann Intern Med 1979;91:459–472.

Spitzer WO. The nurse practitioner revisited: slow death of a good idea. New Engl J Med 1984;310:1049–1051.

Srba L. Nurse Practitioners and Physician Assistants in Substance Abuse Programs. DHHS publication no. (ADM) 81-884. US Department of Health and Human Services, Public Health Service, Alcohol, Drug Abuse, and Mental Health Administration, Rockville, MD, 1981. 17 pp. GPO Item No. 467-A-1.

Stalker T. The explosive IOM primary care report. Health Pract Physician Assist 1978a;2(9):25–34.

Stalker T. PAs—making prison health care better. Health Pract 1978b;2(1):16–18.

Stanhope WD. The roots of the AAPA. J Am Acad Physician Assist 1992;5(9):671–678.

Starfield B. Primary Care: Concept, Evaluation, and Policy. Oxford University Press, New York, 1992.

Stark R, Mann R, DeJoseph JF, Emery M. The women's health care training project–an alternative for training midwives. J Nurse-Midwifery 1984;29(3):191–196.

Starr P. The Social Transformation of American Medicine. Basic Books, New York, 1982.

Stead EA. Conserving costly talents—providing physician's new assistants. JAMA 1966;198(10): 182–183.

Stead EA. Training and use of paramedical personnel. N Engl Med 1967a;277(15):800–801.

Stead EA. The Duke plan for physician assistants. Med Times 1967b; 95:40–48.

Stead EA. What's in a name (Editorial)? Physician's Associate 1971;1(2):9.

Stead EA. New roles for personnel in hospitals: physician extenders. Bull N Y Acad Med 1979;55(1):41–45.

Steinwachs DM, Shaprio S, Yaffe R, et al. The role of new health practitioners in a prepaid group practice. Med Care 1976;14(2):95–120.

Steinwachs DM, Weiner JP, Shapiro S, et al. A comparison of the requirements for primary care physicians in HMOs with projections made by the GMENAC. N Engl J Med 1986;314(4):217–222.

Stoddard JJ, Kindig DA, Libby D. Graduate medical education reform: service provision and transition costs. JAMA 1994;272:53–58.

Storey PB. The Soviet Feldsher as a Physician's Assistant. DHEW Publication No. (NIH) 72–58. Government Printing Office, Washington, DC, 1972.

Storms D, Fox J. The public's view of physician's assistants and nurse practitioners. Med Care 1979;17(5):526–535.

Storms DM. Training and Use of Auxiliary Health Workers: Lessons From Developing Countries. American Public Health Association, Washington, DC, 1979.

Strunk H. Patient attitudes toward physician assistants. Calif Med 1973;118:73–77.

Stuart R, Blair J. Army physician's attitudes about physician's assistants. Mil Med 1974;139(6): 470–472.

Stumpf SH, Bottom WD. Evaluation of admission interviews in physician assistant programs. J Am Acad Physician Assist 1989;2(2):122–126.

Sturmann, KM, Ehrenberg K, Salzberg MR. Physician assistants in emergency medicine. Ann Emerg Med 1990;19(3):304–308.

Stoddard JJ, Kindig DA, Libby D. Graduate medical education reform: service provision and transition costs. JAMA 1994;272:53–58.

Storey PB. The Soviet Feldsher as a Physician's Assistant. DHEW Publication No. (NIH) 72–58. Government Printing Office, Washington, DC, 1972.

Storms D, Fox J. The public's view of physician's assistants and nurse practitioners. Med Care 1979;17(5):526–535.

Storms DM. Training and Use of Auxiliary Health Workers: Lessons From Developing Countries. American Public Health Association, Washington, DC, 1979.

Strunk H. Patient attitudes toward physician assistants. Calif Med 1973;118:73–77.

Stuart R, Blair J. Army physician's attitudes about physician's assistants. Mil Med 1974;139(6):470–472.

Stumpf SH, Bottom WD. Evaluation of admission interviews in physician assistant programs. J Am Acad Physician Assist 1989;2(2):122–126.

Sturmann, KM, Ehrenberg K, Salzberg MR. Physician assistants in emergency medicine. Ann Emerg Med 1990;19(3):304–308.

Styles MM. Nurse practitioners creating new horizons for the 1990s. Nurse Pract 1990;15(2):48–57.

Sylvester PA. Forensic medicine—for, and about PAs. J Am Acad Physician Assist 1996;9(5):53–65.

Synowiez PM. Utilization of physician assistants in group practices. Coll Rev 1986;3(2):57–67.

T

Terris M. False starts and lesser alternatives. Bull N Y Acad Med 1977;53:129–140.

Thompson T. Radiologists look at physician's assistants in radiology. Radiology 1971;100:199–202.

Thompson T. Utilization of specialty-trained physician's associates. Physician's Associate. 1972; 2(4):153–156.

Thompson T. The evaluation of physician's assistants in radiology. 1974;111:603–606.

Thompson T. Before we cheer (editorial). Physician Assist 1996;20:55.

Thorpe KE. House staff supervision and working hours: implications of regulatory change in New York state. JAMA 1990;263(23):3177–3181.

Tideiksaar R. Geriatric medicine—the place for PAs? Physician Assistant and Health Practitioner. 1982;6(6):67–68.

Tideiksaar R. The PA's role in the nursing home. Physician Assist 1984;8(11):28–30.

Tideiksaar R. The changing market and nursing home care. Physician Assist 1986a;10(11):13–14.

Tideiksaar R. The physician assistant and geriatrics: what does the future hold? Physician Assist 1986b;10(6):111–112.

Tiger S. A brief history of Physician Assistant: an editor's retrospective. Physician Assist 1992:15(1):54–55.

Tiger S. Roots and radicals (Editorial). Physician Assist 1993;17(8):8,11.

Timmer S. Call for uniform guidelines for postgraduate surgical residency programs. J Am Acad Physician Assist 1991;4(6):453–454.

Tirado NC, Guzman M, Burgos FL. Workload contributions of a physician assistant in an ambulatory care setting. Veterans Administration Medical Center, San Juan, PR. Puerto Rico Health Sci J 1990;9(2):165–167.

Todd MC. The physician's assistant in perspective. J Am Acad Physician Assist 1992;5(3):206–208.

Tompkins R, Wood R, Wolcott B, et al. The effetiveness and cost of acute respiratory illness medical care provided by physicians and algorithm-assisted physician's assistants. Med Care 1997;15(12):991–1003.

Toth PS, Pickrell KL, Thompson LK. Role of the physician's assistant and the plastic surgeon. South Med J 1978;71(4):430–431.

Trigg ME. PA utilization on a pediatric bone marrow transplant unit. Physician Assist 1990;14(3):64,67–68,70 passim.

U

U.S. News and World Report. Not enough doctors: what's being done. U.S. News and World Report. February 17, 1973, p. 53.

V

Valentine P. A national survey of minority physician assistants. J Am Acad Physician Assist 1994;7(1):14–20.

Vause RC, Beeler A, Miller-Blanks M. Seeking a practice challenge? PAs in federal prisons. J Am Acad Physician Assist 1997;10(2):59–62.

Velie L. Where the jobs are—health careers unlimited. Readers Digest, August 1965, pp. 108–112.

Vital Signs: The state of African Americans in higher education. J Blacks Higher Educ 1993;1:1.

Von Seggen W, Hinds A. Physician Assistants in North Carolina. N C Med J 1993;54:276–280.

W

Wallace KW. Physician assistants in orthopedic surgery. Surg Physician Assist 1995;1(1):52.

Wallen J, Davidson SM, Epstein D, Connelly JP. Non-physician health care providers in pediatrics. Pediatrician 1982;11(3–4):225–239.

Walters R. Geisinger Medical Center tertiary care perspective. In Zarbock S, Harbet K (eds): Physician Assistants: New Models of Utilization. Praeger, New York, NY, 1986.

Warren DC. Legal perspectives on hospital privileges. In Carter RD, Perry HB (eds): Alternatives in Health Care Delivery. Warren Green Co, St. Louis, MO, 1984.

Washington Consulting Group. Survey of Certified Nurse Practitioners and Clinical Nurse Specialists: December 1992 Final Report. Report to the Bureau of Health Professions, Department of Health and Human Services under Contract No. 240-91-0055. Rockville, MD, 1994.

Webster BS, Snook SH. The cost of compensable low back pain. J Occup Med 1990;32(1):13–15.

Weiner JP, Steinwachs DM, Williamson JW. Nurse practitioner and physician assistant practices in three HMOs. Implications for future U.S. health manpower needs. Am J Public Health 1986; 76(5):507–511.

Weiner JP. Forecasting the effects of health reform on US physician workforce staffing patterns: evidence from HMO staffing patterns. JAMA 1994; 272(3):222–230.

Weiner JP, McLaughlin CJ, Gamliel S. Extrapolating HMO staffing to the population at large. The US Health Workforce: Power, Politics, and Policy. In Osterweis M, McLaughlin CJ, Manasse HR, et al (eds): The Association of Academic Health Centers, Washington, DC, 1996.

Weisenberger B. Occupational medicine's new resource. J Occup Med 1974;16(10):676–677.

Weissman GS, Winawer SJ, Baldwin MP, et al. Multicenter evaluation of training of non-endoscopists in 30-cm flexible sigmoidoscopy. CA Cancer J Clin 1987;37:26–30.

Wen CP, Hays CW. Medical education in China in the post-cultural revolution era. 1975;292: 998–1005.

Weston JL. Distribution of nurse practitioners and physician assistants: implications of legal constraints and reimbursement. Public Health Rep 1980;95:253–256.

White GL, Egerton CP, Myers R, Holbert RD. Physician Assistants and Mississippi. J Mississippi State Medical Association, December 1994.

White KL, Connelly J. The Medical School's Mission and The Population's Health. Springer-Verlag, New York, NY,1992.

White RI Jr, Rizer DM, Shuman KR, et al. Streamlining operation of an admitting service for interventional radiology. Radiology 1988;168:127–130.

White RI Jr, Denny DF Jr, Osterman FA, et al. Logistics of a university interventional radiology practice. Radiology 1989;170(3 Pt 2):951–954.

Whiting W, Beyer R. An innovation in health care delivery in workman's compensation. J Occup Med 1973;15(6):499–500.

Williams WH, Kopchak J, Yearby LG, Hatcher CR. The surgical physician assistant as a member of the cardiothoracic surgical team in the academic medical center. In Carter RD, Perry HB (eds): Alternatives in Health Care Delivery. Warren Green Co., St. Louis, MO, 1984.

Willis JB. PA salary distribution. AAPA News 1989; 10(12):1–5.

Willis JB. Prescriptive practice patterns of physician assistants. J Am Acad Physician Assist 1990a;3: 39–56.

Willis JB. Analysis of the influence of gender on PA salaries. J Am Acad Physician Assist 1990b;3(4): 269–276.

Willis JB. Is the PA supply in rural America dwindling? J Am Acad Physician Assist 1990c;3: 433–435.

Willis JB. Explaining the salary discrepancy between male and female PAs. J Am Acad Physician Assist 1992;5:280–288.

Willis JB, Pylitt, LL. Physician assistants and hospital practice. J Am Acad Physician Assist 1993a;6: 115–122.

Willis JB. Barriers to PA practice in primary care and rural medically underserved areas. J Am Acad Physician Assist 1993b;6:418–422.

Wilson HT. The present status of the physician's assistant program of the Bowman Gray School of Medicine. North Carolina Med J 1974;36:202–204.

Wilson WM, White GL, Murdock RT. Physician assistants in ophthamology: a national survey. Physician Assist 1990;14(1):57–59,62,64.

Wilson WM, Pederson DM, Ballweg R, et al. Shaping a model clinical therapeutics curriculum. J Am Acad Physician Assist 1995;9(5):51–56.

Wolinksy FD. The Sociology of Health. Ed 2. Wadsworth Publishing, Belmont, MA, 1988.

World Health Organization. Expert Committee on Professional and Technical Education of Medical and Auxillary Personnel. Training of medical assistants and similar personnel. World Health Organization Technician Report Service 1968;385:5–29.

World Health Organization. The Primary Health Worker. World Health Organization, Geneva, 1980.

World Health Organization Study Group. Report on the Community-based Education of Health Personnel. World Health Organization. Geneva, 1987a.

World Health Organization Study Group. The Primary Care Worker. World Health Organization, Geneva, 1987b.

Wright D, Kane R, Snell G, Woolley FR. Costs and outcomes for different primary care providers. JAMA 1977;238:46–50.

Wright WK, Hirsch CS. The physician assistant as forensic investigator. J Forensic Sci 1987;32(4): 1059–1061.

Y

Yanni F, Backman P, Potash J. Physicians attitudes on the physician's assistant. Physician's Associate 1972;2(1):6–10.

Young GP. Status of clinical and academic emergency medicine at 111 Veterans Affairs Medical Centers. Ann Emerg Med 1993;22(8):1304–1309.

Yturri-Byrd K, Glazer-Waldman H. The physician assistant and care of the geriatric patient. Gerontol Geriatr Educ 1984;5(1):33–41.

Z

Zarbock S, Harbet K (eds): Physician Assistants: New Models Of Utilization. Praeger, New York, 1986.

Zechauser R, Eliastam M. The productivity potential of the physician assistant. J Hum Resour 1974;9: 5–116.

Zimmerly JG, Normans JC. Physicians assistants and malpractice liability. Physician Assist Consultations Jan/Feb 1985:11–13.

Index

Page numbers followed by *f* indicate figures; those followed by *t* indicate tables.